Handbook of Swine Health and Diseases

Handbook of Swine Health and Diseases

Edited by Willow Adams

hayle
medical

New York

Hayle Medical,
750 Third Avenue, 9th Floor,
New York, NY 10017, USA

Visit us on the World Wide Web at:
www.haylemedical.com

ISBN: 978-1-63241-823-4

Cataloging-in-Publication Data

Handbook of swine health and diseases / edited by Willow Adams.
    p. cm.
Includes bibliographical references and index.
ISBN 978-1-63241-823-4
1. Swine--Diseases. 2. Swine--Health. 3. Animal health. 4. Animals--Diseases.
5. Veterinary medicine. I. Adams, Willow.
SF971 .H36 2019
636.408 96--dc23

Table of Contents

Preface

Swine diseases are caused by bacterial and viral pathogens, nutritional and genetic factors. Some of the diseases caused by bacterial agents are bordetelosis, colitis, exudative epidermitis, listeriosis, swine dysentery, etc. Some viral swine diseases are African swine fever, blue eye disease, porcine respiratory coronavirus infection, swine vesicular disease, etc. Nutritional deficiencies in pigs may occur due to iron, vitamin E, calcium, vitamin D and biotin deficiencies, among others. A number of parasites such as Ascaris suum, Cryptosporidium, red stomach worm, Metastrongylus spp, etc. cause diseases in pigs. These diseases can lead to significant economic losses due to reduced productivity. The management of health issues in large swine population requires a major focus on biosecurity. Vaccination is the chief management tool to enhance immunity in swines. By using the combined strategy of minimizing disease challenge and augmenting individual and herd immunity by vaccinations, many swine diseases can be controlled. This book is a compilation of chapters that discuss the most vital concepts and emerging trends in the field of swine health and disease. It explores all the important aspects of swine health in the present day scenario. It is a collective contribution of a renowned group of international experts.

Various studies have approached the subject by analyzing it with a single perspective, but the present book provides diverse methodologies and techniques to address this field. This book contains theories and applications needed for understanding the subject from different perspectives. The aim is to keep the readers informed about the progresses in the field; therefore, the contributions were carefully examined to compile novel researches by specialists from across the globe.

Indeed, the job of the editor is the most crucial and challenging in compiling all chapters into a single book. In the end, I would extend my sincere thanks to the chapter authors for their profound work. I am also thankful for the support provided by my family and colleagues during the compilation of this book.

Editor

1

Influence of spray dried porcine plasma in starter diets associated with a conventional vaccination program on wean to finish performance

Joan Pujols[1], Joaquim Segalés[2,3], Javier Polo[4], Carmen Rodríguez[4], Joy Campbell[5] and Joe Crenshaw[5*]

Abstract

Background: Conventional vaccination programs using a single injection of a combined vaccine against porcine circovirus type 2 (PCV2) and Mycoplasma hyopneumoniae (MHYO) can promote a strong immune response that reduces feed intake for 24 to 48 h post injection. Often such vaccines are given around the time of weaning during a critical stress period in which feed intake is already compromised. Spray dried porcine plasma (SDPP) is a protein source used in starter diets that increases post-weaning feed intake of pigs. The objectives of this study were to determine the effects of a conventional vaccination program along with feeding SDPP in a starter diet on antibody development and wean to finish performance of pigs.

Results: Pigs fed the starter diet with SDPP had improved body weight, average daily weight gain and average daily feed intake during the initial 14 d after weaning along with improved feed efficiency during the initial 7 d after weaning and these responses were independent of vaccination. Vaccination at 3 d after weaning had no significant effect on performance during the initial 14 d after weaning. Cumulative mortality was reduced for pigs fed the starter diet with SDPP, while vaccinated pigs had reduced mortality from d 48 to 145. Both vaccinated pigs and those fed the starter diet with SDPP had heavier carcass weight. One pig per pen was challenged with PCV2 at d 63. A higher percentage of vaccinated pigs were sero-positive for antibodies against PCV2 and MHYO at d 35, 63 and 78. Antibody values against PCV2 were higher for vaccinated pigs at d 35 and 63, but lower at d 146. Percentage of positive samples for PCV2 genome in serum was reduced for vaccinated pigs at d 117 and 146. Antibody values against MHYO were increased for vaccinated pigs at d 35, 63 and 78.

Conclusions: Vaccination supported a long term antibody response against PCV2 and a moderate but weaker antibody response against MHYO for early finishing pigs challenged with PCV2. Using SDPP in the starter diet along with vaccination supported the best long-term beneficial effects on survival to market and carcass weight.

Keywords: Spray dried plasma, Mycoplasma hyopneumoniae, Porcine circovirus type 2, Pigs, Vaccination, Weaning stress, Antibody, Carcass

* Correspondence: joe.crenshaw@functionalproteins.com
[5]APC Inc., 2425 SE Oak Tree Court, Ankeny, IA 50021, USA
Full list of author information is available at the end of the article

Background

Spray dried porcine plasma (SDPP) or spray dried bovine plasma (SDBP) has been used in nursery pig diets due to its documented beneficial effects on post-weaning growth, feed intake, morbidity indices and survival [1, 2]. In past studies, under field conditions, pigs suffering from porcine circovirus type 2-systemic disease (PCV2-SD, formerly known as post-weaning multi-systemic wasting syndrome) had improved performance and survival when fed diets containing SDPP [3, 4]. PCV2 is the essential causative agent of PCV2-SD, a multifactorial disease with a severe economic impact worldwide. PCV2-SD is characterized by wasting, decreased weight gain, lymphadenopathy and dyspnea, affecting mainly pigs from 6 weeks of age to market [5].

Mycoplasma hyopneumoniae (MHYO) is the main etiological agent of enzootic pneumonia, a chronic respiratory disease that affects mainly growing and finishing pigs. MHYO and PCV2 are potential etiological contributors of the porcine respiratory disease complex, which involves bacterial as well as viral agents [6].

Experimental co-infection with MHYO and PCV2 resulted in a more severe clinical disease in growing [7, 8] and adult [9] animals, although not always [10]. In all cases, PCV2 and MHYO vaccines have demonstrated good results in eliciting antibody responses, reduction of clinical signs and better productive outcome [11–13]. In general, manufacturers recommend the application of these vaccines around the time of weaning.

However, pigs at weaning are subjected to complex changes that can affect pig adaptation and growth. Vaccination against PCV2 and MHYO at weaning may result in a transitory reduced feed intake and growth rate [14–16]. For such a reason, products containing spray dried plasma proteins and digestible energy given in drinking water to weaned pigs have been used to overcome the undesirable effects on growth performance after injection with a PCV2/MHYO vaccine [15]. There is growing evidence in pigs and other species that nutrition before and after weaning can have long-term effects on gut, microbiota interaction and immune development [17]. Therefore, for the present study our objectives were to determine the effects of SDPP in a starter diet fed to pigs injected at 3 d after weaning with a single combined vaccine against PCV2 and MHYO on wean to finish performance, carcass parameters, and detection of pathogen genome and antibody development against PCV2 and MHYO.

Results

Treatment groups consisted of vaccinated (V) or saline (S) injected pigs on d 3 after weaning, which were fed starter diets with (P) or without (C) SDPP for the initial 14 d post-weaning. Pigs were assigned to 4 treatment groups (1 VC, 2 VP, 3 SC, 4 SP) with a 2 × 2 factorial arrangement of treatments to determine the effects on wean to finish performance and carcass results and serological results over various time periods. Three orthogonal treatment comparisons were used to test for the main effects of vaccination (vaccine vs saline injected pigs; treatment groups 1 VC + 2 VP vs treatment groups 3 SC + 4 SP), starter diet (pigs fed 0 % vs 6 % SDPP in starter diets; treatment groups 1 VC + 3 SC vs treatment groups 2 VP + 4 SP), and the interaction of the main effects of vaccination and starter diet (treatment groups 1 VC + 4 SP vs treatment groups 2 VP + 3 SC).

Nursery performance results

Average pen performance variables by treatment group and periods of the experiment while pigs were housed at the *Institut de Recerca i Tecnologia Agroalimentàries* (IRTA) nursery facilities are presented in Table 1. The treatment comparison for the main effect of starter diet indicated that average daily weight gain (ADG) was higher for pigs fed starter diet with SDPP during d 0–7 and 0–14 post-weaning. Average daily feed intake (ADFI) was higher for pigs fed starter diet with SDPP during d 0–7, 7–14 and 0–14. Feed efficiency (GF) was improved for pigs fed starter diet with SDPP during d 0–7; but GF was reduced during d 7–14. Treatment comparisons for the main effect of vaccination and the interaction of vaccination and starter diet were not significant for ADG, ADFI or GF during the initial 14 d after weaning or during any other time periods while pigs were housed in nursery facilities. After d 14 when all pigs were fed a common diet to the end of the nursery phase (d 14–48) and for the entire nursery period (d 0–48), there were no significant effects on ADG, ADFI or GF due to treatment comparisons for the main effect of starter diet, vaccination or interaction of starter diet by vaccination.

Mortality and morbidity

Mortality rate of pigs (Table 2) during the initial 14 d after weaning was not significant for any of the treatment comparisons. During d 14–48 and 0–48, mortality rate was reduced for groups of pigs fed starter diet with SDPP. During d 48–145, vaccinated pigs had reduced mortality rate compared to non-vaccinated groups. Over the entire wean to finish period (d 0–145), mortality rate was reduced for groups of pigs fed the starter diet with SDPP. There were no significant interactions of vaccination and starter diet on mortality rate during any periods of the study. Female pigs had lower ($P < 0.01$) mortality rate d 14–48 (1.7 % vs 8.3 %), d 0–48 (2.2 % vs 8.3 %) and d 0–145 (3.8 % vs 11.1 %) compared to male pigs (data not shown).

Table 1 Nursery performance of vaccinated pigs fed starter diet with porcine plasma[a]

Variable	Day[b]	Treatment group				SEM	Probability F-test			
		1 VC	2 VP	3 SC	4 SP		Trt	Vac	Diet	VxD
ADG, g	0–7	57.6	105.8	70.0	104.4	6.57	<0.01	0.41	<0.01	0.31
ADFI, g	0–7	83.1	111.6	86.9	107.0	4.77	<0.01	0.94	<0.01	0.38
GF	0–7	0.730	0.941	0.805	0.965	0.063	<0.01	0.34	<0.01	0.64
ADG, g	7–14	176.9	180.9	183.4	189.1	8.47	0.77	0.39	0.57	0.92
ADFI, g	7–14	222.2	245.6	223.9	249.3	9.10	0.08	0.76	0.01	0.91
GF	7–14	0.812	0.742	0.811	0.761	0.029	0.22	0.76	0.04	0.73
ADG, g	0–14	117.3	143.3	126.7	146.8	5.28	<0.01	0.23	<0.01	0.58
ADFI, g	0–14	152.7	178.6	155.4	178.2	5.67	<0.01	0.84	<0.01	0.78
GF	0–14	0.763	0.804	0.812	0.827	0.024	0.27	0.14	0.24	0.57
ADG, g	14–48	440.8	448.4	449.8	433.8	8.95	0.57	0.75	0.64	0.20
ADFI, g	14–48	651.9	656.1	650.6	647.0	13.5	0.97	0.70	0.98	0.78
GF	14–48	0.678	0.684	0.694	0.672	0.009	0.39	0.82	0.37	0.14
ADG, g	0–48	346.4	359.4	355.5	350.1	6.83	0.55	0.99	0.58	0.19
ADFI, g	0–48	506.3	516.8	506.2	510.3	10.5	0.87	0.75	0.48	0.76
GF	0–48	0.687	0.696	0.705	0.688	0.009	0.45	0.59	0.67	0.14

[a]Values are least squares mean of the pen average performance variable analyzed for block and treatment group (Trt) using orthogonal treatment comparisons for the effect of vaccination (Vac), starter diet (Diet) and interaction of vaccination and starter diet (VxD). Initial BW (5.83 ± 0.1 kg) was included as a covariant. Starter diets were fed for the initial 14 d after weaning, and then all pigs were fed common diets from d 14 to 48. There were 13 pens per treatment group. Treatment groups were a single injection at d 3 post-weaning with PCV2/MHYO vaccine (V) or saline (S) and starter diet with 0 % (C) or 6 % spray dried porcine plasma (P)
[b]Day or period of experiment

Although the mortality rate was high, it was similar to that of the source farm and was mainly consistent with bacterial infections. Approximately 70 % of the mortality occurred between d 14 and 48 after pigs were fed a common diet without SDPP, but before challenge with PCV2 inoculum at d 63. Nearly all mortality cases during d 48 to 145 were described as chronic bacterial infections associated with tail-biting or due to euthanasia because of hind limb paralysis.

Necropsies were performed when feasible, but in some cases it was not possible due to the advanced autolysis state of the body. Most deaths were compatible with systemic bacterial infections showing fibrinous polyserositis and arthritis and, less frequently, colisepticemia-like diarrhea and enteritis. A proportion of animals had a chronic course displaying weight loss; those that died showed fibrous polyserositis and pericarditis, craneo-ventral pulmonary consolidation and/or arthritis. Infections by *Haemophilus parasuis*, *Mycoplasma hyorhinis* and *Escherichia coli* could have been involved together with other agents, but specific laboratory investigations were not performed.

The source farm of the herd was sero-positive for PRRSV, and circulation of this virus could potentially have been a predisposing factor for subsequent bacterial infections. However, IDDEX ELISA results for 100 samples taken at d 146 of the study indicated low (12 %) prevalence of samples sero-positive for PRRSV, suggesting PRRSV had not been circulating earlier in the study.

The experimental starter diets and all other diets were non-medicated with the exception of the common transition diet fed from d 48 to 58 when pigs were moved from the nursery to the pre-fattening facility. This diet contained 200 ppm amoxicillin, 24 ppm oxbendazol, and 120 ppm colistin.

Pigs were monitored daily by visual inspection and animal caretakers applied prescribed treatments after veterinarian clinical inspection. Individual pig treatment for polyserositis, arthritis and pneumonia included a product based on Bencylpeniciline procaine 200,000 UI, dihydrostreptomycin (sulfate) 200 mg and dexamethasone (sodium phosphate) 0.5 mg at the recommended dose according to body weight. The percentage of pigs given individual medications (ranged from 9.9 to 16.6 % across treatment groups) was not significantly different for the various treatment group comparisons. At d 26 of the study when several cases of arthritis appeared, Amoxicillin (trihydrate) 70 % at 0.3 g/L was added to drinking water for 5 days.

Individual pig BW

Results of individual pig BW data by day of experiment from wean to finish (Table 2) indicated that pigs fed the starter diet with SDPP had heavier average BW at d 7, 14 and 21 compared to pigs fed the control diet. However, at all other time periods there were no significant differences due to the main effect of starter diet. Also

Table 2 Mortality, BW and carcass data of vaccinated pigs fed starter diets with porcine plasma[a]

Variable	Day[b]	Treatment group				SEM	Probability F-test			
		1 VC	2 VP	3 SC	4 SP		Trt	Vac	Diet	VxD
Pigs, n	0	91	91	91	90	–	–	–	–	–
Mortality, %	0–14	1.09	0.00	0.00	0.00	0.55	0.41	0.32	0.32	0.32
	14–48	8.89	4.37	5.53	1.11	2.26	0.11	0.14	0.05	0.98
	0–48	9.95	4.37	5.53	1.11	2.32	0.06	0.10	0.03	0.80
	48–145	1.32	0.00	4.77	3.36	1.66	0.17	0.03	0.40	0.98
	0–145	11.06	4.37	9.95	4.44	2.74	0.17	0.85	0.03	0.82
BW, kg	0	5.84	5.83	5.82	5.84	0.10	0.99	0.96	0.97	0.89
	7	6.24	6.58	6.32	6.57	0.06	<0.01	0.52	<0.01	0.44
	14	7.49	7.84	7.60	7.90	0.09	<0.01	0.36	<0.01	0.73
	21	9.17	9.62	9.53	9.66	0.14	0.06	0.15	0.04	0.27
	35	15.06	15.64	15.39	15.55	0.25	0.38	0.62	0.22	0.57
	48	22.47	23.14	22.90	22.70	0.44	0.63	0.98	0.53	0.24
	63	33.32	34.56	34.90	34.09	0.54	0.46	0.84	0.22	0.29
	83	49.64	50.48	49.46	49.92	0.73	0.76	0.60	0.36	0.79
	114	73.40	75.20	72.22	72.14	1.12	0.16	0.06	0.44	0.39
	145	100.7	102.3	98.67	100.8	1.20	0.18	0.13	0.11	0.83
Carcass, n[c]	159	70	74	72	76	–	–	–	–	–
BW, kg[d]	145	101.7	104.2	98.60	101.8	1.14	<0.01	0.01	0.01	0.77
Carcass, kg	159	86.43	88.70	84.05	86.90	0.94	<0.01	0.03	<0.01	0.75
Lean, %	159	57.97	57.38	58.00	57.48	0.36	0.47	0.85	0.11	0.92

[a]Values are least squares mean of percentage mortality, individual pig body weight (BW) and carcass variable by day or period of experiment analyzed for the effects of sex (S), treatment group (Trt), and interaction of Trt and sex (TxS), using orthogonal treatment comparisons for the main effect of vaccination (Vac), starter diet (Diet) and interaction of vaccination and starter diet (VxD). Initial BW (5.83 ± 0.1 kg) was included as a covariant. Starter diets were fed for the initial 14 d after weaning, and then all pigs were fed common diets from d 14 to 145. Treatment factors were a single injection at d 3 post-weaning with PCV2/MHYO vaccine (V) or saline (S) and starter diet with 0 % (C) or 6 % spray dried porcine plasma (P)
[b]Day or period of experiment
[c]Number of carcasses classified at abattoir differed from number of pigs finished due to culling or lost carcass identification
[d]Live BW of pigs at d 145 that subsequently had carcasses classified on d 159

treatment comparisons for the main effect of vaccination or interaction of starter diet and vaccination were not significant at any time periods of the study. Significant effects for sex (data not shown) indicated female pigs were heavier (P <0.03) than male pigs at d 7 (6.51 vs 6.35 kg), d 14 (7.84 vs 7.58 kg) and d 35 (15.67 vs 15.13 kg); but by d 145, males (102.1 kg) were heavier (P <0.01) than females (99.1 kg).

Carcass results
Due to mortality of 27 pigs, lost carcass identification of 36 pigs, and culling or rejection of eight pigs at slaughter, only 292 of the original 363 pigs started on the experiment were used for carcass data (Table 2). Of the eight pigs that were culled at the abattoir, four pigs were culled due to hernias and the other four were culled due to low BW.

There were no significant interactions for the effects of starter diet by vaccination status for any of the carcass parameters. The treatment comparison for the main

effect of starter diet indicated that pigs fed the SDPP diet had heavier average carcass weight and average BW at d 145 for pigs that were classified at slaughter compared to the groups fed the control starter diet. Vaccinated pigs had heavier carcass weight and average BW at d 145 for pigs classified at slaughter compared to non-vaccinated pigs. Carcass lean percentage was not significant for the treatment comparisons of the main effects for vaccination or starter diet. Also males had heavier d 145 BW of pigs classified at slaughter (103.1 kg vs 100.1 kg), heavier carcass weight (87.7 kg vs 85.3 kg), and higher carcass lean percentage (58.2 % vs 57.3 %) compared to females (data not shown).

ELISA values and genome results for PCV2
ELISA results for PCV2 S/P ratio and percentage of sero-positive samples by treatment group and day of experiment are presented in Fig. 1. The S/P results >17 were considered positive. The treatment comparisons for the main effect of starter diet or interaction of starter

diet and vaccination were not significant at any time period for any of the ELISA results for PCV2. The main effect of vaccination was significant for S/P ratio and percentage sero-positivity for PCV2. Vaccinated pigs had higher percentages of sero-positive samples at d 35, 63 and 78 compared to non-vaccinated pigs. Vaccinated pigs had higher S/P ratio against PCV2 on d 35 and 63, but lower S/P ratio on d 146 compared to non-vaccinated pigs.

Percentage of sero-positive samples for PCV2 genome (Fig. 2) was lower for vaccinated pigs at d 117 and 146 compared to non-vaccinated pigs, but no other significant differences were detected at other days of the experiment or for the main effect of starter diet or interaction of starter diet and vaccination.

ELISA values and genome results for MHYO

ELISA results for MHYO inhibition values and percentage of sero-positive samples are presented in Fig. 3. MHYO inhibition results >65 were interpreted as positive. There were no significant effects of starter diet or interaction of starter diet and vaccination on MHYO inhibition values or percentage of sero-positive samples at any time periods. Vaccinated pigs had higher MHYO inhibition value and percentage of sero-positive samples at d 35, 63 and 78 compared to non-vaccinated pigs.

There were no significant effects of starter diet, vaccination, or interaction of diet and vaccination on PCR analysis of nasal swabs for MHYO genome at any time period (Fig. 4). Nasal swabs were not sampled on days 0 and 35 of the study.

Discussion

Weaning of pigs is a period associated with multiple stressors that contribute to reduced growth, feed intake, and feed efficiency and increased morbidity and mortality [18]. Reduced feed intake post-weaning is associated with compromised intestinal barrier function [19]. Weaning stress induces intestinal barrier dysfunctions associated with increased permeability and inflammation that can impact present and future mucosal barrier function [20–22].

Vaccines are useful for helping pigs develop resistance to exposure to pathogens they encounter during their lifetime. However, certain vaccines may stimulate an immune response that results in a measurable reduction of feed intake and growth [12]. When such a vaccine is given around weaning time, this added stress may further exacerbate the reduction in feed intake that is already compromised by weaning stress.

Spray dried plasma has an important role in starter diets as a functional protein source to provide nutrition to support pigs to better transition through the negative effects of weaning stress. The beneficial effects of starter diets containing spray dried plasma on post-weaning pig growth, feed intake, and health are well known [1, 2]. Intestinal barrier dysfunctions associated with weaning stress were reduced when pigs were provided starter diets containing 5 % SDPP fed for 14 d after weaning compared to 0 or 2.5 % SDPP, suggesting diets supplemented with 5 % SDPP support and maintain intestinal barrier function [23]. Therefore, in the present study, 6 % SDPP was used in the starter diet with the intention to assure adequate

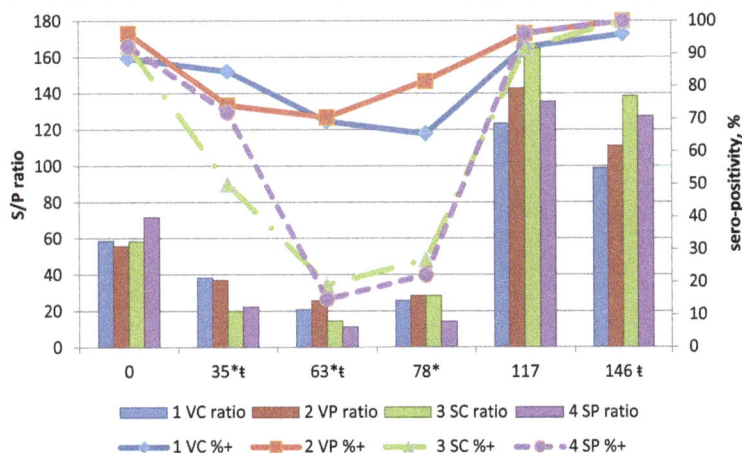

Fig. 1 PCV2 ELISA results by treatment and day of experiment. Values are least squares means of treatment group by day of experiment for serum S/P ratio (ratio, bars, left vertical scale) and percentage positive samples (% +, lines, right vertical scale) against PCV2 (26 samples per treatment by day). S/P ratio >17 considered positive. Treatment groups were vaccinated (V) or saline (S) injected pigs on d 3 after weaning that were fed starter diets with (P) or without (C) spray-dried porcine plasma for the initial 14 d post-weaning. One pig per pen was challenged with PCV2 inoculum on d 63 after weaning. Data was analyzed for the effects of sex, treatment group and interaction of treatment group and sex using orthogonal treatment comparisons for the main effects of vaccination (1 VC + 2 VP vs 3 SC + 4 SP), starter diet (1 VC + 3 SC vs 2 VP + 4 SP) and interaction of vaccination and starter diet (1 VC + 4 SP vs 2 VP + 3 SC). ŧ Main effect of vaccination for day 35, 63 and 146 of the experiment for S/P titer (P <0.05). *Main effect of vaccination for day 35, 63 and 78 of the experiment for % positive samples (P <0.05)

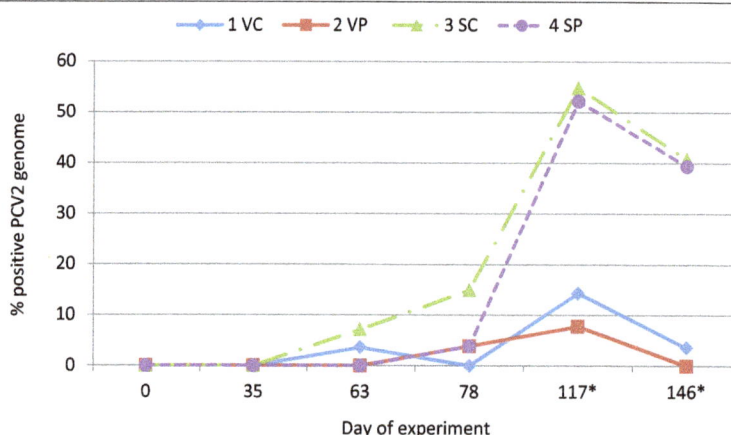

Fig. 2 Serum samples positive for PCV2 genome. Values are least squares means of treatment group by day of experiment for percentage of serum samples positive for PCV2 genome (n = 26 samples per treatment by day). Treatment groups were vaccinated (V) or saline (S) injected pigs on d 3 after weaning that were fed starter diets with (P) or without (C) spray-dried porcine plasma for the initial 14 d post-weaning. One pig per pen was challenged with PCV2 inoculum on d 63 after weaning. Data was analyzed for the effects of sex, treatment group and interaction of treatment group and sex using orthogonal treatment comparisons for the main effects of vaccination (1 VC + 2 VP vs 3 SC + 4 SP), starter diet (1 VC + 3 SC vs 2 VP + 4 SP) and interaction of vaccination and starter diet (1 VC + 4 SP vs 2 VP + 3 SC). *Main effect of vaccination for day 117 and 146 of the experiment (P <0.05)

SDPP was available to support intestinal barrier function during this critical period of post-weaning stress.

In the present study, 6 % SDPP in the starter diet improved short-term post-weaning growth, feed intake and feed efficiency, regardless of vaccination status. Although vaccination at d 3 post-weaning had no significant effect on growth and feed intake, vaccinated pigs fed the control diet had the lowest daily weight gain, feed intake, and gain to feed ratio suggesting a mild short-term effect

of the vaccination on growth and feed efficiency during the initial week of the study.

The early growth advantage for pigs fed SDPP during the initial 14 d after weaning was not maintained through the end of the nursery phase (d 48), but by the end of the study both vaccinated pigs and pigs fed starter diet with SDPP had heavier BW and carcass weight. Pigs previously fed SDPP in the starter diet had reduced mortality to d 48 and this reduction of mortality

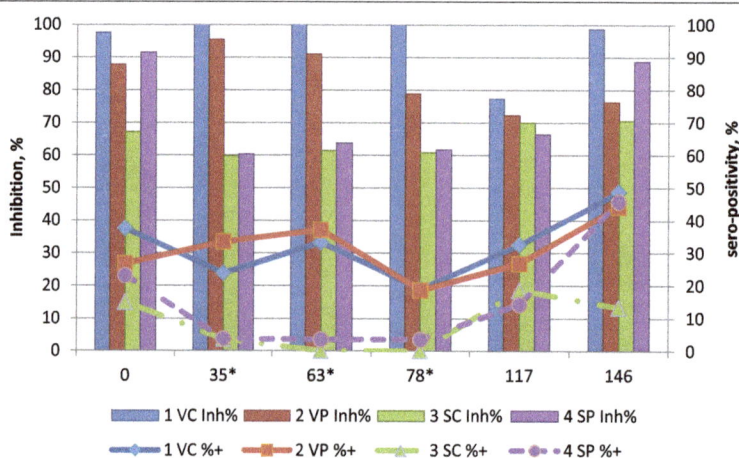

Fig. 3 MYHO ELISA results by treatment and day of experiment. Values are least squares means of treatment group by day of experiment for serum inhibition titer (Inh%, bars, left vertical scale) and percentage positive samples (%+, lines, right vertical scale) against MHYO (26 samples per treatment by day). Inhibition percentage >65 was considered positive. Treatment groups were vaccinated (V) or saline (S) injected pigs on d 3 after weaning that were fed starter diets with (P) or without (C) spray-dried porcine plasma for the initial 14 d post-weaning. One pig per pen was challenged with PCV2 inoculum on d 63 after weaning. Data was analyzed for the effects of sex, treatment group and interaction of treatment group and sex using orthogonal treatment comparisons for the main effects of vaccination (1 VC + 2 VP vs 3 SC + 4 SP), starter diet (1 VC + 3 SC vs 2 VP + 4 SP) and interaction of vaccination and starter diet (1 VC + 4 SP vs 2 VP + 3 SC). *Main effect of vaccination for day 35, 63, and 78 of the experiment (P <0.05) for both inhibition titer and percentage of positive samples

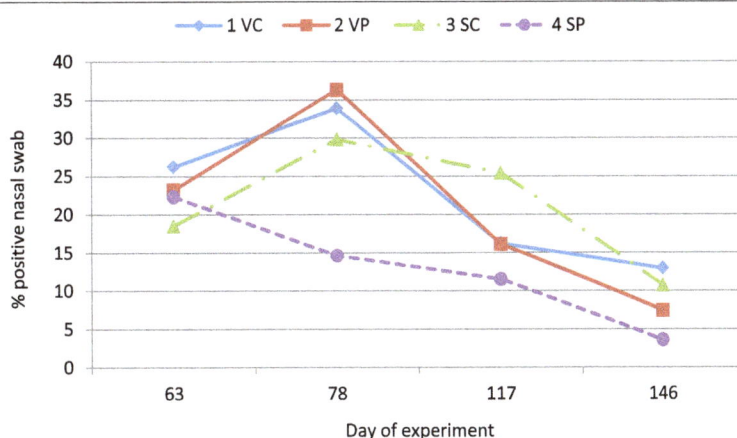

Fig. 4 Nasal swab samples positive for MHYO genome. Values are least squares means of treatment group by day of experiment for percentage of nasal swab samples positive for MHYO genome ($n = 26$ samples per treatment by day). Treatment groups were vaccinated (V) or saline (S) injected pigs on d 3 after weaning that were fed starter diets with (P) or without (C) spray-dried porcine plasma for the initial 14 d post-weaning. One pig per pen was challenged with PCV2 inoculum on d 63 after weaning. Data was analyzed for the effects of sex, treatment group and interaction of treatment group and sex using orthogonal treatment comparisons for the main effects of vaccination (1 VC + 2 VP vs 3 SC + 4 SP), starter diet (1 VC + 3 SC vs 2 VP + 4 SP) and interaction of vaccination and starter diet (1 VC + 4 SP vs 2 VP + 3 SC). There were no significant differences detected among treatment groups at any sampling time

was also maintained to the end of the study. Approximately 70 % of the mortality occurred between d 14 and 48 after pigs were fed a common diet without SDPP, and most of this mortality was associated with lesions compatible with infection caused by *Haemophilus parasuis, Streptococcus suis* or *Mycoplasma hyorhinis* or other potential pathogens. Vaccinated pigs also had reduced mortality from d 48 to 145. Nearly all mortality cases during d 48 to 145 were described as chronic bacterial infections associated with tail-biting or due to euthanasia because of hind limb paralysis.

Past studies have reported reduced mortality associated with PCV2-SD afflicted nursery and grower pigs fed diets with SDPP [3, 4], and this reduced mortality was extended well beyond the feeding period of diets with SDPP [3]. Also, reduced lung lesions have been reported in pigs fed diets with SDPP and experimentally-infected with swine influenza virus [24]. Furthermore, intestinal permeability of pigs previously fed a diet with 5 % SDPP for 14 d post-weaning was reduced when subsequently challenged with *Salmonella typhimurium* and fed diets without SDPP [25]. Collectively, these past results suggest SDPP in starter diets has a longer-term impact on animal resilience to subsequent stress, and this may be related to the reduction of intestinal barrier dysfunction associated with early life stress.

Infectious pressure for PCV2 (Fig. 2) was <10 % for all treatment groups up to d 63; but for MYHO genome (Fig. 4), it was 18 to 26 % positive across treatment groups at d 63. In order to increase the infectious pressure for PCV2, one pig per pen was inoculated with

PCV2 at d 63. Serum PCV2 genome slowly progressed to a higher percentage of positive samples (>50 %) for non-vaccinated pigs by d 117; however, there was little increase in serum PCV2 genome for vaccinated pigs, suggesting vaccination helped reduce subsequent incidence of PCV2 viremia (Fig. 2).

Vaccination supported a strong PCV2 antibody response (Fig. 1) and a modest MHYO antibody response (Fig. 3) and these results are consistent with others [26–30]. A high percentage of pigs at weaning (d 0) had antibodies to PCV2 likely due to the ubiquitous nature of the virus and its widespread sero-prevalence. Under normal conditions pigs acquire antibodies via colostrum that may last up to 10 weeks of age. Therefore, the observed antibody values for PCV2 at weaning are consistent with maternally derived immunity.

Several factors may affect the seroconversion to MHYO under field conditions, such as a variable proportion of infected animals, elongated time to elicit an immune response, or poor correlation of seroconversion with protection that result in no differences in seroconversion between vaccinated and non-vaccinated pigs [31].

Vaccination also reduced the presence of PCV2 genome in serum, after the challenge with PCV2 and this confirms previous research [32, 33]. These serology results may partially explain the reduced mortality of vaccinated pigs during d 48 to 145 of the study when pigs were challenged with PCV2. Starter diet had no significant effects on antibody or genome results. Under the conditions of this study, vaccination and feeding SDPP in the starter diet resulted in pigs with heavier final BW and carcass weight; however most of the reduced mortality was associated with pigs fed the starter diet with SDPP.

Conclusions

Vaccination supported a long term antibody response against PCV2 and a weaker antibody response against MHYO for early finishing pigs challenged with PCV2. SDPP in the starter diet along with vaccination supported the best long-term beneficial effects on survival to market and final BW and carcass weight. Both early life vaccination and nutrition supplemented with SDPP should be considered for reducing risks of longer term mortality and morbidity in later life stages.

Methods

Animals and housing

Pigs ([Large White × Landrace] × Pietrain) weaned at 21 ± 2 d of age were selected from a conventional sow farm managed in a three-week batch farrowing system and transported to an experimental farm at IRTA. The sow farm was seropositive against PRRSV at the time pigs were weaned. Pigs were assigned to 4 treatment groups (1 VC, 2 VP, 3 SC, 4 SP) in a 2 × 2 factorial arrangement of treatments with the effects of injection at d 3 post-weaning with a PCV2/MHYO combined vaccine (V) versus saline (S) or a starter diet with 0 % (C) versus 6 % (P) SDPP as the primary treatment factors. Maternal origin, sex, and weaning

weight were used as blocking factors, according to normal procedures at IRTA. Sow parity was not directly used as a blocking factor; however, parity was balanced across treatment groups within block, since it was associated with maternal origin as a blocking factor. After final allotment there were 13 pens with six pens of males, six pens of females, and one pen of mixed sex per treatment group. There were seven pigs per pen, except one pen assigned to treatment four (SP) had only six pigs for a total of 363 pigs started on experiment. Pigs were kept in two rooms at the weaning facility for 48 d and individual pig BW and feed data per pen were recorded at specific intervals (Table 3). Each room had two rows of pens with a central corridor (26 pens per room) with complete slatted floors and pen dividers that allowed for direct pig contact between pens. The experimental pigs were the only pigs located at the weaning facility during the time of the study. At d 48, the seven pigs from the original pens at the weaning facility were moved as an intact group to a single pen located in one of three different rooms in a grower facility at the experimental farm and kept there until d 83. The grower facility also had pen dividers that allowed for direct pig contact between pens, however the experimental pigs were the only pigs kept at the grower facility during the time of the study. After day 83, pigs were moved again and finished at a commercial farm until d 159 post-weaning before being transported to a commercial abattoir. The commercial farm had no other pigs located at the finishing facility

Table 3 Schedule for data collection, sampling and other experimental events

Day[a]	Pig age, d	Pig weight	Starter diet	Vaccine[b]	Challenge[c]	Blood sample[d]	Nasal swab[e]
0	21	√	√			√	
3	24		√	√			
7	28	√	√				
14	35	√	√				
21	42	√					
35	56	√				√	
48[f]	69	√					
63	84	√			√	√	√
78	99					√	√
83[g]	104	√					
114	135	√					
117	138					√	√
145	166	√					
146[h]	167					√	√

[a]Day of experiment
[b]Pigs were injected with either vaccine or saline
[c]One pig per pen was inoculated intranasally with PCV2 culture
[d]Blood samples were collected from two pigs per pen for ELISA analysis for antibodies against PCV2 and MHYO and PCR for PCV2
[e]Nasal swab samples were collected from two pigs per pen for PCR for MHYO
[f]All pigs were moved from nursery to grower facility at IRTA on d 48
[g]All pigs were moved from grower facility at IRTA to a commercial finishing farm d 83
[h]Carcass data was recorded d 159 for pigs classified at the abattoir

during this time; however it was necessary to distribute pigs within treatment group into 10 to 12 pigs per pen with all pens located in the same room. Pens at the commercial finisher had solid pen dividers that did not allow for pig contact between pens. From d 48 to 145 only individual pig body weight data was recorded at specific intervals (Table 3). Carcass weight and lean percentage classification was recorded at the abattoir for 292 of the original 363 pigs started on experiment. Experimental procedures for animals were approved by the *Departament de Medi Ambient i Habitatge de la Generalitat de Catalunya.*

Experimental starter diets

Two experimental non-medicated diets were fed during the initial 14 d after weaning and were typical of commercial starter diets for weaned pigs in Spain. SDPP was included at 6 % of the test diet (P) and replaced soy protein concentrate used in the control diet (C) on an equal lysine basis. Both starter diets were formulated to contain 1.45 % total lysine and met or exceeded nutrient requirements recommended by IRTA (Table 4). Common non-medicated commercial diets by phase of production were fed from d 14 to d 159 of the study to all pigs, with the exception that the diet fed from d 48 to 58 of the study contained 200 ppm amoxicillin, 24 ppm oxybendazol and 120 ppm colistin.

Vaccines

A combined PCV2 and MHYO vaccine was used by mixing two vaccines Ingelvac-Circoflex™ and Ingelvac-Mycoflex™ (Combo-Flex) prepared 1:1 according to the manufacturer's recommendations (Boehringer Ingelheim Vetmedica GmbH, Ingelheim am Rhein, Germany). The mixed vaccines were given as a single injection (2 ml) by intramuscular route in the neck at d 3 post-weaning. These vaccines were selected as the common products used under commercial conditions in the USA and Europe. Non-vaccinated pigs were injected with 2 ml saline solution at d 3 post-weaning.

PCV2 inocula

Due to low infectious pressure of PCV2 at d 63 post weaning (12 weeks of age), one pig in each pen was challenged with a field strain (SP-10-7-54-13) of PCV2b virus (titer $10^{5.24}$TCID$_{50}$/ml) replicated in PK-15 cells free of pestiviruses, *Porcine circovirus type 1*, and *Torque teno sus viruses 1* and *2* [34]. PCV2 was inoculated by intranasal route by applying 1 ml of virus culture on each nostril using an intranasal mucosal atomization device (LMA® MAD300 nasal, Teleflex Medical, NC).

Table 4 Ingredient and calculated nutrient composition of experimental starter diets

Ingredient, %	Control	Test
Barley	49.34	49.34
Wheat	1.58	0.00
Extruded whole soybeans	15.11	15.12
Soybean meal (47 % CP)	2.48	6.99
Spray dried porcine plasma[a]	0.00	6.00
Soy protein concentrate	9.50	0.00
Dried sweet whey	13.72	13.72
Animal fat	5.24	6.09
Dicalcium phosphate	1.84	2.09
Calcium carbonate	0.00	0.04
Salt	0.28	0.00
Vitamin-trace mineral premix[b]	0.25	0.25
L-lysine	0.36	0.21
DL-methionine	0.19	0.15
L-threonine	0.11	0.02
Total, %	100.0	100.0
Calculated nutrients		
Dry matter, %	89.97	89.55
Crude protein, %	21.08	21.08
Metabolizable energy, kcal/kg	3425	3425
Lactose, %	10.00	10.00
Ether extract, %	9.56	10.48
Ash, %	6.05	6.57
Calcium, %	0.73	0.80
Phosphorus, %	0.76	0.85
Digestible phosphorus, %	0.42	0.55
Sodium, %	0.22	0.34
Chloride, %	0.55	0.53
Lysine, %	1.45	1.45
Methionine, %	0.50	0.44
Methionine + Cysteine, %	0.87	0.89
Threonine, %	0.94	0.94
Tryptophan, %	0.26	0.29

[a]AP820™, APC Europe, Granollers, Spain
[b]Provided the following per kg of diet: vitamin A (E-672) 10000 UI; vitamin D$_3$ (E-671) 2000 UI; vitamin E (alpha-tocopherol) 25 mg; vitamin B$_1$ 1.5 mg; vitamin B$_2$ 3.5 mg; vitamin B$_6$ 2.4 mg; vitamin B$_{12}$ 20 µg; vitamin K$_3$ 1.5 mg; calcium panthotenate 14 mg; nicotinic acid 20 mg; folic acid 0.5 mg; biotin 50 µg; Fe (E-1) (from FeSO$_4$·H$_2$O) 120 mg; I (E-2) (from Ca(I$_2$O$_3$)$_2$) 0.75 mg; Co (E-3) (from 2CoCO$_3$·3Co(OH)$_2$·H$_2$O) 0.6 mg; Cu (E-4) (from CuSO$_4$·5H$_2$O) 150 mg; Mn (E-5) (from MnO) 60 mg; Zn (E-6) (from ZnO) 110 mg; Se (E-8) (from Na$_2$SeO$_3$) 0.37 mg

Sampling and analytical procedures

Blood samples and nasal swabs were collected from two pigs per pen (104 total pigs; 28.7 % of all study pigs) at selected intervals throughout the study (Table 3). The same pigs were sampled throughout the experiment to detect infection and seroconversion. A substitute pig from the same pen was sampled if a previously sampled pig had died. All blood by sampling day were centrifuged at 600 g for 15 min at 4 °C and the serum was analyzed for MHYO and PCV2 antibodies using respectively a monoclonal blocking ELISA Oxoid™ Mycoplasma hyopneumoniae (Oxoid LTD, UK) and an indirect ELISA Ingezim Circo IgG 1.1 PCV.K1 (Ingenasa, Spain), following manufacturers' instructions. The Oxoid™ ELISA detects antibodies against the 74kD outer external protein of MHYO and is considered more sensitive than and at least as specific as other tests [35]. The Oxoid™ ELISA is less useful to measure antibody levels (it measures percentage of inhibition), but in our study working with conventional pigs that may have unspecific serum reactions for other Mycoplasma species [36], the Oxoid™ ELISA kit was selected. For the Oxoid™ ELISA test an inhibition value >65 was considered positive, while for the PCV2 ELISA an S/P ratio >17 was considered positive.

Nasal swabs were re-suspended in 1000 μL of sterile phosphate-buffered saline (PBS) and vigorously vortexed, and 200 μL of the suspension was used for MHYO DNA extraction. DNA was extracted from nasal and serum swab suspensions using BioSprint 96 DNA Blood Kit (Quiagen Hilden, Germany) based on automated magnetic bead extraction system. To assess for potential contamination during the extraction procedure a negative control was included using PBS as an extraction substrate. Serum samples were analyzed for the presence of PCV2 genome by means of a real time quantitative PCR (qrt-PCR) as previously described [37]. Viral concentrations were expressed as PCV2 DNA copy numbers per ml of serum, as described previously [38]. Nested PCR (nPCR) for MHYO were tested by means of a previously described technique [31, 39].

Statistical analysis

Pen was used as the experimental unit when analyzing the effect of weight block and treatment group. Orthogonal treatment comparisons for the main effects of vaccination (treatment groups 1 VC + 2 VP vs treatment groups 3 SC + 4 SP), starter diet (2 VP + 4 SP vs 1 VC + 3 SC), and interaction of vaccination and starter diet (1 VC + 4 SP vs 2 VP + 3 SC), along with the covariance of initial BW were included in the analysis of variance model (SAS 9.2, SAS Inst. Inc., Cary, NC). Individual pig BW and mortality rate at various intervals from wean to finish and individual pig carcass data were analyzed for treatment group, sex, and interaction of treatment and sex, along with the covariance of initial BW and the orthogonal treatment comparisons previously described. Serology and nasal swab data were analyzed the same as individual pig body weight and carcass data. Results were considered significant at P <0.05.

Competing interests
Joan P and Joaquim S declare they have no competing interests. Javier P, Carmen R, Joy C and Joe C are employed by APC Inc who manufactures and sells spray dried plasma.

Authors' contributions
Joan P, Javier P and JS designed and monitored the study, co-wrote the paper. CR, Joy C and Joe C provided statistical analysis and co-wrote the paper. All authors contributed to revisions and read and approved the final manuscript.

Acknowledgements
The authors thank the ownership of the commercial farm for housing animals during the final finishing stages and the collaboration of the abattoir for assistance in collection of carcass information.

Author details
[1]IRTA, Centre de Recerca en Sanitat Animal (CReSA, IRTA-UAB), Campus de la Universitat Autònoma de Barcelona, 08193 Bellaterra, Barcelona, Spain. [2]UAB, Centre de Recerca en Sanitat Animal (CReSA, IRTA-UAB), Campus de la Universitat Autònoma de Barcelona, 08193 Bellaterra, Barcelona, Spain. [3]Departament de Sanitat i Anatomia Animals, Universitat Autònoma de Barcelona (UAB), 08193 Bellaterra, Barcelona, Spain. [4]APC EUROPE, S.A. Avda. Sant Julià 246-258, Pol. Ind. El Congost, E-08403 Granollers, Spain. [5]APC Inc., 2425 SE Oak Tree Court, Ankeny, IA 50021, USA.

References
1. Coffey RD, Cromwell GL. Use of spray-dried animal plasma in diets for weanling pigs. Pig News & Information. 2001;22:39–48.
2. Torrallardona D. Spray dried animal plasma as an alternative to antibiotics in weanling pigs – a review. Asian-Aust J Anim Sci. 2010;23:131–48.
3. Messier S, Gagne-Fortin C, Crenshaw J. Dietary spray-dried porcine plasma reduces mortality attributed to porcine circovirus associated disease síndrome. Orlando: Proc AASV; 2007. p. 147–50.
4. Morés N, Ciacci-Zanella JR, Amara AL, Cordebella A, Lima GJMM, Miele M, et al. Spray dried porcine plasma in nursery and grower feed reduces the severity of Porcine Circovirus associated diseases. Proc Allen D Leman Swine Conf Recent Res Rep St Paul, MN. 2007;34 Suppl:3.
5. Segalés J, Allan GM, Domingo M. Porcine circovirus diseases. Animal Health Res Rev. 2005;6:119–42.
6. Thacker EL. Mycoplasmal disease. In: Straw B, Zimmerman J, D'Allaire S, Taylor DJ, editors. Diseases of Swine. 9th ed. Ames: Blackwell Publishing; 2006. p. 701–17.
7. Opriessnig T, Thacker EL, Yu S, Fenaux M, Meng XJ. Experimental reproduction of postweaning multisystemic wasting syndrome in pigs by dual infection with Mycoplasma hyopneumoniae and porcine circovirus type 2. Vet Pat. 2004;41:624–40.
8. Zhang H, Lunney JK, Baker RB, Opriessnig T. Cytokine and chemokine mRNA expression profiles in tracheobronchial lymph nodes from pigs singularly infected or coinfected with porcine circovirus type 2 (PCV2) and Mycoplasma hyopneumoniae (MHYO). Vet Immunol Immunopathol. 2011; 140:152–8.
9. Opriessnig T, Madson DM, Schalk S, Brockmeier S, Shen HG. Porcine circovirus type 2 (PCV2) vaccination is effective in reducing disease and PCV2 shedding in semen of boars concurrently infected with PCV2 and Mycoplasma hyopneumoniae. Theriogenology. 2011;76:351–60.
10. Sibila M, Fort M, Nofrarías M, Pérez de Rozas A, Galindo-Cardiel I, Mateu E, et al. Simultaneous porcine circovirus type 2 and Mycoplasma hyopneumoniae co-inoculation does not potentiate disease in conventional pigs. J Comp Pathol. 2012;147(2-3):285–95.
11. Maes D, Segalés J, Meyns T, Sibila M, Pieters M, Haesebrouck F. Control of Mycoplasma hyopneumoniae infections in pigs. Vet Microbiol. 2008;126(4): 297–309.
12. Segalés J. Best practice and future challenges for vaccination against porcine circovirus type 2. Expert Rev Vaccines. 2015;14(3):473–87.
13. Payne B, Cline G. The effect of commercial combination PCV2/Mycoplasma hyopneumoniae vaccination products on wean to finish performance. Proc

Allen D Leman Swine Conf. St Paul, MN. 2012;39:203. Retrieved from the University of Minnesota Digital Conservancy, 2012; http://purl.umn.edu/151607

14. Kane EM, Potter ML, Bergstrom JR, Dritz SS, Tokach MD, DeRouchey JM, et al. Effects of diet source and timing of porcine circovirus type 2 (PCV2) and *Mycoplasma hyopneumoniae* vaccines on post-weaning nursery pig performance. J Anim Sci. 2009;87(E-Suppl 3):7.

15. Myers AJ, Bergstrom JR, Tokach MD, Dritz SS, Goodband RD, DeRouchey JM, et al. Effects of Liquitein on weanling pigs administered a porcine circovirus type 2 and *Mycoplasma hyopneumoniae* vaccine strategy. Kansas State University Swine Day. 2011;62-69. http://hdl.handle.net/2097/13480.

16. Potter ML, Kane EM, Bergstrom JR, Dritz SS, Tokach MD, DeRouchey JM, et al. Effects of diet source and vaccination for porcine circovirus type 2 and Mycoplasma hyopneumoniae on nursery pig performance. J Anim Sci. 2012;90:4063–71.

17. Lallès JP, Bosi P, Janczyk P, Koopmans SJ, Torrallardona D. Impact of bioactive substances on the gastrointestinal tract and performance of weaned piglets: a review. Animal. 2009;1:1–19.

18. Campbell JM, Crenshaw JD, Polo J. The biological stress of early weaned piglets. J Anim Sci Biotech. 2013;4:19–22.

19. Spreeuwenberg MAM, Verdonk JMAJ, Gaskins HR, Verstegen MWA. Small intestine epithelial barrier function is compromised in pigs with low feed intake at weaning. J Nutr. 2001;131:1520–7.

20. Smith F, Clark JE, Overman BL, Tozel CC, Huang JH, Rivier JEF, et al. Early weaning stress impairs development of mucosal barrier function in the porcine intestine. Am J Physiol Gastrointest Liver Physiol. 2010;298:G352–63.

21. McKay DM, Baird AW. Cytokine regulation of epithelial permeability and ion transport. Gut. 1999;44:282–9.

22. Píe S, Lallès JP, Blazy F, Laffite J, Sève B, Oswald IP. Weaning is associated with an upregulation of expression of inflammatory cytokines in the intestine of piglets. J Nutr. 2004;134:641–7.

23. Peace RM, Campbell J, Polo J, Crenshaw J, Russell L, Moeser A. Spray-dried porcine plasma influences intestinal barrier function, inflammation and diarrhea in weaned pigs. J Nutr. 2011;141:1312–7.

24. Campbell J, Crenshaw J, Polo J. Impact of feeding spray-dried plasma to pigs challenged with swine influenza virus. Barcelona: Proc Intl Symp Emerging and Re-emerging Pig Diseases; 2011. p. 269.

25. Boyer PE, D'Costa S, Edwards LL, Milloway M, Susick E, Borst LB, et al. 2015. Early-life dietary spray-dried plasma influences immunological and intestinal injury response to later-life *Salmonella typhimurium* challenge. Brit J Nutr. 2015. doi:10.10.1017/S00071145140422X.

26. Fachinger V, Bischoff R, Jedidia SB, Saalmüller A, Elbers K. The effect of vaccination against porcine circovirus type 2 in pigs suffering from porcine respiratory disease complex. Vaccine. 2008;26(11):1488–99.

27. Kixmöller M, Ritzmann M, Eddicks M, Saalmüller A, Elbers K, Fachinger V. Reduction of PMWS-associated clinical signs and co-infections by vaccination against PCV2. Vaccine. 2008;26(27-28):3443–51.

28. Fraile L, Grau-Roma L, Sarosola P, Sinovas N, Nofrarías M, López-Jimenez R, et al. Inactivated PCV2 one shot vaccine applied in 3-week-old piglets: Improvement of production parameters and interaction with maternally derived immunity. Vaccine. 2012;30(11):1986–92.

29. Martelli P, Saleri R, Cavalli V, De Angelis E, Ferrari L, Benetti M, et al. Systemic and local immune response in pigs intradermally and intramuscularly injected with inactivated *Mycoplasma hyopneumoniae* vaccines. Vet Microbiol. 2014;168(24):357–64.

30. Huang Y, Ladinig A, Ashley C, Haines DM, Harding J. Innate and adaptive responses of snatch-farrowed porcine-colostrum-deprived pigs to *Mycoplasma hyopneumoniae* vaccination. BMC Vet Res. 2014;10:219.

31. Sibila M, Calsamiglia M, Vidal D, Badiella LI, Aldaz A, Jensen JC. Dynamics of Mycoplasma hyopneumoniae infection in 12 farms with different production systems. Can J Vet Res. 2004;68(1):12–8.

32. Fort M, Sibila M, Allepuz A, Mateu E, Roerink F, Segalés J. Porcine circovirus type 2 (PCV2) vaccination of conventional pigs prevents viremia against PCV2 isolates of different genotypes and geographical origins. Vaccine. 2008;26(8):1063–71.

33. Opriessnig T, Gerber PF, Xiao C-T, Halbur PG, Matzinger SR, Xiang-Jin M. Commercial PCV2a-based vaccines are effective in protecting naturally PCV2b-infected finisher pigs against experimental challenge with a 2012 mutant PCV2. Vaccine. 2014;32(34):4342–8.

34. Fort M, Sibila M, Nofrarías M, Perez-Martin E, Olvera A, Mateu E, et al. Porcine circovirus type 2 (PCV2) Cap and Rep proteins are involved in the development of cell-mediated immunity upon PCV2 infection. Vet Immunol Immunopathol. 2010;137:226–34.

35. Ameri-Mahabadi M, Zhou E-M, Hsu WH. Comparison of two swine Mycoplasma hyopneumoniae enzyme-linked immunosorbent assays for detection of antibodies from vaccinated pigs and field serum samples. J Vet Diagn Invest. 2005;17:61–4.

36. Feld NC, Qvist P, Ahrens P, Friis NF, Meyling A. A monoclonal blocking ELISA detecting serum antibodies to Mycoplasma hyopneumoniae. Vet Microbiol. 1992;30:35–46.

37. Olvera A, Sibila M, Calsamiglia M, Segalés J, Domingo M. Comparison of porcine circovirus type 2 load in serum quantified by a real time PCR in postweaning multisystemic wasting syndrome and porcine dermatitis and nephropathy syndrome naturally affected pigs. J Virol Methods. 2004;117(1):75–80.

38. Grau-Roma L, Hjulsager CK, Sibila M, Kristensen CS, López-Soria S, Enøe C, et al. Infection, excretion and seroconversion dynamics of porcine circovirus type 2 (PCV2) in pigs from post-weaning multisystemic wasting syndrome (PMWS) affected farms in Spain and Denmark. Vet Microbiol. 2009;135(3-4):272–82.

39. Calsamiglia M, Pijoan C, Trigo A. Application of a nested polymerase chain reaction assay to detect Mycoplasma hyopneumoniae from nasal swabs. J Swine Health Prod. 1999;7:263–8.

2

Characteristics and risk factors for severe repeat-breeder female pigs and their lifetime performance in commercial breeding herds

Satomi Tani[1*], Carlos Piñeiro[2] and Yuzo Koketsu[1]

Abstract

Background: Repeat-breeder females increase non-productive days (NPD) and decrease herd productivity and profitability. The objectives of the present study were 1) to define severe repeat-breeder (SRB) females in commercial breeding herds, 2) to characterize the pattern of SRB occurrences across parities, 3) to examine factors associated with SRB risk, and 4) to compare lifetime reproductive performances of SRB and non-SRB females. Data included 501,855 service records and lifetime records of 93,604 breeding-female pigs in 98 Spanish herds between 2008 and 2013. An SRB female pig was defined as either a pig that had three or more returns. The 98 herds were classified into high-, intermediate- and low-performing herds based by the upper and lower 25th percentiles of the herd mean of annualized lifetime pigs weaned per sow. Multi-level mixed-effects logistic regression models with random intercept were applied to the data.

Results: Of 93,604 females, 1.2% of females became SRB pigs in their lifetime, with a mean SRB risk per service (± SEM) of 0.26 ± 0.01%. Risks factors for becoming an SRB pig were low parity, being first-served in summer, having a prolonged weaning-to-first-mating interval (WMI), and being in low-performing herds. For example, served gilts had 0.81% higher SRB risk than served sows ($P < 0.01$). Also, female pigs in a low-performing herd had 1.19% higher SRB risks than those in a high-performing herd. However, gilt age at-first-mating ($P = 0.08$), lactation length ($P = 0.05$) and number of stillborn piglets ($P = 0.28$) were not associated with becoming an SRB female. The SRB females had 14.4–16.4 fewer lifetime pigs born alive, 42.8–91.3 more lifetime NPD, and 2.1–2.2 lower parities at culling than non-SRB females ($P < 0.05$).

Conclusions: We recommend that producers closely monitor the female pig groups at higher risk of becoming an SRB.

Keywords: Severe repeat-breeding, Lifetime performance, Herd productivity groups

Background

Approximately 7% of first-served female pigs are re-served in commercial herds [1]. Furthermore, a study of 539 U.S.A. herds reported that 17–20% of the re-served females had a second re-service, and also that 22–27% of the second-return females had a total of three or more re-service occurrences [2]. A recent study also indicated that culling guidelines for third-returned females are not always strictly implemented [3], and so a substantial number of severe repeat-breeder (SRB) female pigs may exist in commercial herds, thus increasing non-productive days (NPD) and affecting herd productivity [4]. Meanwhile, there is no clear and consistent definition for repeat-breeder females in previous studies. Repeat-breeding has been defined as one return [5, 6], while SRB has been defined as one to four returns and culled [7]. Furthermore, there is little information about SRB females in commercial herds, such as their lifetime performance, nor how the reproductive performance in parities before a re-service occurrence differs from that of non-SRB females.

---

* Correspondence: composition.013@gmail.com
[1]School of Agriculture, Meiji University, Higashi-mita 1-1-1, Tama-ku, Kawasaki, Kanagawa 214-8571, Japan
Full list of author information is available at the end of the article

Re-servicing has been associated with lower parity and summer serving [8–10]. Other factors that have been associated with lower farrowing rate and more returns are higher pre-service outdoor temperature and prolonged weaning-to-first-mating interval (WMI; [9, 11, 12]). Additionally, a high abortion risk, which is one of the reasons for return occurrences, is also associated with an increased number of stillborn piglets [13]. However, risk factors for SRB females have not been quantified, nor has the pattern of SRB females across parities been examined in detail. Therefore, the objectives of this study were 1) to define SRB females in commercial breeding herds, 2) characterize SRB females across parities, 3) to quantify factors associated with SRB risk, 4) to compare lifetime reproductive performances of SRB and non-SRB females, and 5) to compare reproductive performance of SRB and non-SRB sows in the parity before the SRB sows had their SRB occurrence.

Methods
Study herds
A consultancy firm (PigCHAMP Pro Europa S.L. Segovia, Spain) has requested all client producers to mail their data files since 1998. At the end of 2013, 98 out of the 120 Spanish client herds (82%) allowed their herd data to be used for research purposes. In 2013 the database included approximately 0.7% of all herds in Spain, one of the major pig producing regions in Europe. There are 2,568,450 female pigs in 19,630 breeding herds in Spain [14].

These herds use natural or mechanical ventilation in their farrowing, breeding and gestation barns. The lactation and gestation diets are formulated using cereals (barley, wheat and corn) and soybean meal. Also, all the herds use artificial insemination; double or triple inseminations of sows during an estrous period are practiced for breeding management. Replacement gilts in the herds were either purchased from breeding companies or were home-produced through internal multiplication programs.

Study design, data collection and exclusion criteria
The present study was designed as a retrospective cohort study coordinating by-parity service records from herd entry to removal for female pigs entered the herds from 2008 to 2010, using the PigCHAMP recording system at the end of 2013. Service record were collected from January 2008 to June 2013, because the female pigs lived up to 3 years. At the time the records were collected, 4842 (4.8%) of the 99,533 female pigs had not yet been removed from the herds and so these records were excluded when lifetime records were analyzed. Thus, the initial data contained 517,222 service records in 465,947 parity records and lifetime records of 94,691 females in

the 98 herds. Female pigs were excluded if they had NPD of more than 289 days (99th percentile; 949 records), because these data were likely to be incorrectly recorded.

Service records of sows were excluded if they met any of the following criteria: total number of pigs born was 0 pigs or 26 pigs or more (215 records; [15]); lactation length of either 0–9 days or greater than 41 days (3756 records; [16]); WMI of 36 days or more (3779 records; [16]); re-service intervals of 151 days or more (479 records). Hence, the data included 501,855 service records in 454,058 parity records of 93,604 female pigs. Additionally, records with no gilt age at first-mating (AFM) or with an AFM of either less than 160 days or more than 401 days (6767 females; [16]) were excluded when the combined gilts and sows model was used. Two datasets were created from the data, containing lifetime performance (Dataset 1) and service records for consecutive parities (Dataset 2).

Definitions and categories
An SRB female pig was defined as a pig that had had three or more returns within the same parity, based on a modification of the definition used for RB cows [17]. The SRB risk (%) was defined as the number of SRB females divided by the number of first-served females. A re-served female pig was defined as a pig that had more than one service event within the same parity. The first, second and third returns were defined as the first, second and third returns-to-service within the same parity, respectively. A service included one or more inseminations or natural matings during an estrus period. Re-service intervals were categorized into four groups: early, regular, irregular, and late returns, with respective re-service intervals of 11 to 17, 18 to 24, 25 to 38 and 39 to 150 days post-service [8].

Annualized lifetime pigs weaned per sow was defined as the lifetime number of weaned pigs divided by the sum of the reproductive herd life days × 365 days. Reproductive herd life days was defined as the number of days from the date that the gilts was first-inseminated to its removal [18]. Lifetime NPD was defined as the number of days when a female was neither gestating nor lactating during her reproductive herd life. Lifetime pigs born alive was defined as the sum of the number of pigs born alive in a sow's lifetime.

Three categories of herd productivity were defined on the basis of the upper and lower 25th percentiles of the herd means of annualized lifetime pigs weaned per sow: high-performing herds (> 24.7 pigs), intermediate herds (24.7 to 21.2 pigs) and low-performing herds (< 21.2 pigs). Mean (± SEM) herd size between 2008 and 2013 was 699 ± 64.3 females with a range between 81 and 3222 females.

Removal types included culling and death. Culling due to reproductive failure included culling due to being found not pregnant, repeats and abortion. Reasons for culling were recorded by producers when female pigs were culled. Served month was categorized into four seasonal groups (January to March, April to June, July to September and October to December). Three WMI groups were formed: 0 to 6 days, 7 to 12 days and 13 days or more.

Statistical analysis

Descriptive statistics were performed using SAS version 9.3 (SAS Inst. Inc., Cary, NC). A linear mixed-effects model was applied to the two datasets using the MIXED procedure with a Tukey-Kramer multiple comparisons test. Models 1 and 2 were applied to examine the association between production factors and lifetime performances in Dataset 1 (Model 1), or previous reproductive performance by parity groups in Dataset 2 (Model 2). These models included female groups (SRB or non-SRB females), the four seasonal service groups, the three herd productivity groups and entry year as fixed effects. A random herd effect was also included in both models. A chi-square test was conducted using SAS software to compare the relative frequency (%) of re-service intervals between SRB females and non-SRB females. Also, herd size was compared between the herd groups using ANOVA.

Models 3 and 4 were used to analyze service records for gilts and sows (Model 3) and sows only (Model 4) to determine whether or not a female pig was SRB (i.e., SRB risk per service). Models 3 and 4 were also used to account for the 3-level hierarchy of individual service records within a female and for females within a herd. The models were constructed by applying multilevel generalized linear models for SRB risks with a logit link function to Dataset 2 using MLwiN version 2.29 (University of Bristol, Bristol, UK). However, initial analyses showed that the estimated variances at the sow level were very close to zero (<0.0001). Therefore, the sow level was omitted from the models for the SRB risks [19, 20]. Parameter estimation was performed using the second-order penalized quasi-likelihood method and the iterative generalized least squares algorithm in MLwiN. The models contained the four seasonal service groups, the three herd productivity groups and entry year as fixed effects. Model 3 included AFM, whereas Model 4 contained sow specific factors such as the number of stillborn piglets, the three WMI groups and lactation length. All the continuous variables were centered at their grand mean values. Non-significant variables ($P > 0.05$) were eliminated from each model. The quadratic expressions of continuous variables were examined and non-significant quadratic expressions were removed

($P \geq 0.05$). Random herd effect was also included in the models. The adequacy of the model assumptions for the random effects was assessed by visual inspection of normal-probability plots [21].

Intraclass correlation coefficient

The intraclass correlation coefficients (ICC) were calculated by the following equation [22] to assess the variance in SRB risk that could be explained by the herd:

ICC (records within the same herd) $= \sigma_v^2 / \left(\sigma_v^2 + (\pi^2/3) \right)$, in which σ_v^2 is the between-herd variance and $\pi^2/3$ is the variance at the assumed individual record level.

Results

Mean SRB risk per service ($\pm$ SEM) was 0.26 $\pm$ 0.01% (Table 1). The SRB risks were greater in low parities, with 0.57 and 0.30% SRB risks for parity 0 and 1 females, respectively, compared with only 0.07–0.21% in parity 2 or higher sows (Table 2). The SRB female pigs had more regular returns than non-SRB female pigs ($P < 0.05$; Fig. 1) but the mean ($\pm$ SEM) re-service interval for SRB females was 30.8 $\pm$ 0.31 days because 20% of SRB females had late re-service intervals of 39–150 days. Also, the proportions of SRB females having regular returns at the first, second and third re-service were 50, 57 and 59%, respectively ($P < 0.05$). Third returns occurred in 92% of the 98 herds. Larger herd size was associated with herd productivity groups; low-performing herds (Mean $\pm$ SEM: 482 $\pm$ 60 females) and intermediate herds (617 $\pm$ 83 females) had smaller herd sizes than high-performing herds (1095 $\pm$ 169 pigs; $P < 0.01$).

With regard to lifetime performance, 1150 (1.2%) of the 93,604 females became SRB pigs in their lifetime (Table 3). The SRB females had 3.0–4.3 fewer annualized lifetime pigs weaned, 14.4–16.4 fewer lifetime pigs born alive, 42.8–91.3 more lifetime NPD and 2.1–2.2 lower parities at culling than non-SRB females ($P < 0.01$; Table 3). Additionally, females that became SRB in parity 1 had 5.2% lower farrowing rates in their previous parity than non-SRB females ($P < 0.01$; Table 4). However, there was no difference between SRB and non-SRB female groups for WMI ($P \geq 0.07$).

In both the first-served female (sows and gilts) model and the sows only model, an SRB risk was associated with low parity (i.e., parities 0 and 1), being first-served in summer and being fed in low-performing herds ($P < 0.01$; Table 5). Also, in the sows only model an SRB risk was associated with sows having prolonged WMI. For example, served gilts had 0.43 to 0.81% higher SRB risk than served sows ($P < 0.01$; Table 6). Additionally, females in a low-performing herd had 0.73 to 1.19% higher SRB risks than those in a high-performing herd.

Table 1 Reproductive data for female pigs in 98 commercial herds from 2008 to 2013

Measurements	N	Mean ± SEM	Range Minimum	Maximum
Lifetime records				
Parity at removal	93,604	4.6 ± 0.01	0	13
Gilt age at first-mating, days old[a]	86,837	251.6 ± 0.15	160	400
Number of lifetime pigs born alive	86,749	58.7 ± 0.11	0	202
Lifetime non-productive days of female pigs	93,604	84.9 ± 0.16	0	289
Female life days	88,972	942.8 ± 1.26	28	1703
SRB females, %	93,604	1.2 ± 0.03	–	–
Parity records				
Parity at service	454,058	2.6 ± 0.01	0	12
Records with two returns or more, %	454,058	1.37 ± 0.01	–	–
SRB risk for first served females, %	454,058	0.26 ± 0.01	–	–
Number of pigs born alive	360,454	12.1 ± 0.01	0	25
Number of stillborn piglets	360,454	0.9 ± 0.01	0	19
Lactation length, days	360,454	23.4 ± 0.01	10	41
Weaning-to-first-mating interval, days	360,454	5.8 ± 0.01	0	35
Service records				
Number of services	501,855	1.1 ± 0.01	1	9
Re-service intervals for RB females, days	4258	30.8 ± 0.31	11	145

SRB severe repeat-breeder
[a]The remaining records (93,604-N) were regarded as missing records

Also, the SRB risk of sows that had a WMI of 7–12 days was 0.10% higher than that of sows which had a shorter WMI of only 0–6 days (*P* < 0.05; Table 6). However, AFM (*P* = 0.08), lactation length (*P* = 0.05) and fewer stillborn piglets (*P* = 0.28) were not associated with being an SRB female. With regard to the ICC, the random herd effect explained 25.5% and 30.1% of total variance values for SRB risk in the female (gilts and sows) model and the sow only model, respectively (Table 5).

Discussion

Our study showed that one fifth of the 1.2% of first-served females that became RB pigs had re-service intervals of 39–150 days which would greatly increase NPD. Also, re-serving is one of the risk factors for abortion [13] and further increasing NPD. Re-service intervals and culling intervals account for 70% of NPD [4] which must be minimized to improve sow productivity. Additionally, the fact that SRB females had more regular re-service intervals (18–24 days) than non-SRB females

Table 2 Severe repeat-breeder (SRB) risks in served female pigs by parity group

Measurements	Parity 0	1	2	3	4	5	6 or later
Number of serviced records	93,604	78,243	70,596	62,258	53,371	43,634	52,352
Number of first return records	11,458	8734	5625	4730	3772	2694	2614
First return occurrences, %	12.2	11.2	8.0	7.6	7.1	6.2	5.0
Number of second return records	2325	1324	834	695	490	297	290
Number of culled records after the second return[a]	246	142	87	105	68	55	49
Number of removed records after the second return[b]	394	232	168	136	90	68	64
Number of SRB females[c]	532	235	145	104	70	34	38
SRB risk for first-served females, %	0.57	0.30	0.21	0.17	0.13	0.08	0.07

[a]Number of females culled due to reproductive failure
[b]Other removed records included females removed due to non-reproductive problems (e.g., lameness, diseases or death)
[c]The 8 pigs (1158-1150) had twice SRB in their lifetime

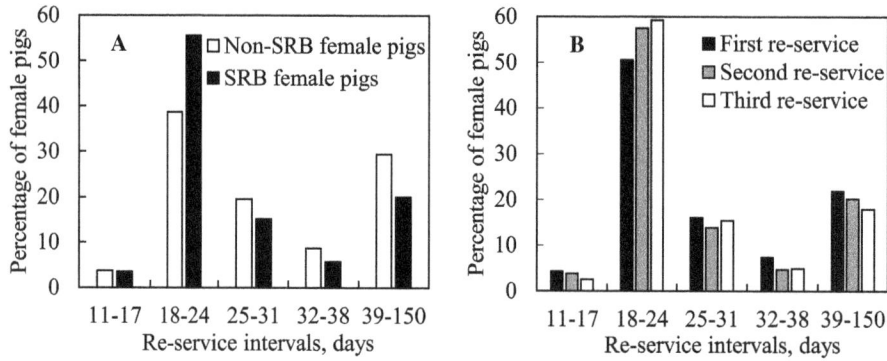

Fig. 1 Relative frequencies (%) of re-service intervals for re-service records. **a** Re-service intervals for 5968 re-service records of severe repeat-breeder (SRB) females and 41,401 re-service records of non-SRB females. **b** Re-service intervals for 2469 first, 2008 s and 1491 third re-service records of SRB females

indicates that SRB females are more likely to have either conception failure or failure of maternal recognition [8]. Other factors may also have contributed to the greater likelihood of SRB females having regular re-service, such as semen quality and storage [23], as well as timing of insemination [24].

In our study we found clear parity effects on the likelihood of females becoming SRB, with a higher risk in low parity females. One possible reason for the higher SRB risks in low parity females is that culling pressure for low parity females is not as high as that for aged sows, because gilts and parity 1 sows are still growing animals and producers want to recover the initial cost of a replacement gilt [5, 25]. Also, some sows with a reproductive problem may be culled before parity 2. Furthermore, recent data from Spanish, Portuguese and Italian herds showed that 41 and 36% of respective first-returned gilts and parity 1 sows had a return recurrence in the same or later parity [20]. Therefore, it is critical to

have more accurate estrus detection and strict selection criteria for gilts in order to decrease both the number of SRB gilts and parity 1 sows and NPD in breeding herds. However, in our study low parity SRB females had shorter estrus duration than equivalent non-SRB females (Fig. 1), and it has also been reported that low parity females have subtle estrus behavior that is more difficult to detect [26]. Therefore, these differences in estrus characteristics make it difficult to identify the correct insemination timing in SRB females. One way to improve gilt development would be to include a boar stimulation protocol [27], which would help to distinguish between gilts that would become fertile females in breeding herds and those that are more likely to become SRB females.

In our study, females that were served in summer had a 0.1% higher SRB risk than those served in winter. Therefore, it appears that high temperature or low lactational feed intake in summer can increase conception failure or pregnancy loss in served females. Other

Table 3 Comparisons of lifetime performance between three female return-to-service groups

Lifetime performance measurements	Female return groups					
	Non-return		Return once or twice, but not SRB		SRB	
	N	Mean (± SE)	N	Mean (± SE)	N	Mean (± SE)
Annualized lifetime number of pigs born alive	56,803	27.6 (0.15)[a]	29,093	25.7 (0.15)[b]	853	21.4 (0.26)[c]
Annualized lifetime number of pigs weaned	56,803	23.6 (0.10)[a]	29,093	22.3 (0.10)[b]	853	19.3 (0.20)[c]
Lifetime non-productive days	61,348	74.0 (1.26)[c]	31,106	122.5 (1.26)[b]	1150	165.3 (1.74)[a]
Lifetime pigs born alive	56,803	58.9 (0.80)[b]	29,093	60.9 (0.80)[a]	853	44.5 (1.35)[c]
Gilt age at first-mating, days old	57,022	254.6 (3.18)[ab]	28,771	253.7 (3.18)[b]	1044	254.7 (3.33)[a]
Number of parity at removal	61,348	4.7 (0.07)[b]	31,106	4.9 (0.07)[a]	1150	2.9 (0.10)[c]
Number of parity at culling	51,496	4.9 (0.08)[b]	27,389	5.0 (0.08)[a]	1052	2.8 (0.11)[c]
Number of parity at death	9852	3.2 (0.07)[c]	3717	4.1 (0.07)[a]	98	3.5 (0.24)[b]
Female life days	58,482	950.2 (10.28)[b]	29,407	1029.5 (10.28)[a]	1083	807.7 (14.99)[c]
Total cumulative re-service intervals, days	61,348	0.0 (0.00)	31,106	56.0 (1.05)[b]	1150	111.3 (1.52)[a]

SE standard error, *SRB* severe repeat-breeder
[a-c]Mean values within a row followed by different letters differ (*P* < 0.05)

Table 4 Comparisons of reproductive performances[1] between severe repeat-breeder (SRB) and non-SRB sows

| | Female pigs | |
| | Non-SRB | SRB |
Parity	Mean (± SE)	Mean (± SE)
Farrowing rate for first service in the previous parity, %		
Parity 1	87.6 (0.54)[a]	82.4 (2.07)[b]
Parity 2	88.6 (0.49)	84.6 (2.51)
Parity 3	92.4 (0.38)	96.5 (2.45)
Parity 4	92.9 (0.34)	89.5 (2.88)
Parity 5	93.2 (0.36)	93.2 (3.96)
Parity 6	94.5 (0.31)	93.4 (4.24)
Weaning-to-first-mating interval in the previous parity, days		
Parity 2	8.3 (0.19)	7.5 (0.73)
Parity 3	6.4 (0.10)	6.8 (0.59)
Parity 4	6.1 (0.10)	6.3 (0.67)
Parity 5	5.9 (0.10)	5.2 (0.88)
Parity 6	5.7 (0.09)	5.6 (0.98)

[1]Reproductive performances are measured at the previous parity before the SRB females became SRB
[a,b]Mean values within a row fallowed by different letters differ ($P < 0.05$)

research has also shown that parity 1 sows are more sensitive than parity 2 or higher sows to high temperature for increasing returns to re-service [8]. It has been suggested that a pregnancy loss in summer is related to a combination of low GnRH secretion, decreased LH release impaired ovarian follicle development and consequently degraded corpora lutea functions that produce low progesterone concentrations [28].

The WMI effect on sows becoming SRB could be related to low gonadotropin secretion and possibly impaired endocrine systems. For example, prolonged WMI in sows is thought to be due to low LH secretion caused by low feed intake during lactation [29]. Therefore, in this study we found that the main risk factors for SRB were low parity (0 or 1), being first-served in summer and having WMI 7–12 days. These findings are consistent with previous studies in the U.S.A., Sweden and Japan reporting a higher re-service risk associated with the same three factors [8, 10, 30].

We also found that herd productivity affected SRB risk. This result suggests that heat detection, pregnancy diagnosis, as well as culling policy and implementation were not good enough in the low-performing herds, probably because small-sized low-performing herds do not have sufficient resources for advanced production systems, sufficient gilt pool, equipment or professional workers. Also, herds with more SRB females will have decreased reproductive productivity and so would become low-performing herds. In contrast, large-sized high-performing herds are likely to be able to employ more skilled workers and have better facilities than small-to mid-sized low-performing herds [31]. Finally, the lack of any association in our study between SRB risks and either lactation length, AFM or the number of

Table 5 Estimates of factors in the final logistic regression models of the severe repeat-breeder risks

| Fixed effects and variance | Gilts and sows | | Sows only | |
	Estimate (± SE)	P-value	Estimate (± SE)	P-value
Intercept[a]	− 8.584 (0.283)	<0.01	− 8.836 (0.325)	<0.01
Parity groups		<0.01		<0.01
Parity 0	2.170 (0.149)		–	
Parity 1	1.534 (0.155)		1.562 (0.155)	
Parity 2–5	0.827 (0.151)		0.862 (0.151)	
First-served month group		<0.01		<0.01
Apr.-Jun.	0.028 (0.075)		0.009 (0.101)	
Jul.-Sep.	0.302 (0.071)		0.338 (0.094)	
Oct.-Dec.	− 0.015 (0.076)		− 0.003 (0.102)	
Herd productivity groups		<0.01		<0.01
Intermediate-performing herds	1.636 (0.288)		1.856 (0.339)	
Low-performing herds	2.473 (0.324)		2.764 (0.377)	
WMI groups				0.03
WMI 7–12 days	–		0.280 (0.111)	
WMI 13 days or more	–		− 0.063 (0.134)	
Herd variance	1.12 (0.18)		1.42 (0.24)	
ICC (records within the same herd), %	25.5		30.1	

SE standard error, *ICC* intraclass correlation coefficient, *WMI* weaning-to-first-mating interval

Table 6 Comparisons between factors for severe repeat-breeder (SRB) risks per service

Explanatory variables	Gilts and sows	
	N	SRB risk (99% CI)
Parity groups		
0	93,604	0.92 (0.67–1.26)[a]
1	78,243	0.49 (0.35–0.68)[b]
2–5	229,859	0.24 (0.17–0.34)[c]
6 or more	52,352	0.11 (0.07–0.18)[d]
First-served month group		
Jan.-Mar.	113,178	0.29 (0.21–0.42)[b]
Apr.-Jun.	114,322	0.30 (0.21–0.44)[b]
Jul.-Sep.	112,615	0.40 (0.27–0.56)[a]
Oct.-Dec.	113,943	0.29 (0.20–0.41)[b]
Herd productivity groups		
Low-performing herds	65,565	1.30 (0.73–2.22)[a]
Intermediate-performing herds	196,848	0.57 (0.37–0.85)[b]
High-performing herds	191,645	0.11 (0.06–0.21)[c]
WMI groups[1]		
WMI 0–6 days	315,071	0.26 (0.19–0.39)[b]
WMI 7–12 days	22,633	0.36 (0.23–0.57)[a]
WMI 13 days or more	22,750	0.27 (0.15–0.42)[ab]

CI confidence interval, WMI weaning-to-first-mating interval
[a-c]Mean values within a group with different letters are different ($P < 0.05$)
[1]The WMI groups were compared in the model containing sows only (N = 360,454)

stillborn piglets indicates that SRB risks were not greatly influenced by these factors in the studied herds.

Regarding lifetime reproductive performance, the fact that SRB females had 90 more NPD than non-SRB females suggests that producers' culling guidelines were not strictly implemented for returned females in the studied herds. Keeping SRB females too long in a herd increases NPD and decreases efficiency of the sows, because the SRB females produce pigs 30% (21.4/ 27.6 annualized lifetime pigs born alive) less efficiently than non-SRB females, and their mean re-service interval of 55 days increase NPD.

The present study shows that low parity SRB sows had a lower farrowing rate in their previous parity than non-SRB sows in the same parity. It is likely that some of the low parity SRB sows had a latent reproductive problem that caused them to have a lower farrowing rate in the earlier parity, even though it had not yet become serious enough for them to require a re-service. One possible reproductive problem in low parity sows is ovary cysts, and a recent study reported that sows with ovary cysts had 20% more returns to estrus than sows without ovary cysts [32]. In contrast, the lack of any difference between parity 1 or higher SRB and non-SRB sows for farrowing rate and WMI sows indicates that the reason that the

sows in parity 1 or higher became SRB was due to problems such as lactation and post weaning period. Finally, in the present study, the relatively high ICC for herd variance of 25.5% for the gilts and sows model and 30.1% for the sows only model indicates that there was a substantial effect of the herds on SRB, for example due to differences in heat detection programs or culling policy.

There are some limitations that should be noted when interpreting the results of the present study. This was an observational study performed using commercial herd data. Health status, nutritional programs, genotype, semen quality, proportions of double and triple inseminations, cysts and early or late abortion were not considered in the analyses. However, even with such limitations, this research provides valuable information for pig producers and veterinarians about SRB females in commercial herds, and the relationships between the risk of having SRB females and production factors.

Finally, our definition of SRB pigs is different from previous reports about repeat-breeding which sometimes is defined as one return [5, 6] and sometimes as one to four returns [7]. In our study, the objective was to examine severe repeat-breeder females, so we defined SRB females as having three or more returns in the same parity.

Conclusions
We recommend that producers closely monitor high risk female groups to reduce their returns-to-service. The high risk groups include mated gilts and parity 1 sows, females being served in summer, and females having prolonged WMI, especially those in low performing herds.

Abbreviations
NPD: Non-productive days; AFM: Gilt age at first-mating; ICC: Intraclass correlation coefficients; SRB: Severe repeat-breeder; WMI: Weaning-to-first-mating interval

Acknowledgements
The authors gratefully thank the swine producers for their cooperation in providing their valuable data for use in this study. We also thank Dr. I. McTaggart for his critical review of this manuscript.

Funding
This work was supported by the Research Grant Kiban-A (2012–2016) and Graduate School GP-2016 from Meiji University.

Authors' contributions
ST and YK were responsible for the study design. CP was responsible for data acquisition and participated in the study design. ST carried out the statistical analysis and drafted the manuscript. All authors read and approved the final manuscript.

Competing interests
The authors declare that they have no competing interests.

Author details
[1]School of Agriculture, Meiji University, Higashi-mita 1-1-1, Tama-ku, Kawasaki, Kanagawa 214-8571, Japan. [2]PigCHAMP Pro Europa S.L., c/Santa Catalina 10, 40003 Segovia, Spain.

References

1. PigCHAMP. PigCHAMP benchmarks. 2015.http://www.pigchamp.com/Portals/0/Documents/Benchmarking%20Summaries/USA%202015.pdf. Accessed 15 Jun 2016.
2. Koketsu Y. Re-serviced females on commercial swine breeding farms. J Vet Med Sci. 2003;65:1287–91.
3. Sasaki Y, Koketsu Y. A herd management survey on culling guidelines and actual culling practices in three herd groups based on reproductive productivity in Japanese commercial swine herds. J Anim Sci. 2012;90:1995–2002.
4. Koketsu Y. Six component intervals of nonproductive days by breeding-female pigs on commercial farms. J Anim Sci. 2005;83:1406–12.
5. Vargas AJ, Bernardi ML, Paranhos TF, Gonçalves MA, Bortolozzo FP, Wentz I. Reproductive performance of swine females re-serviced after return to estrus or abortion. Anim Reprod Sci. 2009;113:305–10.
6. Horvat G, Bilkei G. Exogenous prostaglandin F2α at time of ovulation improves reproductive efficiency in repeat breeder sows. Theriogenology. 2003;59:1479–84.
7. Kauffold J, Melzer F, Berndt A, Hoffmann G, Hotzel H, Sachse K. Chlamydiae in oviducts and uteri of repeat breeder pigs. Theriogenology. 2006;66:1816–23.
8. Iida R, Koketsu Y. Interactions between climatic and production factors on returns of female pigs to service during summer in Japanese commercial breeding herds. Theriogenology. 2013;80:487–93.
9. Tummaruk P, Lundeheim N, Einarsson S, Dalin A-M. Effect of birth litter size, birth parity number, growth rate, backfat thickness and age at first mating of gilts on their reproductive performance as sows. Anim Reprod Sci. 2001;66:225–37.
10. Tummaruk P, Tantasuparuk W, Techakumphu M, Kunavongkrit A. Influence of repeat-service and weaning-to-first-service interval on farrowing proportion of gilts and sows. Prev Vet Med. 2010;96:194–200.
11. Bloemhof S, Mathur PK, Knol EF, van der Waaij EH. Effect of daily environmental temperature on farrowing rate and total born in dam line sows. J Anim Sci. 2013;91:2667–79.
12. Iida R, Koketsu Y. Lower farrowing rate in female pigs associated with higher outdoor temperatures in humid subtropical and continental climate zones in Japan. Anim Reprod. 2016;13:63–8.
13. Iida R, Koketsu Y. Climatic factors associated with abortion occurrences in Japanese commercial pig herds. Anim Reprod Sci. 2015;157:78–86.
14. European commission. Pig: number of farms and heads by agricultural size of farm (UAA) and size of pig herd, 2016. http://appsso.eurostat.ec.europa.eu/nui/submitViewTableAction.do. Aaccessed 30 Dec 2016.
15. Lundgren H, Canario L, Grandinson K, Lundeheim N, Zumbach B, Vangen O, et al. Genetic analysis of reproductive performance in Landrace sows and its correlation to piglet growth. Livest Sci. 2010;128:173–8.
16. Hoving L, Soede N, Graat E, Feitsma H, Kemp B. Reproductive performance of second parity sows: Relations with subsequent reproduction. Livest Sci. 2011;140:124–30.
17. Ferreira R, Ayres H, Chiaratti M, Ferraz M, Araújo A, Rodrigues C, et al. The low fertility of repeat-breeder cows during summer heat stress is related to a low oocyte competence to develop into blastocysts. J Dairy Sci. 2011;94:2383–92.
18. Koketsu Y, Tani S, Iida R. Factors for improving reproductive performance of sows and herd productivity in commercial breeding herd. Porcine Health Manag. 2017;3:1.
19. Vigre H, Dohoo IR, Stryhn H, Busch ME. Intra-unit correlations in seroconversion to Actinobacillus pleuropneumoniae and Mycoplasma hyopneumoniae at different levels in Danish multi-site pig production facilities. Prev Vet Med. 2004;63:9–28.
20. Tani S, Piñeiro C, Koketsu Y. Recurrence patterns and factors associated with regular, irregular, and late return to service of female pigs and their lifetime performance on southern European farms. J Anim Sci. 2016;94:1924–32.
21. Rasbash J, Steele F, Browne WJ, Goldstein H. A User's Guide to MLwiN Version 2.26. UK: University of Bristol; 2012.
22. Dohoo IR, Martin SW, Stryhn H. Veterinary Epidemiologic Research. 2nd ed. Charlottetown: VER Inc.; 2009.
23. Nutthee A, Tantasuparuk W, Manjarin R, Kirkwood RN. Effect of site of sperm deposition on fertility when sows are inseminated with aged semen. J Swine Health Prod. 2011;19(5):295–7.
24. Soede NM, Wetzels CCH, Zondag W, de Koning MAI, Kemp B. Effects of time of insemination relative to ovulation, as determined by ultrasonography, on fertilization rate and accessory sperm count in sows. J Reprod Fertil. 1995;104:99–106.
25. Sasaki Y, Koketsu Y. Reproductive profile and lifetime efficiency of female pigs by culling reason in high-performing commercial breeding herds. J Swine Health Prod. 2011;19:284–91.
26. Steverink D, Soede N, Groenland G, Van Schie F, Noordhuizen J, Kemp B. Duration of estrus in relation to reproduction results in pigs on commercial farms. J Anim Sci. 1999;77:801–9.
27. Patterson JL, Beltranena E, Foxcroft GR. The effect of gilt age at first estrus and breeding on third estrus on sow body weight changes and long-term reproductive performance. J Anim Sci. 2010;88:2500–13.
28. Bertoldo MJ, Holyoake PK, Evans G, Grupen CG. Seasonal variation in the ovarian function of sows. Reprod Fertil Dev. 2012;24:822–34.
29. Koketsu Y, Dial GD, Pettigrew JE, Marsh WE, King VL. Influence of imposed feed intake patterns during lactation on reproductive performance and on circulating levels of glucose, insulin, and luteinizing hormone in primiparous sows. J Anim Sci. 1996;74:1036–46.
30. Koketsu Y, Dial GD, King VL. Returns to service after mating and removal of sows for reproductive reasons from commercial swine farms. Theriogenology. 1997;47:1347–63.
31. King VL, Koketsu Y, Reeves D, Xue JL, Dial GD. Management factors associated with swine breeding-herd productivity in the United States. Prev Vet Med. 1998;35:255–64.
32. Castagna CD, Peixoto CH, Bortolozzo FP. Wentz I, Neto GB, Ruschel Fc. Ovarian cysts and their consequences on the reproductive performance of swine herds. Anim Reprod Sci. 2004;81:115–23.

3

Antimicrobial use in Swedish farrow-to-finish pig herds is related to farmer characteristics

Annette Backhans[1]* (iD), Marie Sjölund[1,2], Ann Lindberg[3] and Ulf Emanuelson[1]

Abstract

Background: Antimicrobial resistance is an increasing problem and reducing AM use is critical in limiting its severity. The underlying causes of antimicrobial use at pig farm level must be understood to select effective reduction measures. We previously showed that antimicrobial use on Swedish pig farms is comparatively low but varies between farms, although few farms are high users. In the present survey of a convenience sample of 60 farrow-to-finish herds in Sweden, we investigated farmers' attitudes to antimicrobials and the influence of information provided by veterinarians about antimicrobial resistance. Farm characteristics were also recorded. We had previously quantified antimicrobial use for different age categories of pigs during one year, as well as external and internal biosecurity. Risk factors based on hypothetical causal associations between these and calculated treatment incidence (TI) for the different age categories were assessed here in a linear regression model.

Results: There were no significant associations between biosecurity and TI for any pig age category. Increasing farmer age was associated with higher TI for suckling piglets and fatteners. For suckling piglets, the age group with the highest frequency of treatment, TI was also significantly associated with farmer and education of the staff, where female farmers, and university educated staff was associated with a higher TI. Larger farms were associated with a higher TI in fatteners.

Conclusions: In the investigated Swedish pig farms, factors that influenced antimicrobial usage were more related to characteristics of the individual farmer and his/her staff than to biosecurity level, other management factors or farmers' attitudes to antimicrobials.

Keywords: Antimicrobial, Biosecurity, Pig, Farmer attitudes

Background

Antimicrobial (AM) use in animal production in Sweden is among the lowest in Europe [1]. This is explained partly by absence of diseases such as porcine reproductive and respiratory syndrome (PRRS) together with a long tradition of implementing preventative measures against livestock diseases [2] and a ban on the use of AM as growth promoters since 1986, which decreased AM use by 65 % [3]. Within the European research project MINAPIG, we recently showed that AM use in Swedish pig herds mainly consists of individual treatments and that most herds apply AM prudently, with rather low use of fluoroquinolones and no use of third-generation cephalosporins [4]. Investigation of the biosecurity level in the same herds showed that, in general, the biosecurity was good, but varied between herds [5]. Thus, Swedish pig production has come a long way in reducing AM use, but the great variation between farms indicates that some farms could reduce use even further.

The presence of infectious diseases in an area has an impact on the health status of pigs, but various biosecurity measures can be applied to prevent pathogens entering or spreading within a herd, thereby improving animal health [6–9]. Thus, improvements in biosecurity could be useful to reduce the need for AM in pig herds. Furthermore, the process by which the farmer decides how to apply treatments has been shown to be influenced by their attitudes and beliefs regarding antimicrobials [10].

---
* Correspondence: Annette.Backhans@slu.se
[1]Department of Clinical Sciences, Swedish University of Agricultural Sciences, SE-750 07 Uppsala, Sweden
Full list of author information is available at the end of the article

Previous studies have shown that farmers generally have little awareness of the risks of AM resistance [11–13], and that they are more concerned about financial issues [14, 15]. To date, very few studies have taken into account both preventive measures and attitudes to AM use [16].

Our recent study showed that the level of AM use varies greatly between pig herds and that there is room for improvement, especially with regard to treatments in suckling piglets [4]. Therefore, the aim of the present study was to investigate the farm, or farmer-related, factors influencing AM use on Swedish farrow-to-finish pig farms, and how biosecurity level, farmers' attitudes to AM and the information provided by the herd veterinarian influence AM use under Swedish conditions. The hypotheses tested were: that a high level of biosecurity is associated with lower AM use; that farmers who are aware of the risks of AM resistance use less AM; and that information provided by veterinarians has an impact on AM use.

Methods

Herds and collection of data

The study was performed within the European research project MINAPIG (Evaluation of alternative strategies for raising pigs with minimal antimicrobial usage). The study design has been described in detail in our previous publications [4, 5]. In brief, 60 Swedish farrow-to-finish herds, with at least 100 sows and 500 finishing pigs per year, were recruited by convenience sampling. The selection criteria were agreed within the MINAPIG project to ensure comparable samples between the participating countries. The herds were visited once during the period April-September 2013, when data on production parameters, biosecurity practices and other herd characteristics were collected by a researcher or the herd veterinarian. A questionnaire on farmers' perceptions on AM use, previously described by Visschers et al. 2015 [15] was filled out before the visit by the person responsible for pig management and collected together with records of the amount of AM used during the year preceding the visit.

Calculation of antimicrobial use

Use of AM was recorded by product, strength of product, administration route and age category. The values were converted to active substance, expressed as mg, and then to treatment incidence (TI) based on Defined Daily Doses for Animal (DDDA) previously agreed within the MINAPIG project [17]. This was done using the online tool ABcheck (available at www.ABcheck. ugent.be), but adapted to the MINAPIG project (www.minapig.eu). The TI was expressed as the number of DDDAs per 1000 pig-days at risk, which is equivalent to the proportion of 1000 pigs that receive a dose of AM each day [18]. The TI values were calculated separately

for suckling piglets (birth to weaning), weaners (weaning to an approximate weight of 30 kg), fatteners (~30 kg to slaughter) and adult pigs (gilts, sows and boars). Further details about these calculations can be found in our previous publication [4].

Assessment of biosecurity

Biosecurity practices applied in the herds were evaluated using the online tool BioCheck (available at www.biocheck. ugent.be) developed by Laanen et al. 2010 [19] and modified for MINAPIG. In brief, BioCheck consists of 109 questions relating to biosecurity measures, grouped into 6 subcategories of each of external and internal biosecurity measures. Examples of external biosecurity measures are "Purchase of animals and semen" and "Transport of animals and removal of manure and dead animals", and of internal biosecurity measures "Disease management", "Biosecurity measures between compartments and the use of equipment" and "Cleaning and disinfection". The score for each subcategory accounts for its estimated importance for the introduction and spread of infectious diseases, with scores ranging between 0, corresponding to "total absence of biosecurity" and 100, corresponding to "perfect biosecurity".

Farmers' attitudes to antimicrobial use and the influence of veterinarians

A questionnaire was developed within the MINAPIG consortium based on semi-structured interviews with 14 pig farmers in Switzerland and Germany (for details see Visschers et al. 2015 [15]). The questionnaire was developed in English, but subsequently translated to Swedish and distributed before the farm visit with a request that it be filled out by the farmer or the person responsible for the pigs (hereafter referred to as 'the farmer'). The questionnaire contained questions about age, gender and years of experience. It also included statements on the benefits and risks of AM use in pig farming, the need to apply AM in pig farming and the information provided by the farm veterinarian regarding AM use. The statements were assessed on a 6-point Likert scale, where higher scores indicated stronger agreement with the respective item, and further combined into four constructs: perceived benefits, perceived risks, perceived need and contribution from veterinarians, each based on a number of individual items. These constructs have been described previously [15, 16] and are presented in Table 1. As all constructs had acceptable to good internal reliability (Cronbach's alpha values between 0.64 and 0.83), the mean for these items per respondent was calculated and used for the constructs in the analyses.

Statistical analyses

A directed acyclic graph (DAG) illustrating the hypothetical causal associations between assumed risk factors and frequency of AM use (expressed as TI) is shown in Fig. 1. Herd characteristics considered for the linear regression models were: number of sows, number of employees, whether the farm was specific pathogen free (SPF) or not, and average reported age at weaning. Individual characteristics were age, gender and years of experience of the farmer, and highest level of education of the staff. Attitudes considered important were the four constructs (perceived benefits of AM, perceived risks of AM, perceived need for AM and information contribution from veterinarians). All candidate risk factors, except gender, level of education and SPF status, were measured on a continuous scale and the assumption of linear associations with the outcome was managed by introducing a quadratic term after centring on the mean, which was retained in the model if it was statistically significant ($p < 0.05$). Multicollinearity between the potential predictor variables was assessed by Spearman rank correlations. SPF status was found to be highly correlated with external biosecurity and was excluded from the model, because external biosecurity was better distributed and was of primary interest in this study. Number of employees was highly correlated with number of sows and only the latter was retained in the regression models. All TI values were log-transformed (natural base) to achieve normally distributed residuals, where 1 was added to all TI values for weaners, fatteners and adults to avoid taking the log of zero.

Results
Farm and farmer characteristics, farmers' attitudes, veterinarians' information contribution, AM use and biosecurity level
Descriptive statistics on herd and individual characteristics, including attitudes to AM and the contribution of veterinarians, are presented in Tables 1 and 2. Three herds were SPF herds, gender distribution was 18 females and 41 males (one farmer did not indicate their gender) and the level of education was 20 farmers with a university degree and 40 without. There was great variation in number of sows, age and years of experience of the farmer and weaning age. Farmers perceived a low need, low-moderate risks and moderate benefits of AM and rated the contribution of their veterinarian's information highly.

The distribution of internal, external and total biosecurity for the participating herds is also presented in Table 2 and the distribution of TI values for the different pig age categories is shown in Table 3.

These data, including detailed information on use of AM substances and biosecurity scores for subcategories, have been published in our two previous papers [4, 5]. As reported there, the TI was highest for suckling piglets and second highest for weaners [4]. However, the TI varied greatly between farms, especially for suckling piglets and weaners. The external biosecurity was higher than the internal biosecurity, but there were few herds with low external biosecurity and few with perfect external biosecurity [5].

Table 1 Statements included in the constructs related to farmers' attitudes to antimicrobial use and to the influence of veterinarians

Construct	Statements	No of answers per score of each statement: 1 (do not agree at al), 6 (fully agree)					
		1	2	3	4	5	6
Perceived risks	AB are associated with risks for the pigs	11	18	13	10	5	2
	AB use in pig farming reduces the effectiveness of ABs in human medicine	5	12	14	11	8	9
	AB are used far too much in pig production	10	15	11	13	5	5
Perceived benefits	AB can be easily and quickly applied	3	5	13	7	15	15
	AB are very cost efficient	3	3	16	10	17	10
	The effect of AB in pigs is very fast	0	0	13	18	14	14
	The animals recover quickly due to AB	0	1	8	16	21	13
	AB highly reduce the number of deaths among pigs	2	11	8	13	15	10
Perceived need of AM	Keeping a large number of pigs is only possible with the intensive use of AB	19	23	6	8	2	1
	Disease incidents caused by the conditions of intensive pig farming can only be cured by AB	23	11	9	8	6	2
Contribution from veterinarians	My veterinarian informs me about the risks of antibiotic use	1	2	3	4	15	33
	My veterinarian informs me about how AB work	0	1	4	5	20	28
	My veterinarian informs me about the impact of alternative strategies and how to use them	1	1	9	11	16	21

AB antibiotic

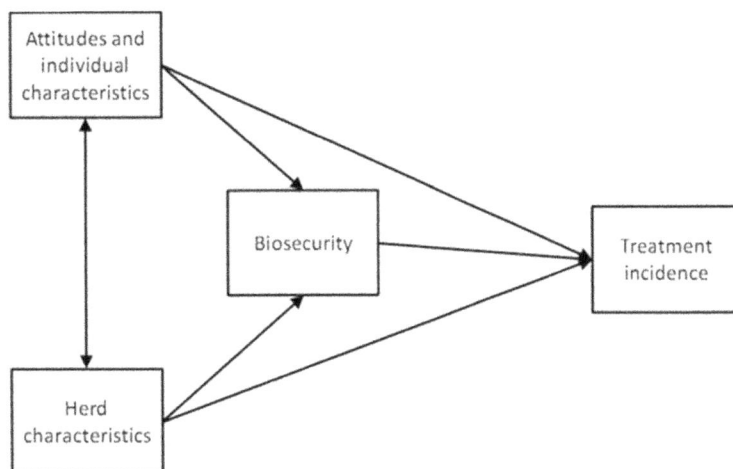

Fig. 1 A directed acyclic graph illustrating the hypothetical causal associations between risk factors (shown as groups) and antimicrobial treatment incidence in Swedish farrow-to-finish herds

Regression analysis

In the regression models including only internal and external biosecurity (results not shown), there were significant associations between internal biosecurity and TI in weaners, fatteners and adults, and between external biosecurity and TI in weaners. However, the linear regression models that also included herd characteristics and individual characteristics and attitudes showed no significant associations between biosecurity and TI for any of the pig age groups (Table 4). The factor most consistently associated with TI was the farmer's age, with higher age being associated with higher TI in suckling piglets and fatteners. In suckling piglets, the age group to which most treatments were applied, TI was significantly associated with age, gender and education, with

higher age, female farmer and university education of the farmer being associated with higher TI. Large farm size, indicated by number of sows, was associated with higher TI in fatteners. The fit of the models was assessed by inspection of the residuals with respect to homoscedasticity and normal distribution, but no deviations were found.

Discussion

Use of AM is lower in pig production in Sweden than in most other European countries [20], but we previously showed that the level varies between farms, with a few farms being high users [4, 5]. The biosecurity level also varies greatly between farms, as do other characteristics such as age, years of experience and education level of

Table 2 Characteristics of the 60 Swedish farrow-to-finish pig herds surveyed

	Mean	Minimum	25th percentile	Median	75th percentile	Maximum
Number of sows	242.7	96	137.5	187.5	275	1200
Number of employees	3.9	2	3	3	4	15
Farmer age	49.7	27	44	49	58	70
Years of experience	22.3	3	15	22	28	50
Pig age at weaning (days)	35	28	33	35	35	49
Total duration (weeks)[a]	26.9	23	25.6	27	28	32
Perceived need for AM[b]	2.3	1	1	2	3	6
Perceived risks of AM[b]	3.1	1	2.3	3	3.8	6
Perceived benefits of AM[b]	4.3	1.8	3.6	4.2	5	6
Veterinarians' information contribution[b]	5	1	4.5	5	6	6
Internal biosecurity[c]	58.8	33	52	61	65.5	80
External biosecurity[c]	68.3	44	61.5	68	76	93

[a]Total duration = entire rearing period from birth to slaughter, data available for 51 herds, AM = Antimicrobial; [b]The original items were assessed on a 6-point Likert scale, where higher scores indicated stronger agreement with the respective item; [c]Scores for internal and external biosecurity range between 0 and 100, where 100 is "perfect biosecurity"

Table 3 Distribution of antimicrobial use for different age groups of pigs, expressed as treatment incidence per 1000 pig-days at risk, in 60 Swedish farrow-to-finish herds

	Mean	Minimum	25th percentile	Median	75th percentile	Maximum
Suckling piglets	75.1	1.6	21.1	54.7	103.2	367.9
Wearers	22.3	0.0	2.1	6.2	20.1	260.5
Fatteners	6.1	0.0	1.6	2.8	6.1	64.9
Adults	10.9	0.0	4.2	8.4	15.4	45.0

the farmer. In this study, two of our starting hypotheses were that a high level of biosecurity is associated with lower AM use (as a result of better pig health), and that farmers who are aware of the risks of AM resistance use less AM. However, the results from the linear regression model showed that the associations between AM use and biosecurity were non-significant when farm and farmer characteristics were included in the model. Furthermore, attitudes to AM were not significantly associated with AM use. Instead, individual characteristics of the farmer were found to be important. For example, older farmers, females and university-educated farmers (any university education) used more AM in suckling piglets, which is the age group to which most treatments are applied [4], and older farmers also used more AM in weaners. We previously reported a link between fewer years of farmer experience, female farmers and higher

biosecurity [5], which led us to expect lower AM use on such farms, but surprisingly gender affected AM use in a different way than expected. Moreover, it could be assumed that a high level of education would lead to more careful use of AM, not more frequent use as found here. However, as discussed in our previous paper [5], females have been shown to have generally higher empathy for animals [21] but also higher medical compliance than men, who tend to show riskier behaviour relating to health issues [22]. The results could therefore be due to females' greater attention to the individual animal's symptoms. The reason why older and more educated farmers had higher AM use than younger and less educated farmers can only be speculated upon, but might be due to similar factors. It could also be speculated whether this means there is over-treatment, especially of suckling piglets, in some herds, or under-treatment in

Table 4 Estimates from a linear regression model of the associations between risk factors and antimicrobial (AM) use (expressed as log-transformed (natural base) treatment incidence (TI) per 1000 pig-days at risk) in different age groups of pigs on 60 Swedish farrow-to-finish herds

Risk factor	Suckling piglets			Weaners			Fatteners			Adults		
	Estimate	Error	p	Estimate	Error	p	Estimate	Error	P	Estimate	Error	p
Intercept	-2.385	3.695		-4.561	4.980		0.569	2.205		3.338	2.138	
Number of sows	0.000	0.001	0.975	0.000	0.001	0.881	0.005	0.003	0.060	0.001	0.001	0.319
Number of sows^{2*}							0.000	0.000	0.042			
Gender - male (n = 41)	-0.877	0.370	0.018	-0.447	0.370	0.226	-0.178	0.370	0.631	-0.003	0.370	0.995
- female (n = 18)	0.000	0.000		0.000	0.000		0.000	0.000		0.000	0.000	
Education - non-uni[a] (n = 39)	-0.725	0.323	0.025	-0.464	0.324	0.152	-0.112	0.331	0.736	-0.159	0.322	0.622
- uni (n = 20)	0.000	0.000		0.000	0.000		0.000	0.000		0.000	0.000	
Age	0.392	0.131	0.003	0.351	0.146	0.016	0.021	0.027	0.439	-0.040	0.026	0.122
Age^{2*}	-0.004	0.001	<0.001	-0.004	0.002	0.013						
Years at work	0.027	0.027	0.310	-0.005	0.028	0.867	-0.016	0.027	0.562	0.014	0.027	0.600
Age at weaning	[b]na			0.032	0.043	0.466						
Need for AM[c]	0.092	0.126	0.4682	-0.047	0.126	0.712	0.044	0.126	0.726	0.028	0.126	0.823
Risks of AM[c]	-0.196	0.143	0.1695	-0.210	0.145	0.148	0.052	0.143	0.719	-0.001	0.143	0.994
Benefits of AM[c]	-0.119	0.155	0.442	0.233	0.155	0.132	0.286	0.156	0.068	0.233	0.154	0.130
Vet's contribution[c]	0.121	0.135	0.372	-0.003	0.135	0.984	-0.134	0.152	0.378	0.141	0.135	0.297
Internal biosecurity[d]	-0.022	0.019	0.237	0.004	0.019	0.823	-0.031	0.019	0.095	-0.024	0.018	0.192
External biosecurity[d]	-0.002	0.021	0.913	-0.033	0.021	0.115	0.011	0.020	0.578	0.001	0.020	0.957

* The quadratic term a*uni* university, *vet* veterinarian, [b]*na* not applicable; [c]Statements were assessed on a 6-point Likert scale, where higher scores indicated higher agreement, combined into four constructs and expressed as the mean score per construct; [d]Scores for internal and external biosecurity range between 0 and 100, where 100 is "perfect biosecurity"

others. The health status in Swedish pig production is generally good, but examples of diseases that are prevalent and often need treatment are arthritis and neonatal piglet diarrhoea in suckling piglets, diarrhoea in weaners, respiratory diseases in fatteners and udder- and leg-related diseases in sows [23–25].

The lack of association between AM use and biosecurity in the present study was unexpected, especially because a negative association between biosecurity level and estimated frequency of treatment for certain clinical signs of disease was reported in a parallel study across four countries [26]. One explanation could be that some of the Swedish herds with otherwise good pig health might have experienced an outbreak of disease, leading to temporarily high AM use. Moreover, herds struggling with health problems might have implemented biosecurity measures to overcome the problem, affecting the results in this limited sample of herds. Both these explanations could result in lack of an association. Furthermore, the most important biosecurity measures, such as all-in all-out systems or lower stocking density than the EU limit [5], might have been implemented already in the majority of our herds. Swedish herds have in general better biosecurity level than herds in other countries [26] and associations with AM use may thus be more difficult to identify. It is also possible that Bio-Check, a tool developed in Belgium, is not entirely appropriate for Swedish conditions. The prevalence of infectious diseases differ between the countries and Sweden is for example declared free from PRRS [2]. Also, pig density is overall considerably lower in Sweden [27]. Consequently, the assumption that a certain biosecurity level (as measured by BioCheck) has the same effect on AM needs may not be valid.

Finally, the associations in the final model, i.e. after accounting for other factors such as herd and farmer characteristics, were marginal, which indicates that biosecurity level is a less important determinant of AM use in Swedish pig herds, perhaps due to an overall better health status. However, it cannot be excluded that the sample size of 60 herds was not sufficient to detect associations when several risk factors were included in the model and the absence of statistically significant associations should not be interpreted as a proof that there is no association. Greater farm size, defined as number of sows, was a significant factor for higher AM use in fatteners, but not in other age groups. Several studies have identified increasing herd size as a risk factor for respiratory disease, which is mainly a problem during the fattening period [28, 29]. The lack of associations with farmers' perceived risks, benefits and need for AM could be due to the relatively narrow distribution of scores, i.e. farmers' attitudes were too similar to be able to identify any differences. Moreover, scores for the information

contribution from veterinarian construct did not differ much between herds. Thus, it cannot be concluded that attitudes are unimportant in explaining AM use, but the results indicate that there is consensus among farmers on their attitudes to AM, perhaps influenced by the issue being a topic debated in society and within pig production. In Sweden, veterinarians are not allowed to sell AM and prescriptions are restricted to named AM products in quantities the veterinarian considers necessary during a limited period, based on regular monitoring of the health status of the pigs and AM use. Moreover, the farmer must undergo special training to administer treatments [30, 31]. These regulations are likely to contribute to awareness about the risks of AM use.

Limitations of the present study to consider are that AM use in the participating herds was lower compared to national AM sales figures for the same period [4], indicating a bias towards farms with lower AM use than the average pig farm. Further, about one third of Swedish herds are farrow-to-finish herds and the study group, a convenience sample of Swedish medium-sized and large herds, represented approximately 22 % of farrow-to-finish herds with >100 sows. Thus actual high users might not have been very well represented in our sample and it is possible that these farmers have different views on AM and their herds have lower biosecurity.

Conclusions

Factors influencing AM use in Swedish farrow-to-finish pig farms were related to individual farmer characteristics such as age, gender and years of experience. However, under Swedish circumstances, biosecurity level had no additional effect on AM use. This indicates the importance of the herd veterinarian's communication skills to ensure correct treatment of sick animals.

Acknowledgements
For the study design of the MINAPIG project, we want to thank the rest of the MINAPIG consortium, in alphabetical order: Catherine Belloc, ONIRIS, France; Lucie Collineau, SAFOSO, Switzerland; Jeroen Dewulf, Ghent University Belgium; Elisabeth Grosse Beilage, TiHo Hannover, Germany; Bernd Grosse Liesner, Boehringer Ingelheim, Germany; Christian Alexander Körk, Boehringer Ingelheim, Germany; Svenja Lösken, TiHo, Hannover Germany; Merel Postma, Ghent University, Belgium; Hugo Seemer, Boehringer Ingelheim, Germany; Katharina Stärk, SAFOSO, Switzerland and Vivianne Visschers, ETHZ, Switzerland.

Funding
The project was part of the European MINAPIG project (Evaluation of alternative strategies for raising pigs with minimal antimicrobial usage: Opportunities and constraints, www.minapig.eu), and was funded through the ERA-NET programme EMIDA (EMIDA19) by the Swedish Research Council Formas.

Authors' contributions
UE study design, statistical analysis, draft of manuscript. AB study design, draft of manuscript, data collection. MS study design, data collection. AL study design. All authors reviewed, edited and approved the final manuscript.

Competing interests
The authors declare that they have no competing interests.

Author details
[1]Department of Clinical Sciences, Swedish University of Agricultural Sciences, SE-750 07 Uppsala, Sweden. [2]Department of Animal Health and Antimicrobial Strategies, National Veterinary Institute, SE-751 89 Uppsala, Sweden. [3]Department of Epidemiology and Disease Control, National Veterinary Institute, SE-751 89 Uppsala, Sweden.

References
1. Grave K, Torren-Edo J, Muller A, Greko C, Moulin G, Mackay D, Fuchs K, Laurier L, Iliev D, Pokludová L, et al. Variations in the sales and sales patterns of veterinary antimicrobial agents in 25 European countries. J Antimicrob Chemother. 2014;69:2284–91.
2. Carlsson U, Wallgren P, Renström LHM, Lindberg A, Eriksson H, Thorén P, Eliasson-Selling L, Lundeheim N, Nörregard E, Thörn C, Elvander M. Emergence of porcine reproductive and respiratory syndrome in Sweden: detection, response and eradication. Transbound Emerg Dis. 2009;56:121–31.
3. Bengtsson B, Wierup M. Antimicrobial resistance in Scandinavia after a ban of antimicrobial growth promoters. Anim Biotechnol. 2006;17:147–56.
4. Sjölund M, Backhans A, Greko C, Emanuelson U, Lindberg A. Antimicrobial usage in 60 Swedish farrow-to-finish pig herds. Prev Vet Med. 2015;121:257–64.
5. Backhans A, Sjölund M, Lindberg A, Emanuelson U. Biosecurity level and health management practices in 60 swedish farrow-to-finish herds. Acta Vet Scand. 2015;57:14.
6. Maes D, Segales J, Meyns T, Sibila M, Pieters M, Haesebrouck F. Control of Mycoplasma hyopneumoniae infections in pigs. Vet Microbiol. 2008;126:297–309.
7. Laanen M, Persoons D, Ribbens S, de Jong E, Callens B, Strubbe M, Maes D, Dewulf J. Relationship between biosecurity and production/antimicrobial treatment characteristics in pig herds. Vet J. 2013;198:508–12.
8. Fraile L, Alegre A, López-Jiménez R, Nofrarías M, Segalés J. Risk factors associated with pleuritis and cranio-ventral pulmonary consolidation in slaughter-aged pigs. Vet J. 2010;184:326–33.
9. Lambert M-È, Arsenault J, Poljak Z, D'Allaire S. Epidemiological investigations in regard to porcine reproductive and respiratory syndrome (PRRS) in Quebec, Canada. Part 2: Prevalence and risk factors in breeding sites. Prev Vet Med. 2012;104:84–93.
10. Alarcon P, Wieland B, Mateus ALP, Dewberry C. Pig farmers' perceptions, attitudes, influences and management of information in the decision-making process for disease control. Prev Vet Med. 2014;116:223–42.
11. Marvin DM, Dewey CE, Rajić A, Poljak Z, Young B. Knowledge of zoonoses among those affiliated with the Ontario swine industry: A questionnaire administered to selected producers, allied personnel, and veterinarians. Foodborne Pathogen Dis. 2010;7:159–66.
12. Moreno MA. Opinions of Spanish pig producers on the role, the level and the risk to public health of antimicrobial use in pigs. Res Vet Sci. 2014;97:26–31.
13. Friedman DB, Kanwat CP, Headrick ML, Patterson NJ, Neely JC, Smith LU. Importance of prudent antibiotic use on dairy farms in South Carolina: A pilot project on farmers' knowledge, attitudes and practices. Zoonoses Public Health. 2007;54:366–75.
14. Visschers VHM, Iten DM, Riklin A, Hartmann S, Sidler X, Siegrist M. Swiss pig farmers' perception and usage of antibiotics during the fattening period. Livest Sci. 2014;162:223–32.
15. Visschers VHM, Backhans A, Collineau L, Iten D, Loesken S, Postma M, Belloc C, Dewulf J, Emanuelson U, Beilage EG, et al. Perceptions of antimicrobial usage, antimicrobial resistance and policy measures to reduce antimicrobial usage in convenient samples of Belgian, French, German, Swedish and Swiss pig farmers. Prev Vet Med. 2015;119:10–20.
16. Visschers VHM, Backhans A, Collineau L, Loesken S, Nielsen EO, Postma M, Belloc C, Dewulf J, Emanuelson U, grosse Beilage E, et al. A comparison of pig farmers' and veterinarians' perceptions and intentions to reduce antimicrobial usage in six european countries. Zoonoses Public Health. 2016: doi:10.1111/zph.12260 [Epub Feb 18].
17. Postma M, Sjölund M, Collineau L, Lösken S, Stärk KDC, Dewulf J, et al. Assigning defined daily doses animal: A European multi-country experience for antimicrobial products authorized for usage in pigs. J Antimicrob Chemother. 2015;70:294–302.
18. Timmerman T, Dewulf J, Catry B, Feyen B, Opsomer G, Kruif A, Maes D. Quantification and evaluation of antimicrobial drug use in group treatments for fattening pigs in Belgium. Prev Vet Med. 2006;74:251–63.
19. Laanen M, Beek J, Ribbens S, Vangroenweghe F, Maes D, Dewulf J. Biosecurity on pig herds. Development of an on-line scoring system and the results of the first 99 participating herds. Vlaams Diergeneeskd Tijdschr. 2010;79:302–6.
20. Sjölund M, Postma M, Collineau L, Lösken S, Backhans A, Belloc C, Emanuelson U, Grosse Beilage E, Stärk KDC, Dewulf J. Quantitative and qualitative antimicrobial usage patterns infarrow-to-finish pig herds in Belgium, France, Germany and Sweden. Prev Vet Med. 2016;130:41–50.
21. Eckardt Erlanger A, Tsytsarev S. The relationship between empathy and personality in undergraduate students' attitudes towards nonhuman animals. Soc Anim. 2012;20:21-38.
22. Courtenay WH, Mccreary DR, Merighi JR. Gender and ethnic differences in health beliefs and behaviors. J Health Psychol. 2002;7:219–31.
23. Engblom L, Lundeheim N, Dalin A, Andersson K. Sow removal in Swedish commercial herds. Livest Sci. 2007;106:76–86.
24. Jacobson M, Fellström C, Jensen-Waern M. Porcine proliferative enteropathy: An important disease with questions remaining to be solved. Vet J. 2010; 184:264–8.
25. Holmgren N, Mattson B, Lundeheim N. Klöv- och benskador hos smågrisar i olika typer av besättningar (Foot and skin lesions among piglets in different types of herds). Swed Vet J (Svensk veterinärtidning). 2008;1:11–17.
26. Postma M, Backhans A, Collineau L, Loesken S, Sjölund M, Belloc C, Emanuelson U, Grosse Beilage E, Stärk KDC, Dewulf J. The biosecurity status and its associations with production and management characteristics in farrow-to-finish pig herds. Animal. 2015; doi:10.1017/S1751731115002487 Published online by Cambridge University Press 16 November 2015.
27. Eurostat, 2014. Pig Farming Sector 2014–statistical Portrait. 2014. http://ec.europa.eu/eurostat/statistics-explained/index.php/Pig_farming_sector_-_statistical_portrait_2014. Accessed 29 June 2016.
28. Beskow P, Lundeheim N, Holmgren N. Pleuritis and pleuropneumonia in fatteners-risk factors and current infectious agents. In Proceedings of the 20th International Pig Veterinary Society Congress; 22-26th June, Durban, South Africa; 2008: 277.
29. Gardner IA, Willeberg P, Mousing J. Empirical and theoretical evidence for herd size as a risk factor for swine diseases. Anim Health Res Rev. 2002;3:43–55.
30. Swedish Board of Agriculture: SJVFS 2013:41. Swedish Board of Agriculture's Regulations on surgical interventions and obligations for animal keepers and animal health care personnel, Saknummer D8, L41. 2013.
31. Swedish Board of Agriculture: SJVFS 2013:42. Swedish Board of Agriculture's Regulations on Medicines and Medicine Use. Saknummer D9.; 2013.

4

Vaccination against parasites – status quo and the way forward

Anja Joachim

Abstract

Although vaccination against various pathogens is integral to health management of swine, vaccines against parasites have not yet been commercialized for the use in pigs. The incentive to develop and commercialize anti-parasitic vaccines in swine are twofold; on the one hand parasitic diseases which are economically important, such as ascarosis and neonatal coccidiosis, could be controlled in a sustainable manner; on the other hand, the transmission of zoonotic parasites, such as *Toxoplasma gondii* or Cysticercus cellulosae, could be effectively interrupted. Although experimental research indicates that vaccination against a number of porcine parasites is feasible, development and commercialization of potential vaccines so far has been very slow, as our knowledge on the host-parasite interplay in porcine parasitic infections is still very limited. In the light of growing concerns regarding consumer health and antiparasitic drug resistance, however, it is timely to re-direct R&D efforts to the development of biological control options.

Keywords: Swine, Vaccine, Immunity, Nematodes, Protozoa

Background - vaccines against parasites

In modern swine medicine, vaccination against various pathogens is an integral part of the health management. However, currently not a single vaccine against parasites of swine is commercially available. Compared to viral and bacterial pathogens, there is a general scarcity for anti-parasite vaccines; only two anti-nematode vaccines, one anti-tick-vaccine and a handful of antiprotozoal vaccines are available for domestic animals. The reasons for such a limited number of anti-parasite vaccines are manifold. For many parasitic infections the development of immunity is slow, and especially in livestock animals, the required time is too short for the vaccine to be of value before animals go to slaughter.

Since parasites, especially helminths, are prime manipulators of the immune system, immunity is often also incomplete and not sufficient to interrupt the life cycle, which aids in the continuation of transmission in a population regardless of vaccination. For host species with a fast turnover the development of anti-parasite vaccines are considered too expensive and especially in intensive pig (or poultry) production chemical control is cheaper, easier to apply and is considered to have a broader market. The only anti-parasite vaccine currently available for use in pigs, the anti-Cysticercus cellulosae-vaccine for the prevention of porcine cysticercosis (which leads to infection of humans with the tapeworm *Taenia solium*), is not yet commercially available although it has a very good efficacy [19]. Simplified and cost-effective application will have to be developed to apply this highly effective vaccine to pigs on a large scale, such as the expression of the recombinant antigen in feed plants [28].

However, the development of vaccines against parasites is still a significant research topic in medical and veterinary sciences. Pathogenic and therefore economically important diseases, especially those which are insufficiently controlled by available chemotherapeutics or have developed resistance against them that cannot be immediately overcome, are still in the focus. In addition, zoonotic parasites represent an attractive target under the One Health aspect, and finally there is a growing public interest in organic production of food free of chemicals, which is fostered by consumer concern about drug residues in meat, eggs or milk.

Which swine parasites are to be considered for vaccines?

The only group of vaccines against parasites that is well developed are the anti-coccidial vaccines for poultry, i.e.

Correspondence: Anja.Joachim@vetmeduni.ac.at
Institute of Parasitology, University of Veterinary Medicine Vienna,
Veterinaerplatz 1, A-1210 Wien, Austria

Eimeria in chicken and turkey. Live virulent and attenuated vaccines are the predominant types on the market; some strains have been used for more than 50 year without significant alterations [39]. Technically, vaccination with life parasites, in this case *Eimeria* oocysts from several relevant species, represents an infection of susceptible animals under controlled conditions. The parasites undergo the complete life cycle and recirculation of oocysts induces a natural booster, rendering chicken immune after several cycles of reproduction. It is assumed that vaccine strains which are susceptible to anticoccidials can displace resistant field isolates when applied repeatedly [5].

In order to be a candidate for vaccine development, parasites have to fulfil several prerequisites. They must be sufficiently pathogenic to induce disease and or/economic losses that can be ameliorated by vaccination, and natural infections must be immunogenic and induce protective immunity and an immunological memory. Amongst the most common swine parasites, some fulfil these criteria. *Sarcoptes scabiei* var. suis, the mange mite of pigs, causes severe economic losses and frequently serious disease in pigs when untreated [6]. Currently, control of porcine sarcoptic mange relies on the application of acaricides and the maintenance of mite-free herds [18]. Immunity against scabies has been described in different species including humans [43]. Vaccination has been attempted in rodent models [11] and other species, and it might also be feasible in pigs.

Strongyloides ransomi is a nematode which is most commonly transmitted with the colostrum after reactivation of hypobiotic larvae in the sow. It causes transient diarrhoea in suckling piglets and induces strong immunity in the adult intestinal stage which leads to rapid expulsion by the host. The immune mechanisms of expulsion have been investigated for other *Strongyloides* species [51], therefore this nematode also fulfils the principle criteria for a vaccination candidate. This is also true for other nematode species of swine that are expelled by action of the gut immune system in pigs, the large roundworm, *Ascaris suum* [24], and the whipworm, *Trichuris suis*. In contrast to these the nodule worm *Oesophagostomum* induces only a weak reaction of the host's immune system [1], making the latter unsuitable for immunological intervention. With regard to the economic importance, porcine nematodes, especially *Strongyloides*, *Trichuris* and the nodule worms, have decreased in prevalence sind the advent of broad-spectrum anthelminthics and modern management, although *A. suum* prevalences can still be considerable, especially in traditional management systems or on organic farms [16, 29–31].

Of the protozoa, *Toxoplasma gondii* is an attractive candidate for vaccine development, as it is the most important foodborne zoonotic parasite on a global scale, and interruption of the life cycle by preventing cyst formation in animals used for meat production would effectively truncate foodborne transmission. A range of promising vaccine designs and candidates has been used in mice [20], and also in pigs (e.g. [3] for recent works). While it is assumed that vaccination of livestock against *Toxoplasma* can prevent infection in humans, the infection in pigs causes only minor production losses or animal health problems and the attractiveness of such a vaccine for pig producers is certainly only limited unless the label "*Toxoplasma*-free pork" has economic advantages. In suckling piglets *Cystoisospora suis* (syn. *Isospora suis*) causes intestinal infections which may cause transient diarrhoea mostly in the second week of life. Due to the peculiarities of the porcine neonatal immune system (see below) and the strong age resistance to *C. suis* in piglets older than three weeks [46, 47], it is currently assumed that only pigs older than six weeks can mount an appropriate immune response. For this and other reasons vaccination of piglets against *C. suis* is not considered feasible. However, alternative approaches have recently been evaluated (see below).

Parasite control in swine production – current status
Currently, antiparasitic treatment schemes for pigs is comprised of a "standard" application scheme for different production branches; they are not "tailor-made" or risk-based and not driven by diagnosis, since metaphylactic application of antiparasitic drugs during the prepatent phase (when parasites cannot readily be detected by routine screening) is preferred to prevent dissemination of environmental stages (especially nematode eggs or coccidia oocysts) and infection of the litter or herd. Complete elimination from a herd is often difficult to achieve due to high prevalences, frequent distribution and durable environmental stages, the best example being eggs of *A. suum* which are almost impossible to inactivate and which can remain infectious for years under suitable conditions [27, 45]. An exception is the control of mange; *S. scabiei* has no long-lived environmental stage and relies on direct contact for transmission, so systematic application of acaricides can effectively reduce infection and stamping out the parasite on a farm is possible when quarantine measures and proper diagnostic screening are in place (e.g. [38]). However, sustainability is jeopardized by the development of acaricide resistance as reported from human scabies [22]. Integrated measures like complete all-in-all-out and disinfection with effective chemicals can relieve the infection pressure of endoparasite infections [15] but eradication is generally considered not feasible. Although resistance against anthelmintics in pig nematodes seems to be restricted to *Oesophagostomum* at low frequencies [2, 9, 41] and resistance to anticoccidials in the control of *C. suis* is currently not reported, the limited number of substances available especially for parasite control in pigs is of concern; especially because no routine tests are available for the detection of parasiticide resistance, and no programs to delay the development of resistance (like shuttle programs

as for chicken coccidiosis prevention [44] or equine cyathostominosis) are in place. Alternative control strategies (for review see [32]) haven been shown to be effective but are currently not commercially available. It must therefore be assumed that, although currently parasites may not be considered as an issue of major concern in pig health and production, in the long run alternatives to the current chemotherapy must be sought to maintain appropriate control and efficacy of available drugs.

Consequences of neonatal enteric infections: parasites and their buddies

At the time of birth the porcine immune system is poorly developed (for review see [47]); intestinal Peyer's patches contain almost no immune cells and the gut epithelium and subepithelial tissues are only completely populated with T- and B-cells and antigen-presenting cells at about six weeks of age, leaving ample time for pathogens to establish and reproduce. At the same time, the gut microbiota are establishing and infections with pathogens at a very early age may have a number of consequences beyond transient parasite infection. Synergistic effects have been described for *C. suis* and toxigenic *Clostridium perfringens* where timely anticoccidial treatment also alleviated the effects of clostridiosis [26], showing that *C. suis* infections promote adhesion of clostridia to the intestinal mucosa, exacerbating the effects of bacterial infection. Preliminary studies also indicated that infections with *C. suis* alter the succession of bacterial communities in neonatal pig gut, delaying the establishment of lactobacilli (as reviewed in [37]). As interactions between microbiota and the immune system are key to the development of a functional immune system [40] such events may have lasting effects on the development of intestinal and immune functions. As such alterations have been described for other intestinal parasitic infections [21], a role of intestinal parasitic infections in gut health should be re-evaluated in pigs, too.

Cystoisospora suis - a candidate for vaccination?

As mentioned above, *C. suis* is an important cause of neonatal diarrhoea; infected animals excrete several million oocysts in the patent phase of infection and the dissemination within and between litters accounts for a rapid spread of the parasite with the consequence of transmission to the majority of piglets within the first week after birth. Although infections are transient with creamy to watery non-haemorrhagic diarrhoea for one to six days, affected animals often develop poorly and stay smaller even until weaning compared to healthy (treated) litter mates [25], which accounts for the financial losses attributed to this disease [17, 33] requiring treatment. In addition, dysbiosis may contribute to increased morbidity (see above) and require antibiotic treatment [7]. Good control of oocyst excretion and coccidiosis-related diarrhoea is achieved by metaphylactic treatment of piglets on the third to fifth day of life with a single dose of toltrazuril (20 mg/kg of body weight) but recently questions about the sustainability of "blanket treatment" of piglets in terms of resistance and drug residues in meat have risen (see [37]), and a call for alterative control strategies has been voiced.

C. suis as a member of the Apicomplexa, which have a strictly intracellular development in the host, was assumed to be under the control of the cellular immune system, mainly NK cells, CD4$^+$ and CD8$^+$ T-cells, while antibodies are probably not protective [47]. Phenotyping of cells after primary infection revealed that several subpopulations of T-cells (especially γδ-T cells and, T_H cells) were decreased in peripheral organs (blood, spleen) but increased in the jejunum upon infection), and after challenge infection (5 months after primary infection) these cell populations also produced interferon-γ (which is crucial for the defence against apicomplexan parasites) and were able to proliferate upon antigen stimulation [8, 48, 49]. Thus, despite considerable individual reactions, it can be assumed that *C. suis* can induce specific primary and adaptive immune reactions in pigs including the induction of an immunological memory.

Since a relative of *C. suis*, *Cryptosporidium parvum* which also inhabits the epithelium of the small intestine, is at least partially controlled by specific antibodies [23], investigations in the possible role of anti-*C. suis* antibodies were made and colostral transfer of antibodies resulting in high serum levels in piglets was described, and IgA levels in the blood of piglets experimentally infected with *C. suis* soon after birth were negatively correlated with diarrhoea [34]. When sows were inoculated before birth with high doses of *C. suis* oocysts, no clinical signs or oocyst excretion were noticed but the levels of immunoglobulins (especially IgA) in their blood, colostrum and milk were correlated with a decrease in diarrhoea and oocyst excretion in their experimentally infected off spring compared to piglets from non-superinfected sows [35], indicating that application of oocysts to sows ante partum can confer at least partial protection against *C. suis* in piglets. It was also concluded that the role of the sow in spreading the parasite is probably minor since even after infection with high doses (100,000 oocysts / sow) no shedding was observed; however in the immunity against *C. suis* the role of the mother in the provision of colostrum containing protective substances is probably pivotal. From this it is currently assumed that immunological control of neonatal porcine cystoisosporosis would have to be conferred as a maternal vaccination which could be applied in time before the infection of the new-born piglets to immunologically mature gilts or sows and could be boostered by natural infections circulating in a herd.

Determination of vaccine candidates – the way forward
Current vaccines against coccidian in chicken are mostly virulent or attenuated live vaccines (see above). This

technology requires the use of animals for production of vaccines with all its disadvantages (biosafety, ethical concerns etc.). Lately, a subunit vaccine against *Eimeria maxima* of chicken was developed and marketed for use in maternal immunization [36, 42]. Although it is also produced in animals and its lasting success in the field still remains to be evaluated, the concept of inactivated vaccines against parasites has received a significant incentive with this development. Until recently, the search for new vaccine candidate molecules was slow and cumbersome due to the lack of cost-effective high yield / high throughput *in vitro* techniques for parasite propagation and screening. New techniques in biotechnology and bioinformatics have enabled rapid and cost-effective screening of genomes and transcriptomes of parasites for vaccine and drug target candidates (as reviewed in [4, 12], and others) including *A. suum* [13], *T. suis* [14], *T. gondii* (www.toxodb.org/) and *C. suis* (Palmieri, submitted). For *C. suis* a genome size of 83 Megabases encoding >8300 genes is estimated, and a recently developed pipeline for the search of vaccine candidates in apicomplexan parasites (Vacceed; [10]) has detected 562 candidates in *C. suis* which now need to be evaluated further *in silico, in vitro* (using a cell culture system supporting the complete life cycle of *C. suis*; [50]) and *in vivo*.

Conclusion

In summary, although vaccines against porcine parasites do not seem to be an immediate issue for pig industry and health, the time to get started has never been better, as new tools and technologies are greatly accelerating the achievements in this field of veterinary medicine.

C. suis would be an attractive candidate for vaccine development, as preliminary data have shown that a protective effect could be achieved by immunisation of sows; however, more basic and applied research will be needed to fully understand the mechanisms that lead to protection.

Joint forces of the veterinary profession, immunology, bioinformatics and biotechnology specialists will be required to develop and test new vaccine concepts and vaccines to be suitable for a competitive market. Combinations of vaccines and optimised delivery systems will have to be developed alongside to incorporate anti-parasite vaccines into the health management systems of pig production.

Abbreviations

A. suum: Ascaris suum; C. suis: Cystoisospora suis; S. scabiei: Sarcoptes scabiei; T. gondii: Toxoplasma gondii

Acknowledgements
Not applicable.

Funding
Not applicable.

Author's contributions
The first author is the sole and corresponding author of this manuscript.

Competing interests
The author declares that she has no competing interests.

References
1. Andreasen A, Skovgaard K, Klaver EJ, van Die I, Mejer H, Thamsborg SM, Kringel H. Comparison of innate and Th1-type host immune responses in *Oesophagostomum dentatum* and *Trichuris suis* infections in pigs. Parasite Immunol. 2016;38(1):53–63.
2. Bauer C, Gerwert S. Characteristics of a flubendazole resistant isolate of *Oesophagostomum dentatum* from Germany. Vet Parasitol. 2002;103(1–2):89–97.
3. Burrells A, Benavides J, Cantón G, Garcia JL, Bartley PM, Nath M, Thomson J, Chianini F, Innes EA, Katzer F. Vaccination of pigs with the S48 strain of *Toxoplasma gondii*–safer meat for human consumption. Vet Res. 2015;46:47.
4. Cantacessi C, Campbell BE, Jex AR, Young ND, Hall RS, Ranganathan S, Gasser RB. Bioinformatics meets parasitology. Parasite Immunol. 2012;34(5): 265–75.
5. Chapman HD, Jeffers TK. Vaccination of chickens against coccidiosis ameliorates drug resistance in commercial poultry production. Int J Parasitol Drugs Drug Resist. 2014;4(3):214–7.
6. Davies PR. Sarcoptic mange and production performance of swine: a review of the literature and studies of associations between mite infestation, growth rate and measures of mange severity in growing pigs. Vet Parasitol. 1995;60(3–4):249–64.
7. Driesen SJ, Fahy VA, Carland PG. The use of toltrazuril for the prevention of coccidiosis in piglets before weaning. Aust Vet J. 1995;72(4):139–41.
8. Gabner S, Worliczek HL, Witter K, Meyer FR, Gerner W, Joachim A. Immune response to *Cystoisospora suis* in piglets: local and systemic changes in T-cell subsets and selected mRNA transcripts in the small intestine. Parasite Immunol. 2014;36(7):277–91.
9. Gerwert S, Failing K, Bauer C. Prevalence of levamisole and benzimidazole resistance in *oesophagostomum* populations of pig-breeding farms in North Rhine-Westphalia, Germany. Parasitol Res. 2002;88(1):63–8.
10. Goodswen SJ, Kennedy PJ, Ellis JT. Vacceed: a high-throughput in silico vaccine candidate discovery pipeline for eukaryotic pathogens based on reverse vaccinology. Bioinformatics. 2014;30(16):2381–3.
11. Gu X, Xie Y, Wang S, Peng X, Lai S, Yang G. Immune response induced by candidate *Sarcoptes scabiei* var. cuniculi DNA vaccine encoding paramyosin in mice. Exp Appl Acarol. 2014;63(3):401–12.
12. Jex AR, Koehler AV, Ansell BR, Baker L, Karunajeewa H, Gasser RB. Getting to the guts of the matter: the status and potential of 'omics' research of parasitic protists of the human gastrointestinal system. Int J Parasitol. 2013; 43(12–13):971–82.
13. Jex AR, Liu S, Li B, Young ND, Hall RS, Li Y, Yang L, Zeng N, Xu X, Xiong Z, Chen F, Wu X, Zhang G, Fang X, Kang Y, Anderson GA, Harris TW, Campbell BE, Vlaminck J, Wang T, Cantacessi C, Schwarz EM, Ranganathan S, Geldhof P, Nejsum P, Sternberg PW, Yang H, Wang J, Wang J, Gasser RB. *Ascaris suum* draft genome. Nature. 2011;479(7374):529–33.
14. Jex AR, Nejsum P, Schwarz EM, Hu L, Young ND, Hall RS, Korhonen PK, Liao S, Thamsborg S, Xia J, Xu P, Wang S, Scheerlinck JP, Hofmann A, Sternberg PW, Wang J, Gasser RB. Genome and transcriptome of the porcine whipworm *Trichuris suis*. Nat Genet. 2014;46(7):701–6.
15. Joachim A, Dülmer N, Daugschies A, Roepstorff A. Occurrence of helminths in pig fattening units with different management systems in Northern Germany. Vet Parasitol. 2001;96(2):135–46.
16. Katakam KK, Thamsborg SM, Dalsgaard A, Kyvsgaard NC, Mejer H. Environmental contamination and transmission of *Ascaris suum* in Danish organic pig farms. Parasit Vectors. 2016;9:80.
17. Kreiner T, Worliczek HL, Tichy A, Joachim A. Influence of toltrazuril treatment on parasitological parameters and health performance of piglets in the field–an Austrian experience. Vet Parasitol. 2011;183(1–2):14–20.
18. Laha R. Sarcoptic mange infestation in pigs: an overview. J Parasit Dis. 2015; 39(4):596–603.

19. Lightowlers MW. Control of *Taenia solium* taeniasis/cysticercosis: past practices and new possibilities. Parasitology. 2013;140(13):1566–77.

20. Lim SS, Othman RY. Recent advances in *Toxoplasma gondii* immunotherapeutics. Korean J Parasitol. 2014;52(6):581–93.

21. Loke P, Lim YA. Helminths and the microbiota: parts of the hygiene hypothesis. Parasite Immunol. 2015;37(6):314–23.

22. Lopatina IuV. Resistance of the itch mites *Sarcoptes scabiei* De Geer, 1778 to scabicides [in Russian]. Med Parazitol (Mosk). 2012;1:49–54.

23. Martín-Gómez S, Alvarez-Sánchez MA, Rojo-Vázquez FA. Oral administration of hyperimmune anti-*Cryptosporidium parvum* ovine colostral whey confers a high level of protection against cryptosporidiosis in newborn NMRI mice. J Parasitol. 2005;91(3):674–8.

24. Masure D, Vlaminck J, Wang T, Chiers K, Van den Broeck W, Vercruysse J, Geldhof P. A role for eosinophils in the intestinal immunity against infective *Ascaris suum* larvae. PLoS Negl Trop Dis. 2013;7(3):e2138.

25. McOrist S, Blunt R, El-Sheikha H, Morillo Alujas A, Ocak M, Deniz A. Evaluation of efficacy of oral toltrazuril (Baycox 5%®) for the improvement of post weaning gut health in pigs. Pig J. 2010;63(12):73–9.

26. Mengel H, Kruger M, Kruger MU, Westphal B, Swidsinski A, Schwarz S, Mundt HC, Dittmar K, Daugschies A. Necrotic enteritis due to simultaneous infection with *Isospora suis* and clostridia in newborn piglets and its prevention by early treatment with toltrazuril. Parasitol Res. 2012;110(4):1347–55.

27. Mejer H, Roepstorff A. *Ascaris suum* infections in pigs born and raised on contaminated paddocks. Parasitology. 2006;133(Pt 3):305–12.

28. Monreal-Escalante E, Govea-Alonso DO, Hernández M, Cervantes J, Salazar-González JA, Romero-Maldonado A, Rosas G, Garate T, Fragoso G, Sciutto E, Rosales-Mendoza S. Towards the development of an oral vaccine against porcine cysticercosis: expression of the protective HP6/TSOL18 antigen in transgenic carrots cells. Planta. 2016;243(3):675–85.

29. Rahbauer M. Prävalenz von *Ascaris suum* in Abhängigkeit von der Art der Haltung und den verwendeten Antihelminthika. [Prevalence of *Ascaris suum* in relation to management and use of anthelminthics.] Diploma thesis Vetmeduni Vienna 2012, 32 pages.

30. Roepstorff A. Transmission of intestinal helminths in Danish sow herds. Vet Parasitol. 1991;39(1–2):149–60.

31. Roepstorff A. Helminth surveillance as a prerequisite for anthelmintic treatment in intensive sow herds. Vet Parasitol. 1997;73(1–2):139–51.

32. Roepstorff A, Mejer H, Nejsum P, Thamsborg SM. Helminth parasites in pigs: new challenges in pig production and current research highlights. Vet Parasitol. 2011;180(1–2):72–8.

33. Scala A, Demontis F, Varcasia A, Pipia AP, Poglayen G, Ferrari N, Genchi M. Toltrazuril and sulphonamide treatment against naturally *Isospora suis* infected suckling piglets: is there an actual profit? Vet Parasitol. 2009;163(4):362–5.

34. Schwarz L, Joachim A, Worliczek HL. Transfer of *Cystoisospora suis*-specific colostral antibodies and their correlation with the course of neonatal porcine cystoisosporosis. Vet Parasitol. 2013;197(3–4):487–97.

35. Schwarz L, Worliczek HL, Winkler M, Joachim A. Superinfection of sows with *Cystoisospora suis* ante partum leads to a milder course of cystoisosporosis in suckling piglets. Vet Parasitol. 2014;204(3–4):158–68.

36. Sharman PA, Smith NC, Wallach MG, Katrib M. Chasing the golden egg: vaccination against poultry coccidiosis. Parasite Immunol. 2010;32(8):590–8.

37. Shrestha A, Abd-Elfattah A, Freudenschuss B, Hinney B, Palmieri N, Ruttkowski B, Joachim A. Cystoisospora suis - A model of mammalian cystoisosporosis. Front Vet Sci. 2015;2:68.

38. Smets K, Neirynck W, Vercruysse J. Eradication of sarcoptic mange from a Belgian pig breeding farm with a combination of injectable and in-feed ivermectin. Vet Rec. 1999;145(25):721–4.

39. Strube C, Daugschies A. Antiparasitäre Vakzinen beim Nutztier: Wunsch und Wirklichkeit [Vaccines against livestock parasites: expectations and reality]. Berl Munch Tierarztl Wochenschr. 2015;128:437–50.

40. Swiatczak B, Cohen IR. Gut feelings of safety: tolerance to the microbiota mediated by innate immune receptors. Microbiol Immunol. 2015;59(10):573–85.

41. Várady M, Bjørn H, Nansen P. In vitro characterization of anthelmintic susceptibility of field isolates of the pig nodular worm *Oesophagostomum* spp., susceptible or resistant to various anthelmintics. Int J Parasitol. 1996; 26(7):733–40.

42. Wallach MG, Ashash U, Michael A, Smith NC. Field application of a subunit vaccine against an enteric protozoan disease. PLoS One. 2008;3(12):e3948.

43. Walton SF. The immunology of susceptibility and resistance to scabies. Parasite Immunol. 2010;32(8):532–40.

44. Witcombe DM, Smith NC. Strategies for anti-coccidial prophylaxis. Parasitology. 2014;141(11):1379–89.

45. Wiwanitkit S, Wiwanitkit V. Inactivation of *Ascaris suum* eggs. Am J Infect Control. 2013;41(9):849.

46. Worliczek HL, Mundt HC, Ruttkowski B, Joachim A. Age, not infection dose, determines the outcome of *Isospora suis* infections in suckling piglets. Parasitol Res. 2009;105 Suppl 1:S157–62.

47. Worliczek HL, Gerner W, Joachim A, Mundt HC, Saalmüller A. Porcine coccidiosis–investigations on the cellular immune response against *Isospora suis*. Parasitol Res. 2009;105 Suppl 1:S151–5.

48. Worliczek HL, Buggelsheim M, Alexandrowicz R, Witter K, Schmidt P, Gerner W, Saalmüller A, Joachim A. Changes in lymphocyte populations in suckling piglets during primary infections with *Isospora suis*. Parasite Immunol. 2010; 32(4):232–44.

49. Worliczek HL, Ruttkowski B, Joachim A, Saalmüller A, Gerner W. Faeces, FACS, and functional assays - preparation of *Isospora suis* oocyst antigen and representative controls for immunoassays. Parasitology. 2010;137(11):1637–43.

50. Worliczek HL, Ruttkowski B, Schwarz L, Witter K, Tschulenk W, Joachim A. *Isospora suis* in an epithelial cell culture system - an in vitro model for sexual development in coccidia. PLoS One. 2013;8(7):e69797.

51. Yasuda K, Matsumoto M, Nakanishi K. Importance of both innate immunity and acquired immunity for rapid expulsion of *S. venezuelensis*. Front Immunol. 2014;5:118.

5

Provision of straw by a foraging tower – effect on tail biting in weaners and fattening pigs

Carolin Holling[1]* , Elisabeth grosse Beilage[1], Beatriz Vidondo[2] and Christina Nathues[2]

Abstract

Background: Straw is one of the most effective rooting materials to reduce tail biting in pigs. A so-called foraging-tower (FT) provides only small quantities of straw compatible with liquid manure systems. The focus of the present study was on the effect of providing straw by FT in order to prevent tail biting in tail docked pigs. Four consecutive batches of 160 pigs, randomly divided into a straw (SG) and a control group (CG) were followed up from weaning to slaughter.

Results: Tail wounds (Score ≥ 2) were detected in 104 out of 12,032 single observations (SG n = 48; CG n = 56) in 9 pens (SG n = 4/32; CG n = 5/32) mainly focused on the fattening period of batch 2 due to a failure in the ventilation system. No significant differences concerning the distribution of Score ≥ 2 in pens of the SG and CG could be identified. Bite marks (Score 1) were documented in 395 observations at animal level (SG n = 197, CG n = 198) in all batches. In the nursery period, the air velocity significantly increased the chance that at least one pig per pen and week showed a tail lesion score ≥ 1 ($p = 0.024$). In the fattening period ammonia concentration was positively associated with tail lesions ($p = 0.007$).

The investigation of blood samples revealed infections with *Mycoplasma hyopneumoniae* in all batches and a circulation of Porcine Reproductive and Respiratory Syndrome Virus (NA-vaccine strain) and Porcine Circovirus Type 2 in two batches each. The average daily straw consumption was 3.5 g/pig (standard deviation (SD) = 1.1) during the rearing period and 31.9 g/pig (SD = 7.7) during the fattening period.

Conclusion: Due to the low prevalence of tail biting in all batches the effect of the FT tower could not be evaluated conclusively. The operation of the FT with an average daily straw consumption of 3.5 g/pig (SD = 1.1) during the rearing period and 31.9 g/pig (SD = 7.7) during the fattening period did not affect the weight gain. Exploratory behaviour seems to cause bite marks (score 1), which do not necessarily result in tail biting. The main outbreak of tail biting was probably triggered by a failure of the ventilation system, which resulted in a number of climatic and air quality changes including higher ammonia concentrations and sudden temperature changes.

Keywords: Environmental enrichment, Welfare, Exploratory behaviour, Ammonia

Background

Tail biting is an abnormal behaviour in the domestic pig causing reduced animal welfare and economic losses in pig production worldwide [1]. Despite the prohibition according to Council Directive 2008/120/EC [2], most pigs in conventional pig production in the EU are tail docked [3, 4]. Only when there is evidence that pigs have previously been injured by tail biting and on condition that inadequate environmental conditions and management systems have been addressed previously, is tail docking exceptionally allowed. The European Food Safety Authority (EFSA) estimates a prevalence of tail biting in docked pigs around 3%, while the prevalence in undocked pigs in Finland, Sweden and Norway, where tail docking is totally banned, is assumed to be between 6 and 10% and as high as up to 30% [3].

Although tail docking is effective in reducing the prevalence of tail biting, it can neither totally solve the

* Correspondence: carolin.holling@tiho-hannover.de
[1]University of Veterinary Medicine Hannover, Field Station for Epidemiology, Büscheler Str. 9, D-49456 Bakum, Germany
Full list of author information is available at the end of the article

problem [5, 6], nor is it consistent with animal welfare [3, 7]. However, victims of tail biting suffer from acute pain, have an increased risk of infections and a reduced weight gain. As a consequence, tail biting is not compatible with welfare and it is in the interest of pig producers to avoid economical losses due to tail biting [1, 8]. Nevertheless, the prevention of tail biting should focus on identifying and eliminating predisposing, possibly interacting risk factors. These include, for example, a lack of manipulable enrichment materials, a high stocking density, poor air quality, poor health, a reduced feed and water quality, restricted feeding and drinking systems as well as genetics [9, 10]. By fulfilling the pigs' natural exploratory behaviour, which consists of rooting, sniffling, biting and chewing various digestible and indigestible items, the provision of rooting material can reduce the risk of tail biting [11]. On this account permanent access to a sufficient quantity of material is also regulated by law to increase animal welfare (Council Directive 2008/120/EC) [2]. In comparison to most enrichment objects (e. g., chains, rubber hoses, balls) rooting materials like straw or wood shavings prevent tail biting more effectively [11, 12]. Assuming a behavioural synchronisation of pigs even the accessibility of materials or objects could play an important role in avoiding aggression due to competitive behaviour [13].

However, in Western Europe most current housing systems have fully slatted floors and liquid manure systems, which could be blocked by offering large amounts of straw [12, 14]. A so-called foraging-tower (FT) provides only small quantities of straw compatible with liquid manure systems. The focus of this study was on the effect of providing straw by FT in order to prevent tail biting in tail docked pigs.

Methods

The study was conducted from June 2013 to August 2014 in a conventional farrow to finish herd in Germany with a history of tail biting in fattening pigs for several years. In the past, the prevalence of tail biting had been estimated as being up to 15% in affected batches, although the tails had been docked.

Animals, housing and management

The piglets, Landrace x Large White x Pietrain crossbreds, were tail docked within the first three days of life and male pigs were castrated within the first week of life. During the suckling period piglets had been vaccinated against Porcine Circovirus Type 2 (PCV2) (Ingelvac CircoFLEX, Boehringer Ingelheim Vetmedica, Inc., D-55216 Ingelheim/Rhein, Germany) and *Mycoplasma hyopneumoniae* (MH) (Porcilis® M Hyo, Intervet Deutschland GmbH, D-85701 Unterschleissheim, Germany). The sows on the farm were regularly vaccinated against Porcine Reproductive and Respiratory Syndrome (PRRS) (Ingelvac PRRS® MLV, Boehringer IngelheimVetmedica, Inc.), Erysipelas and Parvovirus (Porcilis® Ery + Parvo, Intervet Deutschland GmbH) as well as Swine Influenza Virus (SIV) (RESPIPORC FLU3, IDT Biologika GmbH, D-06861 Dessau-Rosslau, Germany). After a suckling period of 26 days, all weaners ($n = 480$) were sorted by weight (low, medium, high) in three groups due to the farmer's routine management. Each weight group was housed in one of the units of the rearing barn containing eight pens (3.2 × 2.5 m) with 20 pigs each. Only the weaners of the medium weight group ($n = 160$) were included in the study.

The floor was fully slatted, consisting of one third concrete and two thirds plastic. The pigs were fed automatically ad libitum with commercial feed (Table 1) by a wet/dry swing feeder (AP Company, DK-7570 Vemb, Denmark) in each pen. Water was available ad libitum via two drinking nipples per pen.

At a weight of approximately 28 to 30 kg pigs were vaccinated against SIV (RESPIPORC FLU3, IDT Biologika GmbH) and moved to the fattening barn in which two equal units, containing 16 pens each, were used for the study. Ten pigs were kept in each pen (3.2 × 2.5 m). All pens were equipped with fully slatted concrete floor and a long trough (length: 3.2 m; animal: feeding place ratio 1:1). The pigs of two adjoining pens were fed restrictively eight times a day with commercial feed (Table 1) by one feeding valve of a liquid feeding system. Water was available ad libitum via one drinking nipple per pen. Artificial light was switched on from 6:30 h to

Table 1 Commercial feeds used in the study from wean to finish

Type of feed	Weight of pigs[a] (kg)	Form of feed	ME[b]/kg	Crude protein (%)	Lysine (%)	Crude fibre (%)	Crude oils and fats (%)
complete feed for piglets	5.5—6.5	small pellets	16.00	23.00	1.65	2.20	8.50
complete feed for piglets	6.5—10	pellets (2.2 mm)	14.00	20.00	1.40	3.30	3.30
complete feed for piglets	10—30	pellets (3.0 mm)	14.00	20.00	1.32	3.50	4.00
complete feed I for fattening pigs	30—50	liquid	13.20	17.00	1.05	4.20	3.70
complete feed II for fattening pigs	50—120	liquid	13.40	14.00	0.95	3.70	3.40

[a]To avoid sudden changes in diet, feed was blended with the following feed for at least one week
[b]metabolizable energy

20:00 h. The ventilation system consists of spray cooling channels, an overhead extraction system and a heating system operated with biogas.

Foraging tower and dummy

The foraging tower (Fig. 1) was developed by the Agricultural Center "Haus Düsse" (D-59505 Bad Sassendorf, Germany) for fattening pigs and consists of a movable plastic tube used as a container (height 130 cm, diameter: 31 cm) and a round concrete base (diameter 70 cm) on which it is fixed. The container was permanently filled with short-chopped wheat straw (length: 5–7 cm) of high quality. The pigs nudge the material from a small adjustable gap (adjusted size in this study:

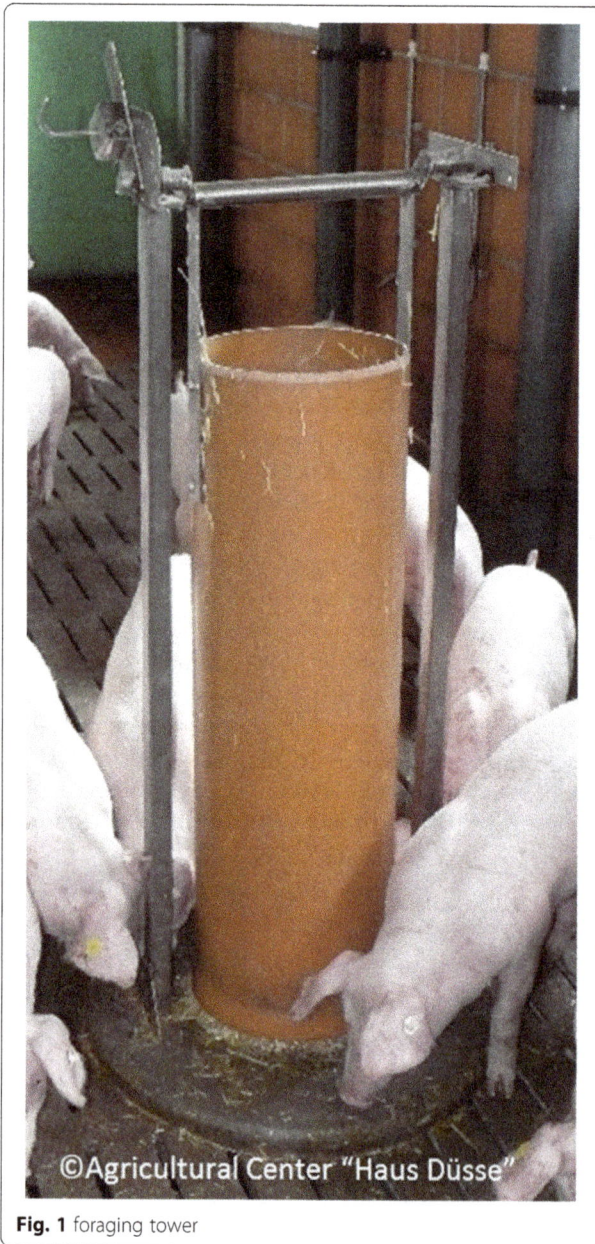

Fig. 1 foraging tower

2.5—4.0 cm) between the container and the concrete base. For usage during the rearing period smaller foraging towers had been manufactured (plastic tube: height 110 cm, diameter 20 cm, concrete base: diameter 65 cm). Prior to the experiment the pens for the straw group (SG) were randomly selected and a foraging tower was installed. The remaining pens for the control group (CG) were equipped with an equally sized dummy consisting of a concrete base and a plastic tube, which was neither movable nor filled with straw.

Experimental design

In total, 640 pigs in 32 rearing pens and 64 fattening pens were followed up from weaning to slaughter in four consecutive batches of 160 pigs each. At weaning 80 castrated male pigs and 80 female pigs of the medium weight group were randomly selected for the straw (SG) or control (CG) group, individually marked with a numbered ear tag and allocated to eight pens (20 pigs per pen) separated by gender. For the fattening period the pigs of each pen were randomly divided into two groups and placed in two neighbouring pens, fed by one feeding valve, in the fattening barn (16 pens, 10 pigs per pen). The unit design in the rearing and fattening barn is shown in Fig. 2.

Data collection

At the beginning and at the end of the rearing and fattening period the weight of the pigs per pen was measured. Once a week the tails of all pigs were scored by the same observer using the parameters "tail lesion" and "blood freshness" (Table 2, modified from Zonderland et al.) [12] and documented for each pen. Scores 2, 3, 4 and 5 were defined as different stages of tail biting. Pigs with tail wounds ≥ Score 2 were individually identified by their ear tag number and recorded. In cases of tail biting the scoring interval was reduced to every second day and slowly increased, if no fresh bleeding tail wounds had occurred any more. The scoring was stopped, when the farmer delivered the first group of pigs to slaughter.

At the same time the ammonia content and the air velocity were measured with a gas detector (Draeger Pac® 7000, Draegerwerk AG & Co. KGaA, D-23558 Luebeck, Germany) and a hot-wire anemometer (testo 491, Testo AG, D-79853 Lenzkirch, Germany) at four (rearing unit) or six (fattening unit) predefined locations, respectively (Fig. 2). The air temperature was recorded continuously by two data loggers (testo 175 T1, Testo AG, D-79853 Lenzkirch, Germany) per unit.

Blood samples from 22 randomly selected pigs were taken at the beginning and at the end of the fattening period of each batch (paired serum samples) and tested by enzyme linked immunosorbent assay (ELISA) for antibodies against PRRSV (IDEXX PRRS X3®, IDEXX

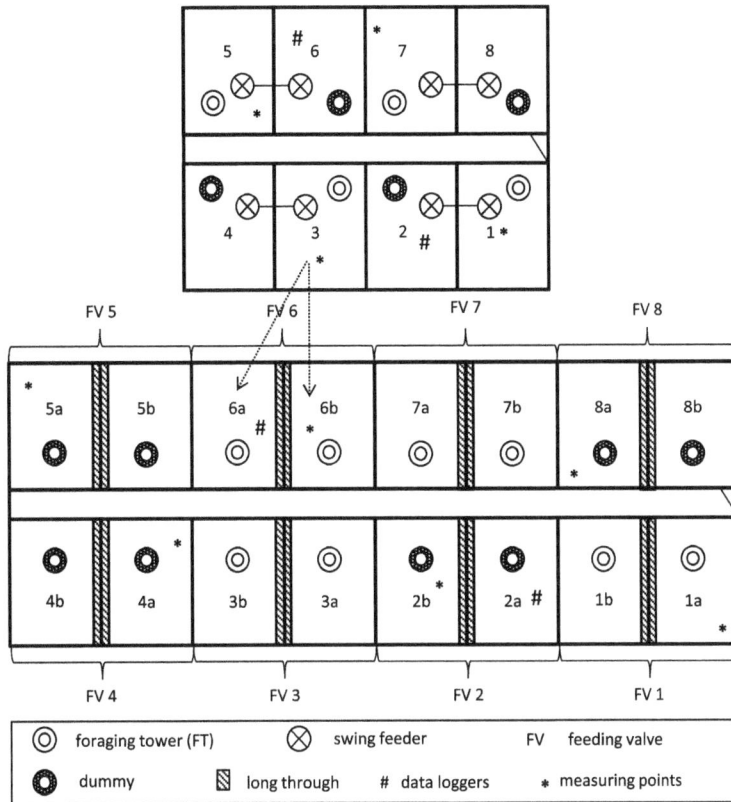

Fig. 2 Illustration of unit design in the rearing (above) and fattening barn (below) used in this study (not true to scale). The *arrows* show an option of dividing pigs of one rearing pen (20 pigs) into two fattening pens (2 × 10 pigs)

Switzerland AG, CH-3097 Liebefeld-Bern, Switzerland) and MH (IDEXX M. hyo®, IDEXX Laboratories, Inc., Westbrook, Maine, 04092 USA). PCR's for PRRSV (EZ-PRRSV™ MPX 4.0 RT-PCR®, Tetracore Inc., Rockville, MD 20850, USA) and PCV2 (according to Brunborg et al. [15]) were performed in eight pool samples with a maximum of three samples per pool from the beginning and eight pool samples from the end of the fattening period per batch.

The feed consumption per feeding valve was recorded by the feeding computer (HOWEMA Gerätebau GmbH & Co. KG, D-49429 Visbek, Gemany). Straw consumption was recorded by the farmer documenting the number of previously weighed 2.5 kg-bags of straw per FT he used for the daily replenishment. The remaining straw of the last bag per FT and the amount of straw in the FT were weighed again and subtracted at the end of each period.

Statistical analysis

Data storage and management was done in Microsoft Excel® (Version 2010, Microsoft Corporation, Redmond, Washington, US) and statistical analyses were performed in R software version 3.3.1 (R Core Team (2016)). The unit of observation was the pen in a given week ("pen-week"). Scorings routinely performed once a week and the scorings that were additionally carried out in case of tail biting were summarized using the highest scores per week and animal. After that, scorings yielded a number of animals per score (0–5) for each pen. For statistical analyses, this information was further combined in a summary score per pen-week, in which each tail lesion score was multiplied by the number of animals exhibiting this score, and the sum of these values taken. If, e.g., in a pen consisting of 20 animals, in a given week two pigs showed tail lesion score 2 and one pig showed tail lesion score 3, the summary score of this pen-week was $2 * 2 + 1 * 3 = 7$. Furthermore, pen-week was dichotomized (at least one pig with score ≥1 = positive vs. no pig with score ≥1 = negative).

To assess the effect of treatment (the foraging tower) on the occurrence of tail biting, a series of mixed effects models were calculated for nursery and fattening period separately, using R package 'lme4'. Preliminary analyses included tests for normality of numerical variables with Kolmogorov-Smirnov-Test and linearity with the outcome variable. All variables were tested for associations with the outcome or correlations between variables, using Chi^2-Tests, Mann-Whitney U-Test and Spearman's

Table 2 Scores for the parameters tail lesion and blood freshness (modified from Zonderland et al., [12])

Parameter	Score	Description
Tail lesion	0	No tail lesion visible
	1	Little lesions/bite marks are visible (size of a pinhead)
	2	Clearly visible wound ≤ cross section of the tail
	3	Clearly visible wound ≥ cross section of the tail without signs of inflammation (redness, swelling, heat)
	4	Clearly visible wound ≥ cross section of the tail with mild signs of inflammation (redness, swelling, heat)
	5	Clearly visible wound ≥ cross section of the tail with severe signs of inflammation (redness, swelling, heat)
Blood freshness	0	No blood visible
	1	Old dried black blood in the form of a scab
	2	Sticky dark red blood, mainly half a day to a day old
	3	Fresh bleeding wound

rank correlation coefficient, depending on the scale of the variables. In the case of a correlation coefficient of $r > 0.6$, the more biologically meaningful variable was used in the multivariable model. Calculated p-values of less than 0.05 were considered statistically significant.

Due to the low occurrence of tail biting over the whole period of observation, with many pen-weeks where no pigs exhibited tail lesion scores above 0, it was not possible to fit a model to all observations with any discrete-scale outcome variable (e.g., the summary score or the number of pigs with score ≥ 2 per pen-week). For this reason, a two-step approach was chosen: In a first step, a generalized linear mixed-effects model including all observations was calculated with dichotomized pen-week as outcome and the treatment group as main effect. To account for the climatic conditions, also the ammonia concentration, the air velocity, the highest day/night temperature range and the average temperature in that week were considered as fixed effects. These temperature variables were chosen because they were deemed to be the most comprehensive and least correlated ones (as opposed to minimum and maximum temperature). Furthermore, to account for the fact that observations in the same pens were made at different times, the week was also included as fixed effect. Lastly, to account for the hierarchical structure of the data of pen-week being nested in pen and pen being nested in batch, and thus to account for the additional influence of pen and batch, a random effect for pen nested in batch was included (random intercept model). In a second step, a linear mixed-effects model was calculated only with the positive pen-weeks (summary score > 0), using the discrete-scale summary score but otherwise with the same set-up as described for the first model. To meet the assumptions necessary for a linear model (i.e., the normality and linearity, tested visually with quantile-quantile-plots), the summary score was log-transformed.

The modelling process consisted of 1) testing each explanatory variable (group, ammonia concentration, air velocity, average temperature and day/night temperature) individually with pen nested in batch as random effect and correcting for week as fixed effect; 2) running the multivariable model with all four explanatory variables; 3) manual backward selection based on the highest p-value, until all explanatory variables retained in the final model had significant p-values.

Furthermore, the effect of treatment on the parameters feed consumption and average weight gain per day per fattening pig was assessed in two linear mixed models with treatment group as fixed effect and batch as random effect (random intercept models). The association between the quantity of straw consumption and feed consumption (outcome variable) in the fattening period within the TG was assessed in a linear mixed model with straw consumption as fixed effect and batch as random effect (random intercept model). Lastly, for nursery pigs, the same model as in fattening pigs was calculated for weight gain, whereas data on feed consumption were not available for the nursery period.

Results

In total, the occurrence of tail lesions was analyzed in 12,032 single observations at animal level (SG $n = 6016$, CG $n = 6016$) and 976 (SG $n = 488$, CG $n = 488$) observations at pen-week level. Tail wounds (score ≥ 2) were detected in 104 single observations (SG $n = 48$; CG $n = 56$) in different 9 pens (SG $n = 4/32$; CG $n = 5/32$). The number of affected pigs per pen and the duration of tail biting are shown in Table 3. The duration was calculated as the number of consecutive weeks in which at least one pig per pen with a fresh bleeding tail wound was present. The occurrence of tail biting was mainly focused on four pens with 15 affected pigs in batch 2 and one pen during the rearing period of batch 4. Bite marks (score 1) were

Table 3 Number of pigs affected by tail biting per batch, pen and period and the duration of tail biting per pen

Batch	Pen	Straw group (affected pigs)	Control group (affected pigs)	Period	Duration of tail biting[b] (weeks)
1	105	1	–	rearing	1
2	205a	–	1	fattening	1
2	205b	–	6	fattening	7
2	207b	4	–	fattening	9
2	208a	–	4	fattening	5
3	305b	–	2	fattening	2
4	405	5	–	rearing	4
4	402a	–	1	fattening	2
4	406a	1[a]	–	fattening	1

[a]The pig was one of the five affected pigs from pen 405 during rearing period
[b]Number of consecutive weeks in which at least one pig with a fresh bleeding was present (Score 3 for blood freshness)

documented in 395 observations at animal level (SG n = 197, CG n = 198). The proportions of pigs with tail wounds (score ≥ 2) and bite marks (score 1) in all pens per week in the SG and CG are shown in Fig. 3 a and b for batch 2 and in the Additional files 1 a, b, 2 and 3 a, b for batch 1, 3 and 4.

In the nursery, 58 of 108 pen-weeks (53.7%) in the SG had at least one pig with score ≥ 1 (= positive pen-week), compared to 52 (58.1%) in the CG. A score of 5 was not seen in any pen-weeks in the nursery, whereas in two pen-weeks the highest score observed in a pig was 4, one pen-week had a highest score of 3 and another one a highest score of 2 (all in the SG).

In the fattening period, the number of positive pen-weeks was 53 of 256 (20.7%) in the SG and 67 (26.2%) in the CG. There were 13 pen-weeks (SG = 6, CG = 7) in which the highest score observed in an animal was 5; in five pen-weeks (SG = 3, CG = 2), the highest score was 4; in 2 pen-weeks (all CG), the highest score was 3 and in 5 pen-weeks (SG = 1, CG = 4), the highest score was 2. The summary scores in positive pen-weeks in the SG and CG are shown in Fig. 4 for each period.

The severest outbreak of tail biting with the highest number of affected pigs (score ≥ 2) was observed in the fattening period of batch 2. Due to a temporary failure in the ventilation system during the fattening period of the second batch the temperature loggers recorded a sudden rise in temperature of 11.5° Celsius [°C] within 27 h (days 62 and 63). The average temperature in the following week (week 10: 25.9 °C) was 5.3 °C higher than in the previous week (week 9: 20.6 °C). The measured ammonia concentrations were 18.5 ppm on day 62 and 29.8 ppm on day 69. During the following weeks ammonia contents increased up to 43.7 ppm. Tail biting started on day 67. Otherwise, no clear temporal patterns in the proportion of pigs showing bite marks (score 1) and tail wounds (score ≥ 2) over the course of the

rearing and fattening period could be observed (Fig. 3 a and b and Additional files 1 a, b, 2 and 3 a, b).

The results of the mixed-effect models to assess the effect of treatment and climate variables on the occurrence of tail biting, accounting for the time, pen and batch, are indicated in Tables 4, 5, 6 and 7. For the treatment, no statistically significant effect could be identified in any of the models. In the nursery period, only the air velocity significantly increased the chance that a pen-week had at least one pig with score ≥1 in the final model (p = 0.024). Among the positive pen-weeks, the day/night temperature range showed a positive (p = 0.014) and the average temperature a negative (p = 0.003) association with the summary score. In the fattening period, in the final model only the day/night temperature range (p = 0.027) had an effect on whether the pen-week was positive or not, whereas ammonia concentration was positively associated with the summary score (p = 0.007).

The results of serology (see Additional files 4 and 5), reveal infections with MH in all batches and with PRRSV in the second and third batch. Performing a PRRSV-PCR, the NA-genotype was found in two of eight pool samples of batch 2 at the end of the fattening period as well as in all eight pools of batch 3 at the beginning of the fattening period. The sequencing of the ORF7 region of the PRRSV strain detected in the third batch resulted in a homology of 99% with the PRRSV-NA vaccine strain. The sequencing of a strain from the second batch was not successful due to a low threshold cycle (Ct)-value. PCV2 was detected by PCR in two out of eight sample pools of the first and the fourth batch at the beginning of the fattening period.

The average daily straw- and feed consumption per pig and the average daily weight gain per pig are shown in Table 8. The average daily straw consumption in the SG was 3.5 g/pig (SD = 1.1) during the rearing period and 31.9 g/pig (SD = 7.7) during the

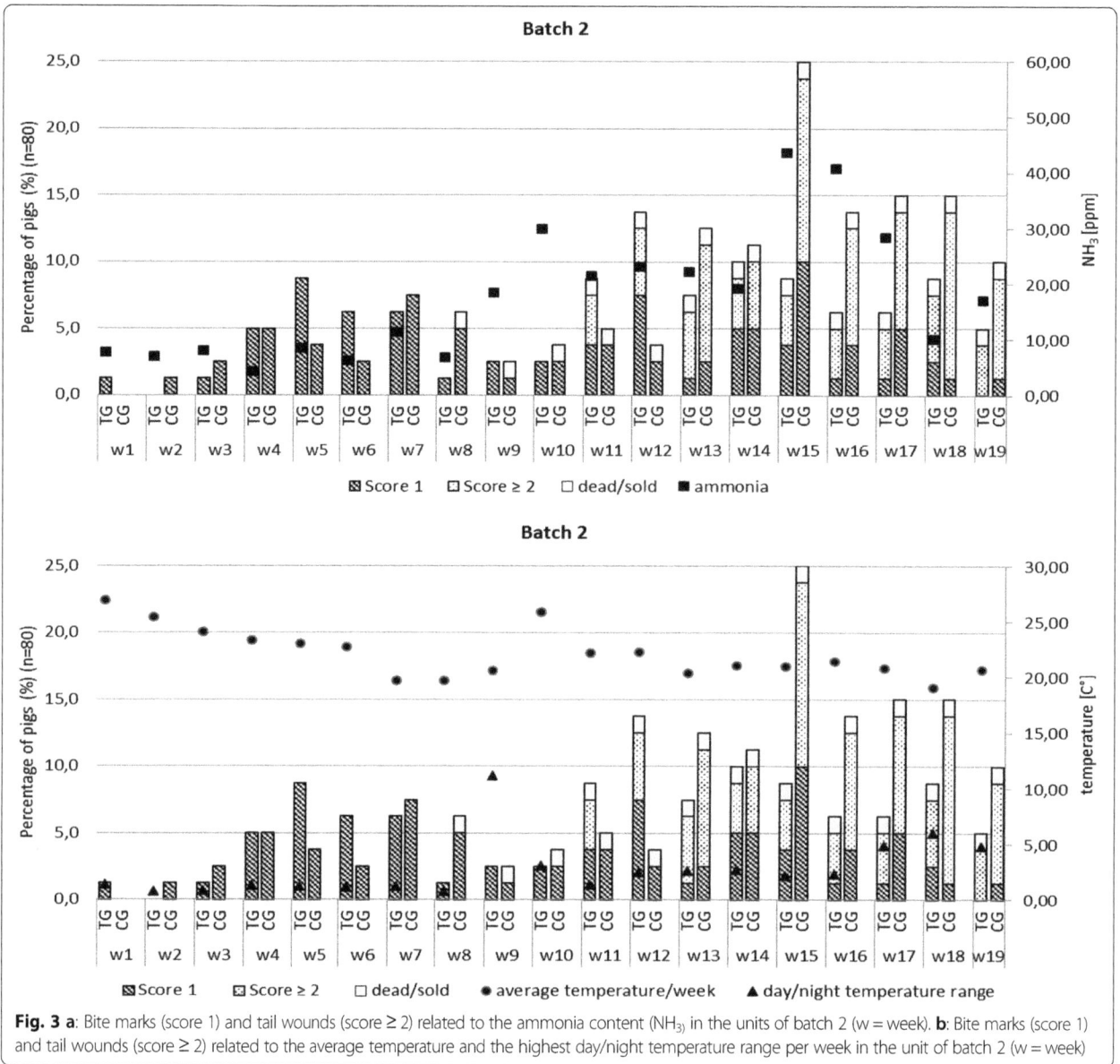

Fig. 3 a: Bite marks (score 1) and tail wounds (score ≥ 2) related to the ammonia content (NH₃) in the units of batch 2 (w = week). **b**: Bite marks (score 1) and tail wounds (score ≥ 2) related to the average temperature and the highest day/night temperature range per week in the unit of batch 2 (w = week)

fattening period. Comparing the average daily weight gain (SG = 809 g, SD = 58); CG = 800 g, SD = 74) during fattening and the average daily feed consumption per pig (SG = 2.1 kg, SD = 0.3; CG = 2.0 kg, SD = 0.3) of the SG and CG no significant differences were detected in the linear mixed-effects models (Table 9). In the SG, feed consumption and straw consumption in fattening were negatively but not significantly correlated.The mean values, minimum values, maximum values and the standard deviations (SD) of the measured temperatures, ammonia concentrations and air velocities as well as of the calculated day/night temperature ranges are presented in Tables 10 and 11 for each batch and period.

Discussion

In this study the occurrence of tail biting was mainly focused on four pens with 15 affected pigs in batch 2, probably triggered by a failure in the ventilation system. Another outbreak of tail biting was registered in one pen during the rearing period of batch 4 with five affected pigs without any apparent cause. Thus, the prevalence of tail biting was much lower than expected from farm history and allows no statistically substantiated evaluation of the FT regarding the occurrence of tail biting in the SG and CG.

Nevertheless, in line with previous studies providing straw in racks [12, 16] the FT was not able to totally prevent tail biting under the conventional housing

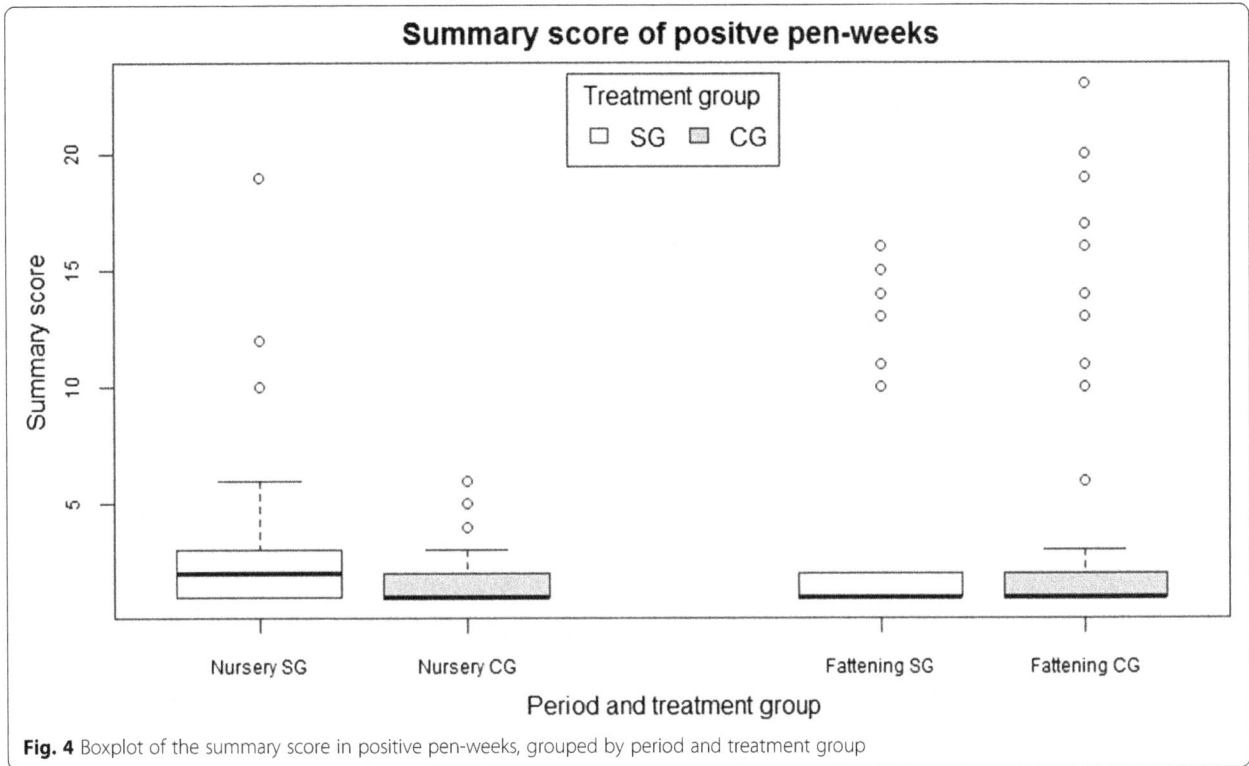

Fig. 4 Boxplot of the summary score in positive pen-weeks, grouped by period and treatment group

conditions in this study. A reason for this could be the quantity of straw provided by the FT, which mainly influences the time during which pigs are occupied by foraging. Jensen et al. [17] figured out that an amount of 250 g straw per pig and day was the point where pigs stopped increasing the oral manipulation of straw. In another study 390 g straw per pig and day were necessary to achieve no further reduction in abnormal behaviour towards pen mates [18]. In contrast to our study, these studies were performed in pens with partly solid concrete floor. Providing comparable amounts of straw in

the present study was not possible due to the fully slatted concrete floor and the liquid manure system. However, small amounts of straw are more effective in preventing tail biting in conventionally housed pigs than non-modifiable enrichment objects or barren environment [12, 16, 19].

Furthermore, the results suggest that a higher straw consumption could reveal a lower feed intake. Assessing this negative correlation, we should keep in mind that the straw consumption per pig was very low and we were not able to define the amount of straw, which fell through the

Table 4 Results of the generalized linear mixed-effects model for the nursery period with dichotomized pen-week (at least one pig with score ≥1 vs. no pig with score ≥1) as outcome variable and pen nested in batch as random effect (random intercept): results of models for each individual explanatory variable, the full model and the final model

Nursery	Individual models		Full model		Final model[a]	
Fixed effect	Estimate	P-value	Estimate	P-value	Estimate	P-value
Week	−0.077	0.045	−0.040	0.679	−0.059	0.529
SG (CG = baseline)	0.331	0.590	0.330	0.539		
day/night temperature range	0.204	0.063	0.150	0.223		
average temperature	−0.167	0.245	model did not converge with this variable included		model did not converge with this variable included	
ammonia concentration	−0.024	0.521	−0.065	0.112		
air velocity	27.265	0.024	26.233	0.055	27.265	0.024

[a]random effect batch:pen (Intercept): variance 1.927

Table 5 Results of the linear mixed-effects model for the nursery period with log-transformed summary score per pen-week as outcome variable and pen nested in batch as random effect (random intercept): results of the models for each individual explanatory variable, the full model and the final model

Nursery	Individual models		Full model		Final model[a]	
Fixed effect	Estimate	P-value	Estimate	P-value	Estimate	P-value
Week	0.072	0.001	−0.078	0.070	−0.041	0.001
SG (CG = baseline)	0.259	0.141	−0.322	0.067		
day/night temperature range	−0.010	0.698	0.157	0.005	0.135	0.014
average temperature	−0.075	0.037	−0.269	0.001	−0.226	0.003
ammonia concentration	−0.005	0.682	0.007	0.637		
air velocity	−0.321	0.936	3.895	0.402		

[a]random effect batch:pen (Intercept): variance 0.1271, residual variance 0.2643

slats and was not eaten by the pigs. Additionally, we found no significant differences in feed consumption and weight gain on comparing the SG and CG.

Bulens et al. [14] offered straw in four different types of application (Funbar, MIK Toy, rack and straw feeder) and found no difference in growth either. In contrast, other studies [16, 20, 21] showed that feed consumption and daily weight gain were higher in straw bedded systems. However, in straw bedded housing systems the amount of digested straw is difficult to measure and pigs are able to control their microenvironment [20] influencing the demand for energy. Therefore, the results are not comparable.

An explanation for the differences between batches concerning straw consumption could be that it was impossible to achieve an equally sized gap of all foraging towers by using the same adjustment due to the hand manufacturing of the foraging towers. Furthermore, some containers seemed to be easier to move than others so that the farmer had to regulate the adjustment based on his own estimation in order to try to provide the same amount of straw to all pigs of the treatment group.

Despite the low prevalence of tail biting, bite marks were frequently detected in all batches and were nearly equally distributed in both groups. The most accepted description of tail biting in literature by Taylor et al. [22] ("Two-stage tail-biting") differentiates between a "pre-damage stage" and a "damage stage". The "pre-damage stage" is suggested to be a precursor of tail biting and is considered as explorative "tail-in-mouth" behaviour without causing any visible damage to the skin. The "damage stage" begins if the tail starts bleeding due to dental manipulation [22, 23]. In contrast to this definition the prevalence and the distribution of bite marks in the present study indicate that these small skin lesions are a consequence of exploratory behaviour, which do not necessarily result in tail biting, at least in pigs with docked tails.

Furthermore, climatic conditions have often been linked to the physical comfort of pigs and seem to have to an influence on the occurrence of tail lesions in this study.

This is in accordance with the evaluation by Dutch pig farmers, who identified climate as the main risk factor for tail biting [24]. The impact of air velocity on the probability that a pen-week had at least one pig with score ≥1, shown in this study, is in line with Scheepens

Table 6 Results of the generalized linear mixed-effects model for the fattening period with dichotomized pen-week (at least one pig with score ≥1 vs. no pig with score ≥1) as outcome variable and pen nested in batch as random effect (random intercept): results of the models for each individual explanatory variable, the full model and the final model

Fattening	Individual models		Full model		Final model[a]	
Fixed effect	Estimate	P-value	Estimate	P-value	Estimate	P-value
Week	0.062	0.429	−0.091	0.037	−0.067	0.087
SG (CG = baseline)	−0.380	0.325	−0.390	0.313		
day/night temperature range	−0.119	0.027	−0.106	0.074	−0.119	0.027
average temperature			−0.108	0.259		
ammonia concentration	0.018	0.174	0.013	0.405		
air velocity	−0.522	0.729	1.162	0.479		

[a]random effect batch:pen (Intercept): variance 1.301

Table 7 Results of the linear mixed-effects model for the fattening period with log-transformed summary score per pen-week as outcome variable and pen nested in batch as random effect (random intercept): results of the models for each individual explanatory variable, the full model and the final model

Fattening	Individual models		Full model		Final model[a]	
Fixed effect	Estimate	P-value	Estimate	P-value	Estimate	P-value
Week	−0.008	0.759	0.059	0.006	−0.724	0.009
SG (CG = baseline)	−0.075	0.724	−0.082	0.681		
day/night temperature range	−0.061	0.032	−0.033	0.303		
average temperature	−0.046	0.278	−0.077	0.088		
ammonia concentration	0.016	0.007	0.017	0.015	0.016	0.007
air velocity	−0.061	0.935	0.939	0.237		

[a]random effect batch:pen (Intercept): variance 0.2492, residual variance 0.3337

et al. [25]. In their study, pigs showed significantly more exploratory and agonistic behaviour on penmates in periods of draught, which were produced with cold air and a high air velocity [25]. Nevertheless, interpreting the measured values for air velocity in our study, we should keep in mind that these values might be subject to strong variation, represent only one point of time per week and might be influenced by movements of the animals as well as the observer. In accordance with our results, temperature changes, have previously been associated to the occurrence of tail biting [26]. However, the average temperature in the nursery period, which was negatively associated with the summary score in this study, had a contrary effect in the study of Smulders et al. [27]. Here a high temperature in the nursery was the most important factor influencing the occurrence of tail biting [27]. Regarding these results, we have to consider, that too high temperatures as well as too low temperatures have a negative impact on the pig's physical comfort. The outbreak of tail biting during the fattening period in batch 2 was probably caused by a failure in the ventilation system, which is the most important factor in reduced air quality [28] and temperature changes.

Pigs are exposed to particulate matter and gases, such as ammonia (NH_3), carbon dioxide (CO_2), hydrogen sulfide (H_2S), methane (CH_4) and nitrous oxide (N_2O) [29]. Particulate matter and ammonia are known to have an impact on animal health and behaviour by adversely influencing the mucosal clearance system and irritation of the respiratory epithelia [28, 29], whereas carbon dioxide and hydrogen sulfide (in usually measured concentrations) are less harmful to animal health [28] and methane and nitrous oxide are related to global climate changes [30].

O'Connor et al. [31] assumed that atmospheric ammonia concentrations of 20 ppm had a negative impact on the pigs' behaviour and physical comfort, while Jones et al. [32] showed that pigs already avoided ammonia concentrations of 10 ppm. Former attempts to induce tail biting by worsening the air quality were only partially successful [26, 33]. In our study, ammonia concentration was positively associated with the summary score (p = 0.007).

In addition to increasing ammonia contents a causal relationship of a risen air temperature should not be neglected. Geers et al. [34] suggested that inadequate temperature should be listed as a possible cause of tail biting. In their study tail biting was positively associated

Table 8 Weight gain, straw consumption and feed consumption per pig and day during the rearing and fattening period

Batch	Group	Rearing period			Fattening period			
		duration [days]	weight gain (pig/day) [g]	straw consumption (pig/day) [g]	average duration [days]	weight gain (pig/day) [g]	straw consumption (pig/day) [g]	feed consumption (pig/day) [kg]
1	SG	61	537	3.3	99.3	827	32.7	2.0
1	CG	61	502	-	101.1	835	–	2.1
2	SG	38	466	3.0	115.2	849	25.0	2.0
2	CG	38	458	–	117.3	800	–	1.9
3	SG	43	446	4.8	123.9	737	36.7	1.9
3	CG	43	412	–	126.1	702	–	1.7
4	SG	50	639	3.7	91.4	826	25.5	2.4
4	CG	50	638	–	91.0	835	–	2.3

Table 9 Results of the four linear mixed-effects models: with treatment group as explanatory variable and 1) average daily weight gain per pig (ADG) in nursery, 2) ADG in fattening and 3) feed consumption in the fattening as outcome, as well as 4) straw consumption as explanatory variable and feed consumption in fattening as outcome; each model with batch as random effect (random intercept)

	Nursery		Fattening	
Outcome ADG				
Fixed effect:	Estimate	P-value	Estimate	P-value
SG (CG = baseline)	−19.350	0.113	−16.560	0.301
Random effect:	Variance	Residual variance	Variance	Residual variance
Batch	8345	1117	2720	4030
Outcome feed consumption				
Fixed effect:			Estimate	P-value
SG (CG = baseline)			−0.079	0.209
Random effect:			Variance	Residual variance
Batch			0.056	0.030
Fixed effect:			Estimate	P-value
Straw consumption			−0.012	0.143
Random effect:			Variance	Residual variance
Batch			0.022	0.038

to an air temperature of 22—24 °C in pigs of 30—40 kg and to a temperature range of 16—18 °C in pigs weighing 40—50 kg. The pigs were housed on 40% partly slatted floors with floor heating at the beginning of the fattening period. With respect to this study the optimal air temperature range depends on the existing housing conditions. Lying, excreting and fouling behaviour are indicators for evaluating the pigs' optimal temperature range [35]. In the absence of bedding, an air temperature of 20—16 °C for pigs of 40—50 kg and a temperature of 18—14 °C for pigs of 60—100 kg is recommended, the temperature reducing with increasing age of the pig [36]. In our study, especially during the week tail biting occurred in batch 2, the average temperature was far too high for the pigs with an assumed weight of

approximately 55—65 kg per pig. Furthermore, pigs had been exposed to high temperature differences in the previous week. For practical reasons we did not record the behaviour of pigs.

D'Eath et al. [37] emphasize relationships between various known or suspected risk factors and the occurrence of tail biting. Among other potential risk factors, malfunction of the ventilation adversely affecting temperature and air quality might entail increasing activity levels and more pig directed exploratory behaviour because pigs compete for lying areas, which could improve their physical comfort. Damaging tail biting proceeds when other pigs tolerate tail manipulation.

Thus, the relationship between high ammonia levels, high air temperature and tail biting is probable in this

Table 10 Air temperature and night/day temperature range during the rearing period (R) and the fattening period (F)

Batch	Period	Air temperature [C°]					Day/night temperature range [C°]				
		n	mean	min	max	SD	n	mean	min	max	SD
1	R	6337	25.91	22.60	35.30	2.23	66	3.62	0.7	8.15	2.06
1	F	6117	22.79	18.40	29.15	1.67	65	3.68	1.20	7.10	1.36
2	R	3595	24.35	21.90	28.90	1.48	42	0.73	0.40	1.35	0.22
2	F	8058	21.24	16.4	29.00	2.21	85	2.12	0.90	11.15	1.52
3	R	4080	23.59	18.30	27.50	1.20	43	1.06	0.45	4.65	0.84
3	F	4057	20.17	17.05	26.30	1.58	43	3.43	1.00	7.95	1.89
4	R	4697	24.64	21.20	29.10	1.34	50	1.71	0.50	5.70	1.25
4	F	7811	23.60	19.00	34.50	2.49	82	4.17	0.90	11.10	2.44

Table 11 Ammonia content and air velocity during the rearing period (R) and the fattening period (F) measured at weekly intervals at four (rearing) or six (fattening) locations in the unit

Batch	Period	Ammonia [ppm]					Air velocity [m/s]				
		n	mean	min	max	SD	n	mean	min	max	SD
1	R	10	9.65	0.00	20.50	7.82	10	0.08	0.05	0.12	0.02
1	F	8	5.58	0.00	10.00	3.94	9	0.18	0.10	0.55	0.14
2	R	6	6.96	4.25	8.50	1.54	6	0.05	0.04	0.08	0.02
2	F	13	22.50	6.83	43.67	11.00	12	0.09	0.06	0.12	0.02
3	R	7	9.39	6.00	14.50	3.57	6	0.05	0.04	0.07	0.01
3	F	12	10.57	5.17	15,83	3.81	12	0.10	0.05	0.19	0.04
4	R	6	9.04	2.75	19.5	5.54	6	0.07	0.05	0.10	0.02
4	F	8	6.29	1.30	11.10	2.89	9	0.15	0.09	0.21	0.04

case. Nevertheless, we have to consider that other parameters for air quality such as particulate matter, carbon dioxide, hydrogen sulfide and air humidity, not measured in this study play a role and might also have had an impact on tail biting.

Another potential risk factor for tail biting, identified by Taylor et al. [10], is the parameter health. In a study by Moinard et al. [9] tail biting was positively associated with respiratory disease. Performing a pathological examination, Munsterhjelm et al. [38] assume that most lung lesions were secondary to infected tail lesions, but disease could not be ruled out as a possible cause of tail biting. In order to assess respiratory diseases as a potential trigger in this study paired serum samples were analysed for the most prevalent pathogens causing primary infections of the respiratory tract in this age group and area – MH, PCV2 and PRRSV. Despite vaccinating the piglets against MH and PCV2 at the end of the suckling period increasing antibody titers against MH during the fattening period (all batches) and the detection of PCV2 by PCR (batches 1 and 4) revealed infections not causing clinical respiratory disease. The PRRS-NA vaccine strain (ATCC VR2332) and strains with a nucleotide identity of 98–100% in ORF 5 were frequently found in herds where only the sows had been vaccinated with Ingelvac® PRRS MLV [39]. The circulating PRRSV-NA strain in batch 2 probably originates from Ingelvac® PRRS MLV used in the sow herd. With regard to tail biting during the rearing period (batch 4), serum samples of this age group were not investigated as serology is unsuitable due to missing discrimination of possibly co-existing maternal antibodies.

Conclusion

Due to the low prevalence of tail biting in all batches the effect of the FT tower could not conclusively be evaluated. Operating the FT with an average daily straw consumption of 3.5 g/pig (SD = 1.1) during the

rearing period and 31.9 g/pig (SD = 7.7) during the fattening period did not affect the weight gain. Exploratory behaviour seems to cause bite marks, which do not result in tail biting. The main outbreak of tail biting was probably triggered by a failure of the ventilation system, which resulted in a number of climatic and air quality changes including higher ammonia concentrations and sudden temperature changes.

Additional files

Additional file 1: a: Bite marks (score 1) and tail wounds (score ≥ 2) related to the ammonia content (NH₃) in the unit of batch 1 (w = week). b: Bite marks (score 1) and tail wounds (score ≥ 2) related to the average temperature and the highest day/night temperature range per week in the unit of batch 1 (w = week). (PDF 76 kb)

Additional file 2: a: Bite marks (score 1) and tail wounds (score ≥ 2) related to the ammonia content (NH₃) in the units of batch 3 (w = week). b: Bite marks (score 1) and tail wounds (score ≥ 2) related to the average temperature and the highest day/night temperature range per week in the unit of batch 3 (w = week). (PDF 54 kb)

Additional file 3: a: Bite marks (score 1) and tail wounds (score ≥ 2) related to the ammonia content (NH₃) in the units of batch 4 (w = week). b: Bite marks (score 1) and tail wounds (score ≥ 2) related to the average temperature and the highest day/night temperature range per week in the unit of batch 4 (w = week). (PDF 66 kb)

Additional file 4: Results of the IDEXX PRRS X3® ELISA. (PDF 289 kb)

Additional file 5: Results of the IDEXX M. hyo® ELISA. (PDF 334 kb)

Abbreviations
ADG: Average daily weight gain; CG: Control group; e. g: exempli gratia (for example); EFSA: European Food Safety Authority; ELISA: Enzyme linked immunosorbent assay; F: Fattening period; FT: Foraging-tower; ME: metabolizable energy; MH: *Mycoplasma hyopneumoniae*; MLV: Modified live vaccine; NA: North American; PCR: Polymerase chain reaction; PCV2: Porcine Circovirus Type 2; PRRS: Porcine reproductive and respiratory syndrome; PRRSV: Porcine reproductive and respiratory syndrome virus; R: Rearing period; SD: Standard deviation; SG: Straw group; SIV: Swine Influenza Virus

Acknowledgements
The farmer and his family are greatly acknowledged for their support during the entire study.

Funding
Not applicable.

Authors' contributions
Elisabeth grosse Beilage designed and supervised the entire study. Carolin Holling assisted in designing the study, performed the data collection and drafted the manuscript. Christina Nathues performed the statistical analysis, supported by Beatriz Vidondo, and drafted the manuscript. All authors read and approved the final manuscript.

Competing interests
The authors declare that they have no competing interests.

Author details
[1]University of Veterinary Medicine Hannover, Field Station for Epidemiology, Büscheler Str. 9, D-49456 Bakum, Germany. [2]Veterinary Public Health Institute, Vetsuisse Faculty, Schwarzenburgstrasse 155, CH-3097 Liebefeld, BE, Switzerland.

References
1. Valros A, Heinonen M. Save the pig tail. Porcine Health Manage. 2015;1:2.
2. European Union. Council Directive 2008/120/EC of 18 December 2008 laying down minimum standards for the protection of pigs (Codified version). Official J Europ Union. 2009;L47:5–13.
3. European Food Safety Authority (EFSA). Scientific opinion of the panel on animal health and welfare on a request from commission on the risks associated with tail biting in pigs and possible means to reduce the need for tail-docking considering the different housing and husbandry systems. EFSA J. 2007;611:1–13.
4. Nannoni E, Valsami T, Sardi L, Martelli G. Tail docking in pigs: a review on its short- and long-term consequences and effectiveness in preventing tail biting. Ital J Anim Sci. 2014;13:9.
5. Chambers C, Powell L, Wilson E, Green LE. A postal survey of tail biting in pigs in South-West England. Vet Rec. 1995;136:147–8.
6. Hunter EJ, Jones TA, Guise HJ, Penny RH, Hoste S. The relationship between tail biting in pigs, docking procedure and other management practices. Vet J. 2001;161:72–9.
7. Simonsen HB, Klinken L, Bindseil E. Histopathology of intact and docked pig tails. Br Vet J. 1991;147:407–12.
8. D'Eath R, Niemi J, Ahmadi BV, Rutherford K, Ison S, Turner S, Anker HT, Jensen T, Busch M, Jensen KK. Why are most EU pigs tail docked? Economic and ethical analysis of four pig housing and management scenarios in the light of EU legislation and animal welfare outcomes. Animal. 2016;10:687–99.
9. Moinard C, Mendl M, Nicol CJ, Green LE. A case control study of on-farm risk factors for tail biting in pigs. Appl Anim Behav Sci. 2003;81:333–55.
10. Taylor NR, Parker RM, Mendl M, Edwards SA, Main DC. Prevalence of risk factors for tail biting on commercial farms and intervention strategies. Vet J. 2012;194:77–83.
11. Studnitz M, Jensen MB, Pedersen LJ. Why do pigs root and in what will they root? A review on the exploratory behaviour of pigs in relation to environmental enrichment. Appl Anim Behav Sci. 2007;107:183–97.
12. Zonderland JJ, Wolthuis-Fillerup M, Van Reenen CG, Bracke MBM, Kemp B, Den Hartog LA, Spoolder HAM. Prevention and treatment of tail biting in weaned piglets. Appl Anim Behav Sci. 2008;110:269–81.
13. Docking CM, de Weerd HAV, Day JEL, Edwards SA. The influence of age on the use of potential enrichment objects and synchronisation of behaviour of pigs. Appl Anim Behav Sci. 2008;110:244–57.
14. Bulens A, Van Beirendonck S, Van Thielen J, Buys N, Driessen B. Straw applications in growing pigs: effects on behavior, straw use and growth. Appl Anim Behav Sci. 2015;169:26–32.
15. Brunborg IM, Moldal T, Jonassen CM. Quantitation of porcine circovirus type 2 isolated from serum/plasma and tissue samples of healthy pigs and pigs with postweaning multisystemic wasting syndrome using a TaqMan-based real-time PCR. J Virol Methods. 2004;122:171–8.
16. Van de Weerd HA, Docking CM, Day JEL, Breuer K, Edwards SA. Effects of species-relevant environmental enrichment on the behaviour and productivity of finishing pigs. Appl Anim Behav Sci. 2006;99:230–47.
17. Jensen MB, Herskin MS, Forkman B, Pedersen LJ. Effect of increasing amounts of straw on pigs' explorative behaviour. Appl Anim Behav Sci. 2015;171:58–63.
18. Pedersen LJ, Herskin MS, Forkman B, Halekoh U, Kristensen KM, Jensen MB. How much is enough? The amount of straw necessary to satisfy pigs' need to perform exploratory behaviour. Appl Anim Behav Sci. 2014;160:46–55.
19. Munsterhjelm C, Peltoniemi OAT, Heinonen M, Hälli O, Karhapää M, Valros A. Experience of moderate bedding affects behaviour of growing pigs. Appl Anim Behav Sci. 2009;118:42–53.
20. Van de Weerd HA, Docking CM, Day JEL, Edwards SA. The development of harmful social behaviour in pigs with intact tails and different enrichment backgrounds in two housing systems. Anim Sci. 2005;80:289–98.
21. Lyons CAP, Bruce JM, Fowler VR, English PR. A comparison of productivity and welfare of growing pigs in 4 intensive systems. Livest Prod Sci. 1995;43:265–74.
22. Taylor NR, Main DC, Mendl M, Edwards SA. Tail-biting: a new perspective. Vet J. 2010;186:137–47.
23. Schroder-Petersen DL, Simonsen HB, Lawson LG. Tail-in-mouth behaviour among weaner pigs in relation to age, gender and group composition regarding gender. Acta Agric Scand Sect A-Anim Sci. 2003;53:29–34.
24. Bracke MBM, De Lauwere CC, Wind SMM, Zonerland JJ. Attitudes of dutch Pig farmers towards tail biting and tail docking. J Agric Environ Ethics. 2013; 26:847–68.
25. Scheepens CJM, Hessing MJC, Laarakker E, Schouten WGP, Tielen MJM. Influences of intermittent daily draught on the behaviour of weaned pigs. Appl Anim Behav Sci. 1991;31:69–82.
26. van Putten G. An investigation into tail-biting among fattening pigs. Br Vet J. 1969;125:511–6.
27. Smulders D, Hautekiet V, Verbeke G, Geerst R. Tail and ear biting lesions in pigs: an epidemiological study. Anim Welf. 2008;17:61–9.
28. Cargill C, Murphy T, Banhazi T. Hygiene and air quality in intensive housing facilities in Australia. Animal Prod Aust. 2002;24:387–93.
29. Michiels A, Piepers S, Ulens T, Van Ransbeeck N, Sacristan RDP, Sierens A, Haesebrouck F, Demeyer P, Maes D. Impact of particulate matter and ammonia on average daily weight gain, mortality and lung lesions in pigs. Prev Vet Med. 2015;121:99–107.
30. Ni JQ, Heber AJ, Lim TT, Tao PC, Schmidt AM. Methane and carbon dioxide emission from two Pig finishing barns. J Environ Qual. 2008;37:2001–11.
31. O'Connor EA, Parker MO, McLeman MA, Demmers TG, Lowe JC, Cui L, Davey EL, Owen RC, Wathes CM, Abeyesinghe SM. The impact of chronic environmental stressors on growing pigs, Sus scrofa (Part 1): stress physiology, production and play behaviour. Animal. 2010;4:1899–909.
32. Jones JB, Burgess LR, Webster AJF, Wathes CM. Behavioural responses of pigs to atmospheric ammonia in a chronic choice test. Anim Sci. 1996;63:437–45.
33. Ewbank R. Abnormal behavior and pig nutrition - unsuccessful attempt to induce tail biting by feeding a high-energy, low fiber vegetable protein ration. Br Vet J. 1973;129:366–9.
34. Geers R, Dellaert B, Goedseels V, Hoogerbrugge A, Vranken E, Maes F, Berckmans D. An assessment of optimal air temperatures in pig houses by the quantification of behavioral and health-related problems. Anim Prod. 1989;48:571–8.
35. Huynh TTT, Aarnink AJA, Gerrits WJJ, Heetkamp MJH, Canh TT, Spoolder HAM, Kemp B, Verstegen MWA. Thermal behaviour of growing pigs in response to high temperature and humidity. Appl Anim Behav Sci. 2005;91:1–16.
36. DIN 18910–1. Wärmeschutz geschlossener Ställe - Wärmedämmung und Lüftung. Teil 1: Planungs- und Berechnungsgrundlagen für geschlossene, zwangsgelüftete Ställe. Berlin: Beuth Verlag; 2004.
37. D'Eath RB, Arnott G, Turner SP, Jensen T, Lahrmann HP, Busch ME, Niemi JK, Lawrence AB, Sandoe P. Injurious tail biting in pigs: how can it be controlled in existing systems without tail docking? Animal. 2014;8:1479–97.
38. Munsterhjelm C, Simola O, Keeling L, Valros A, Heinonen M. Health parameters in tail biters and bitten pigs in a case-control study. Animal. 2013;7:814–21.
39. Grosse Beilage E, Nathues H, Meemken D, Harder TC, Doherr MG, Grotha I, Greiser-Wilke I. Frequency of PRRS live vaccine virus (European and North American genotype) in vaccinated and non-vaccinated pigs submitted for respiratory tract diagnostics in North-Western Germany. Prev Vet Med. 2009;92:31–7.

6

Risk factors for oral antimicrobial consumption in Swiss fattening pig farms

Corinne Arnold[1], Gertraud Schüpbach-Regula[2], Patricia Hirsiger[3], Julia Malik[3], Patricia Scheer[1], Xaver Sidler[3], Peter Spring[4], Judith Peter-Egli[4] and Myriam Harisberger[1]*

Abstract

Background: Antimicrobial consumption in veterinary medicine is of great importance. Increased awareness by the public and media has led to demands for decreased use of antimicrobials in pigs. This study aimed to identify risk factors for regular oral antimicrobial consumption in Swiss fattening pig farms, and to quantify the amount of antimicrobial active substances administered orally to pigs at the farm level.

Results: A case–control study was performed on 99 fattening farms between May 2014 and January 2015. Seventy-two case farms (with oral group treatment of antimicrobials in at least 50 % of pigs) and 27 control farms (with no regular oral group treatment) were visited once during the study. Data about potential risk factors and antimicrobial consumption were collected by questionnaire. Antimicrobial consumption was recorded and treatment incidence (TI) was calculated for all farms over a one year period. Sulphonamides and tetracyclines were the antimicrobials consumed in the greatest quantity. The median TI for oral antimicrobial use in the case group was 224.7. In the control group, the median TI was 0 for oral antimicrobial use, with values ranging from 0 to 140.1. In a multivariable regression model, seven risk factors associated with regular oral antimicrobial group treatment were identified: mixing pigs from different suppliers within the same pen, absence of a work protocol that ensures treating of healthy pigs before sick pigs, distance to next pig farm < 500 metres, external analysis of production parameters, no availability of dirty visitor boots, the farmer not working on other farms, and no application of homoeopathic agents.

Conclusions: The results of this study point out the importance of increasing farmers' awareness of good farming practices and biosecurity. Important recommendations for decreasing oral antimicrobial consumption identified by this study include avoiding mixing pigs from different suppliers in the same pen and strictly handling sick pigs after healthy ones. Improvements in these areas could enhance the overall health of pigs and thereby reduce the consumption of antimicrobials on pig farms.

Keywords: Pigs, Fattening farms, Risk factors, Antimicrobial consumption, Treatment incidence

Background

The amount of antimicrobial agents used in veterinary medicine has been an important topic for many years. The potential risks to public health arising from the high use of antimicrobials in animals have been discussed in various scientific publications as well as in the media [1]. Increased public and media awareness has put increased pressure on farmers and veterinarians to reduce antimicrobial use. In Switzerland, the total quantity of veterinary antimicrobial products sold for use in all animal categories, reached a peak in 2008. Since 2009 the sale of antimicrobials for veterinary use has decreased. In 2013, sales of 53,384 kg of antimicrobials were registered in Switzerland, about two-thirds of which were antimicrobial premixes for administration in feed or water. The total volume sold represents a reduction of 26 % in total Swiss antimicrobial sales compared to 2008 [2].

* Correspondence: mha@suisag.ch
[1]SUISAG, Division SGD, Sempach, Switzerland
Full list of author information is available at the end of the article

Although the exact proportion of antimicrobials used in pigs in Switzerland is not known, pigs and cattle were estimated to account for the majority of the veterinary antimicrobial use in 2012 [3]. Swine in Switzerland have a high health status, as the domestic Swiss swine population is free or almost free from several important diseases such as porcine reproductive and respiratory syndrome and enzootic pneumonia [4]. Despite the high health status, antimicrobial use in Switzerland is still relatively high compared to other countries [5]. In swine production antimicrobials are most often applied as group therapy [6] and mostly by oral administration [7, 8]. Previous Swiss studies have reported that the greatest quantities of antimicrobials used during fattening, were used during the first two weeks of the fattening period [9]. Antimicrobials were most frequently administered prophylactically (about 80 % of total amount) [10]. However, prophylactic antimicrobial use has not been shown to decrease mortality, or to reduce the number of therapeutic treatments [10]. Therefore, it could be speculated that there is substantial potential to reduce antimicrobial usage while maintaining a high animal health status.

High antimicrobial consumption is also a concern in other countries. For example, Denmark has introduced a "yellow card"scheme, which imposes restrictions on farmers who exceed predefined levels of consumption [11]. In Germany, a 2014 amendment to legislation introduced a legal requirement for farmers to report antimicrobial use and the antimicrobial usage data is stored in a central database. In addition the responsible local veterinary service has the authority to impose measures on farmers whose antimicrobial usage exceeds defined levels [12]. In the Netherlands an independent institution sets benchmarks for antimicrobial usage, which are re-evaluated on a yearly basis. Farms that exceed these benchmark levels are obliged to decrease their consumption by implementing measures [13]. Since the introduction of this program in 2012, antimicrobial consumption has been reduced by 56 % compared to consumption in 2007. This has been achieved by a combination of compulsory and voluntary actions. The Netherlands has set a new goal of reducing consumption in 2015 by 70 % compared to 2007 [14]. In Switzerland, there is currently no central antimicrobial consumption database that could be used to set benchmarks for antimicrobial consumption.

The identification of risk factors for antimicrobial group treatment in fattening farms is important for developing on farm strategies for reducing antimicrobial use without impairing animal health. However, only a limited number of risk factors for high antimicrobial use have been reported [15–17]. In a study performed in the Netherlands, the risk factors farm system and number of fattening pigs were found to be associated with antimicrobial use on fattening farms [15]. Hybschmann et

al. performed a risk factor analysis in Denmark on antimicrobial use for gastrointestinal diseases [16]. Herd size, herd health status and herd type were identified as risk factors [16]. Compared to these countries, herd sizes in Switzerland are smaller and many farms produce for specific pork distribution labels. Farms are often specialised in farrowing or fattening and few produce in a closed system. It is likely that risk factors from studies in other countries will not be valid under these housing and management conditions. The identification of further risk factors would be crucial to support reduction of antimicrobial use. For this reason we conducted a risk factor analysis for fattening pig farms in Switzerland. This study will be relevant to Swiss swine producers and can serve as an example to other countries that have small farms and good general pig health.

The aim of this case–control-study was, to identify risk factors for regular oral antimicrobial treatment in Swiss fattening farms, and to quantify the amount of antimicrobials used at a farm level during a 12-month period.

Results
Farm characteristics
A list of 437 potential participants was generated from the Swiss Pig Health Service (SGD) database. Two hundred and sixteen farms were excluded. Of these, 106 farms were excluded before telephone contact, when the list was checked by SGD veterinarians having more current knowledge about these farms, because these farms no longer fulfilled the inclusion criteria. The other 110 farms were excluded after the first telephone interview because they no longer used regular oral antimicrobial group treatments. Of the farms that met the antimicrobial inclusion criteria, 50 % agreed to participate in the study (77 % in the control group, 44 % in the case group). Reasons for not participating included: no interest (total 66 %, control 67 %, case 66 %), farm structure (retirement, ending or already ended pig farming, less than 30 pigs, farmer participates in the study with his other farm) (total 32 %, control 33 %, case 31 %), and other reasons (total 3 %, control 0 %, case 3 %). Eleven of the 110 farms that agreed to participate were excluded retrospectively because they raised pigs for other purposes than fattening.

The final study sample consisted of 99 fattening farms. Ninety-two percent of the farms were members of the SGD. The median weight of pigs at the onset of the fattening period was 25.5 kg (*n* = 97) and the median live weight at slaughter was 109.9 kg (*n* = 87). Herd size varied between 50 and 1300 pig places (median 170). The proportion of total farm revenue represented by swine production varied between 1-100 % (median 25 %). Seventy percent of farmers were between 41 and

60 years old, 14 % were younger than 41, and 16 % older than 60. As a consequence, 68 % of farmers had more than 24 years of experience in pig production. For most farms, the person having the main responsibility for the pigs was the owner of the farm (85 %). Other farms were on a lease arrangement (10 %), partly owned and leased (1 %), or the main responsible person was employed (4 %). Time spent in the pig barn ranged from 0.8 to 28 h per week per 100 pig places with a median of 4.2 h per week per 100 pig places. Daily weight gain of pigs ranged from 675 to 1,014 gram with a median of 808.9 gram ($n = 80$). The median duration of the fattening period was 102 days. Feed conversion (digestible energy pig (DE)/kg) values ranged from 32.5 to 41.0 megajoules DE/kg with a median of 36.0 megajoules DE/kg. However, these data were only available for 70 farms. Mortality rates were less than or equal to 2 % in 69 % of the farms (0–5.5 %, median 1.6 %, $n = 97$).

Antimicrobial use

A total of 500 kg of active antimicrobial substance was administered orally on the 99 study farms during the 12 months prior to the investigation. Active ingredients used were sulphonamides (305 kg, 61 %), tetracyclines (125 kg, 25 %), trimethoprim (42 kg, 8 %), polymyxin E (8 kg, 2 %), amoxicillin (11 kg, 2 %), macrolides (9 kg, 2 %), and pleuromutilins (0.5 kg, 0.1 %). Five of the twenty-seven control farmers also administered oral antimicrobials, but they all reported treating less than 50 % of their pigs. In both case and control farms, all oral antimicrobials were administered in feed. Results of TI calculations for active substances used orally are presented in Table 1. In the case group, the TI for oral antimicrobials ranged from 29.9 to 418.1 (median 224.7, mean 211.7, SD 101.3). The TI for the control group ranged from 0 to 140.1 (median 0, mean 10.5, SD 29.4).

In the case group, 72 % of the farms administered oral antimicrobials to all pigs. The remaining 28 % of case farms orally administered antimicrobials to at least 50 % of pigs during the 12 months prior to the investigation. In the case group, 93 % of the farmers reported that they administered oral antimicrobials mainly for prophylaxis. They usually did not carry out diagnostic examinations prior to treatment, since the treated pigs did not have any abnormal clinical signs. The other 7 % of case farms reported using antimicrobials orally to treat specific conditions (diarrhoea, fever, respiratory symptoms, lameness). Reasons for using oral antimicrobials reported by case group farmers were (multiple answers possible, n in parenthesis): problems occurred during previous fattening period(s) (22), too many different pig suppliers (20), as an insurance policy (16), always used antimicrobials (17), on recommendation (e.g. veterinarian or pig trader) (17) or that an attempt without antimicrobials was not successful (10). All case group farmers were asked if they would also use antimicrobials at the beginning of the production period if they always received pigs from the same single supplier. Forty-four percent answered yes or that they already had only one supplier; forty-eight percent reported that it would probably be possible to work without antimicrobials if they had one supplier, and 8 % were unsure.

The analysis of antimicrobials administered as injection was performed accordingly. The TI for antimicrobial injections ranged between 0 and 23.3 (median 3.3, mean 5.0, SD 5.5) for the control group and between 0 and 68.5 (median 4.0, mean 5.6, SD 12.5) for the case group.

Risk factor analysis

The results of screening analyses of risk factors that were associated with the case or control status of the farm (p-value <0.1), are presented in Table 2. Factors

Table 1 Treatment incidence (TI = Number of animals treated daily with one animal daily dose (ADD) per 1000 pigs) of the active substances for all oral antimicrobials used during the 12 months prior to the investigation of farms. Data are presented for the case group (with oral group treatment of antimicrobials in at least 50 % of pigs) and the control farms (with no regular oral group treatment)

	TI case group ($n = 80$)					TI control group ($n = 30$)				
	Min[1]	Max[2]	Median	Mean	SD[3]	Min	Max	Median	Mean	SD
Sulphonamides	0.0	258.2	101.6	100.6	82.9	0.0	93.4	0.0	4.3	18.1
Tetracyclines	0.0	365.8	0.0	35.5	61.3	0.0	13.5	0.0	0.8	3.0
Trimethoprim	0.0	129.1	34.6	43.9	46.8	0.0	46.7	0.0	1.7	9.0
Polymyxin E	0.0	196.2	0.0	6.9	27.8	0.0	41.1	0.0	2.0	8.2
Amoxicillin (penicillin)	0.0	103.0	0.0	7.8	22.6	0.0	13.3	0.0	0.8	3.0
Macrolides (tylosin)	0.0	117.2	0.0	16.0	31.3	0.0	13.5	0.0	0.8	3.0
Pleuromutilins (valnemulin)	0.0	73.2	0.0	1.0	8.6	0.0	0.0	0.0	0.0	0.0

Min[1] minimum
Max[2] maximum
SD[3] standard deviation

Table 2 All relevant results of the univariable analysis of risk factors ($p < 0.1$) for regular oral antimicrobial group treatment in case farms (more than 50 % of pigs treated) and in control farms (no regular oral group treatment) for Swiss fattening pig farms

Description	Answers	% control group	% case group	p-value (chi^2 or fisher's exact)
		$n = 27$	$n = 72$	
Label	Conventional or no label	51.9	37.5	0.0427
	Label 1 (straw, access to outdoor area)	25.9	33.3	
	Label 2 (bedding, access to outdoor area)	14.8	29.2	
	Label 3 = Organic	7.4	0.0	
Renovation of building (pen)	Yes	25.9	58.3	0.0041
	No	74.1	41.7	
Husbandry education	Education 1 (farmer with a certification of achievement)	33.3	33.3	0.0211
	Education 2 (Apprenticeship and further education as pig farm manager)	59.3	38.9	
	Others/no husbandry education	7.4	27.8	
Working on other farms	Yes	25.9	8.3	0.0398
	No	74.1	91.7	
Analysis of production parameters	By farmer (program, computer, written, none)	66.7	30.6	0.0011
	By others (external)	33.3	69.4	
Most frequent cause of death at the onset	Haemorrhagic intestinal syndrome	55.6	33.3	0.0252
	Unknown cause of death	33.3	36.1	
	Other causes	11.1	30.6	
Visitor boots available	Yes, clean	33.3	43.4	0.0084
	Yes, dirty	33.3	15.2	
	No	33.3	41.4	
Production system all-in/all-out	Yes	48.2	77.8	0.0043
	No	51.9	22.2	
Number of suppliers at the same time	One supplier	51.9	19.4	0.0014
	More than one supplier	48.2	80.6	
Pigs originate from same supplier(s)	Yes	59.3	23.6	0.0008
	No	40.7	76.4	
All pigs vaccinated against Lawsonia	Yes	33.3	13.9	0.0287
	No or unknown	66.7	86.1	
Mixing pigs of different suppliers within same pen	Yes	33.3	66.7	0.0028
	No	66.7	33.3	
Work sequence depending on the age	From younger to older pigs	18.5	11.1	0.0115
	No working order (age not considered)	55.6	30.6	
	All pigs having the same age	25.9	58.3	
Cleaning frequency	After each batch: whole barn	44.4	72.2	0.0191
	After each batch: pen(s)	37.0	15.3	
	Less frequent	18.5	12.5	
Heating of barn (before the onset)	Yes	37.0	56.9	0.0775
	No	63.0	43.1	

Table 2 All relevant results of the univariable analysis of risk factors ($p < 0.1$) for regular oral antimicrobial group treatment in case farms (more than 50 % of pigs treated) and in control farms (no regular oral group treatment) for Swiss fattening pig farms *(Continued)*

Work sequence depending on healthy before sick pigs	Yes	59.3	20.8	0.0002
	No	40.7	79.2	
Distance to the next pig farm	<500 metres	25.9	56.9	0.0060
	≥500 metres	74.1	43.1	
Application of homoeopathic agents	Yes	25.9	5.6	0.0084
	No	74.1	94.4	

P-values of the chi^2 analysis are presented or alternatively for factors with counts ≤5 for a group, results of the fisher's exact testing are shown

with a p-value ≥0.1 in the screening included the following topics: health-related data (e.g. estimated disease frequencies or if diagnostic tests had previously been performed), biosecurity (e.g. details about pest control or hand wash facilities), other management practices (e.g. deworming or feeding practices), housing system (e.g. access to outdoor facility or floor types) as well as farm structure and demographic data (e.g. herd size, age of the animal caretaker or if the caretaker owns the farm or is employed).

Variables that were included in the final multivariable logistic regression model are presented in Table 3. Seven factors associated with regular use of antimicrobials in feed were identified. A farmer mixing pigs from different suppliers within the same pen had a 4 times higher odds of being in the group with regular oral antimicrobial use than farmers that did not mix pigs. Proximity to other pig farms was also found to be a potential risk. The odds of being in the case group were almost 10 times greater among farms having a neighbouring farm within a 500 meter radius. Farmers, who did not follow a specified work sequence that included managing healthy pigs before sick pigs, had approximately 16 times higher odds

of being in the case group than farmers who followed such a sequence. Farmers who did not use homoeopathic agents had about 10 times higher odds of being in the group with regular antimicrobial use than farmers who used homoeopathic agents. Working on other farms had a protective effect, as farmers who worked on other farms were less likely to be in the case group (odds ratio = 0.05). The analysis of performance data by the farmer (program, computer, written, or none) was also found to be protective (odds ratio = 0.12). The presence of dirty visitor boots on farms was protective (odds ratio = 0.06) when compared to the absence of visitor boots.

Discussion

In this study risk factors for regular oral antimicrobial use on Swiss fattening pig farms were identified and the amount of antimicrobials used at a farm level was quantified. Participation rates were 77 % for the control, and 44 % for the case groups (in total 50 %). The difference in participation between the two groups may have been influenced by the study design. All of the case farms were also enrolled in an additional longitudinal study for the FitPig project, which required at least one additional

Table 3 Results of the multivariable logistic regression model for the risk factor analysis for oral antimicrobial use in Swiss fattening pig farms

Description	Answers	p-value model	OR[b]	95 % CI[c]
Work sequence depending on healthy before sick pigs (Ref.[a] Yes)	No	<0.01	16.68	3.4-81.8
Working on other farms (Ref. No)	Yes	<0.01	0.05	0.006-0.4
Distance to the next pig farm (Ref. ≥ 500 metres)	<500 metres	0.01	9.88	1.7-57.1
Visitor boots available (Ref. No boots available)	Yes, clean	0.97	1.03	0.2-4.7
	Yes, dirty	0.01	0.06	0.006-0.5
Analysis of production parameters (Ref. by others (external))	By farmer (program, computer, written, none)	0.01	0.12	0.02-0.6
Application of homoeopathic agents (Ref. Yes)	No	0.02	10.49	1.4-78.8
Mixing pigs of different suppliers within the same pen (Ref. No mixing)	Yes	0.05	4.16	1.0-17.4

[a]Ref.: reference group
[b]OR: odds ratio
[c]CI: confidence interval

farm visit. Therefore, more case than control farmers elected not to participate, because the farmers considered the extra visit(s) to be too time-consuming. For this reason voluntary participation by farmers may have introduced a bias into this study. Having a biased sample may have resulted in an underestimation of antimicrobial consumption. This bias could be stronger in the case farms, because the participation rate was lower in this group.

Antimicrobial use

Sulphonamides and tetracyclines accounted for the major proportion of orally administered substances. This is in agreement with findings reported in an earlier study performed in Switzerland [18]. The usage patterns reported in this study differ from those found in other countries, where tetracyclines are more commonly used than sulphonamides [13, 19, 20]. A possible explanation could be that Swiss pig farmers were discouraged from using certain antimicrobials, including tetracyclines, in the past and SGD members are still discouraged from using certain antimicrobials, including tetracyclines, without carrying out further diagnostics. This is done to prevent antimicrobial administration from masking of clinical signs of economically important diseases such as enzootic pneumonia or swine dysentery which are systematically monitored by the authorities or the SGD health programme (personal communication Y. Masserey, head of regional SGD office).

To allow a standardized comparison of usage among farms, the TI was calculated. The TI has been used in previous studies to describe antimicrobial use [7, 21, 22]. In this study there was a wide range of farm level TI values. This was likely due to the definition of case and control farms used in this study. For this reason, the TI's may not be representative of Swiss fattening farms and generalizing to the population of Swiss fattening farms should be done with caution. On the farms in this study, there was no evidence that the control group had to compensate for the lower use of oral antimicrobials using a larger quantity of parenteral use of antimicrobials.

A comparison to the TI's found in other studies was not carried out, because methods for calculating TI's has not been standardized across countries and the recommended animal daily dose (ADD) varies between countries. An international working group is currently developing a list of ADD's that is valid for international use [23]. However, at this time the list does not include all antimicrobial products used on farms in this study. Other differences between countries include variation in methods for estimating days at risk and for kg of pig treated [7, 21]. In a recent study Moreno 2014 [24] reported that different values were used in almost all studies. Setting standard values is crucial for enabling comparisons between countries.

Five of the twenty-seven control farms used oral antimicrobials. Even though the TI's on these farms were low, there was a small number of control farms that had higher TI values than some of the case farms. On control farms oral administration mostly took place later in the fattening period and for therapeutic treatment of sick animals. These animals had a higher average weight and therefore more active substance was required to treat them. This could not be accounted for in the calculation of the TI used in this study, because the same standard pig weight was used for all farms. Finally, differences in TI may have been due to farmers administering antimicrobials at lower than recommended dosages, or for shorter treatment periods than recommended. There were differences in data quality between farms because some farmers did not report the number of animals treated or the administered dosage. For these reasons it was possible to calculate TI based only on amount of active substance used, rather than calculating daily doses used.

Risk factor analysis

In this study, seven risk factors for increased oral antimicrobial use at the beginning of the fattening period were identified in Swiss fattening farms. A higher risk for oral antimicrobial use was found on farms mixing pigs from different supplying farms within the same pen. It is very likely that pigs from different farms were exposed to different pathogens. Transport in combination with formation of new groups [25] can cause stress for the animals, and can increase the risk of disease occurrence. This first risk factor was associated with the number of supplying farms, and whether the suppliers changed over time. These were also identified as risk factors in other studies [10, 26]. However, these were not in the final multivariable model in this study. A work sequence, in which sick animals were handled before healthy ones, was also a risk factor for regular antimicrobial use. This risk factor could be related to differences in the awareness of the importance of good management practices between case and control farms. The difference in awareness might also explain why other risk factors such as not working on other farms, external analysis of production parameters and no availability of dirty visitor boots were associated with increased oral antimicrobial use. Working on other farms may support the exchange of knowledge and increase the general awareness for good biosecurity. The factor of dirty visitor boots being of a lower risk than no visitor boots cannot be easily explained. It is possible that in a retrospective study design as applied in the present investigation, some factors in statistical analysis could have been found by coincidence. The higher risk for farms located in a radius of less than 500 metres to other pig farms could be due there being a higher probability of pathogen transfer over short distances. This factor was already described by van der Fels-Klerx et al. [15] as potential risk factor. Farms administering homoeopathic agents had a lower risk for regular antimicrobial consumption. It may be possible that farmers in the control group were looking for alternative substances to antimicrobials and used homoeopathic agents instead. An indirect association may be more likely than direct causality for some risk factors. For example external analysis of performance data could be interpreted as indicator for the professional attitude of the farmers. Some of the factors not being part of the multivariable model in this study have been reported as risk factors in other studies. The size of the farm [15, 16] had no significant effect in this study. In another study performed in Switzerland, the sanitary break (time period when no pigs are in the barn or pen, before the next group of pig arrives), and not consequently practicing all-in-all-out were identified as risk factors, but were not part of the multivariable model of this study [10].

Conclusion

In this study, risk factors for increased oral antimicrobial use on Swiss fattening pig farms were identified. An important recommendation to decrease oral antimicrobial consumption would be to avoid mixing pigs from different suppliers in the same pen. Additionally, more attention should be paid to the work sequence. Sick pigs should be handled after handling healthy ones. This study suggests that it would be important to increase the awareness of the farmers of the value of good farming practices, biosecurity and herd health. Improving the overall health of the pigs would help to reduce the consumption of oral antimicrobials on fattening pig farms.

Methods
Data collection
Study design

A case–control study was performed with 99 fattening pig farms in Switzerland. Each farm was visited once. The control group consisted of 27 and the case group of 72 participating farms. The difference in group sizes was due to a follow-up intervention study in which only the farms of the case group participate. The follow-up study is a controlled field trial with the aim to reduce antimicrobial usage in farms with routine use of oral antimicrobials. The sample size for our study was calculated to detect an odds ratio of 3.5 with a power of 80 % and a significance level of 5 %, using the software PASS 12 (Hintze, J. (2013). PASS 12. NCSS, LLC. Kaysville, Utah, USA. www.ncss.com). The following inclusion criteria were used to define and select case farms: oral antimicrobial group treatment taking place at the beginning of the

fattening period had to be administered to at least 50 % of all pigs during the previous twelve months. The control group included farms without routine oral group treatment or, farms where oral antimicrobials were administered to less than 50 % of all pigs in the last 12 months. The minimum farm size was 30 pig places. The person mainly responsible for the pigs had to have adequate German language skills to be able to answer the questionnaire accurately.

Recruitment

A list of potential case and control farms was generated from the database of the SGD, where information on oral antimicrobial treatments was available from January 2011 to August 2014. About 60 % of the Swiss fattening farms are members of the SGD (personal communication HP. Keller, CEO SUISAG). Farmers joining the SGD benefit from a health programme with the main goal of preventing the spread of economically important diseases. The programme mainly consists of certifying farms according to their health status and rules for pig trading. Regular farm visits by a veterinarian are also a key element of the programme. All farms fulfilling the study inclusion criteria were extracted from the SGD database. To achieve a broader representation of the Swiss population of pig fattening farms, an additional effort was made to recruit farmers who were not members of the SGD. Veterinarians of the Swiss Association of Pig Medicine were asked to identify farms fulfilling the inclusion criteria. From the list of both groups of farmers, case and control farms were randomly selected until a sufficient sample size of farms, fulfilling all inclusion criteria, was achieved. Initially, a letter was sent to all farmers, informing them about the upcoming project. Farmers were subsequently contacted by telephone, inclusion criteria were verified, and they were asked to participate. All participants were recruited and visited between May 2014 and January 2015. All visits were performed by 3 veterinarians working on the project.

Materials

Data were collected using two questionnaires. One was sent to the farmers before the farm visit and the second was completed during the farm visit. Questionnaires were designed by a group of experts (pig veterinarian, epidemiologists, and agronomist) to align with the results of former studies [10, 22]. Questionnaires included the following topics: farm structure and details about the farmer, performance data, housing, management, food and water supply, health of pigs, biosecurity and antimicrobial use. Draft questionnaires were evaluated by a social scientist with experience in questionnaire design and the questionnaire was pretested on 2 farms. The results of the pre-test were not included into the final analysis. Questionnaires are available on request from the authors (in German). Data on the antimicrobial consumption within the last twelve months were extracted either from the farm inventory or the treatment journal, prescription forms or, if these were not available, from the veterinarian's invoices.

Data analysis

Statistical analysis was performed using NCSS 9, NCSS, LLC. Kaysville, Utah, USA. Descriptive statistic was carried out for potential risk factors and antimicrobial usage. For antimicrobial consumption, the amount of active substance used was calculated for each substance separately as the product of number of units (e.g. ml, mg) administered and the weight of active ingredient per unit (e.g. mg/ml or mg/kg). To enable a comparison of the antimicrobial use between farms, the TI was chosen as a measure of usage [7, 21, 22]. The TI was calculated by dividing the amount of active substance used (mg) through the product of: the ADD, the days at risk and kg weight of pigs. The outcome was then multiplied by 1000. The TI is a measure of the number of animals treated daily with one ADD per 1000 pigs [21]. Information about the ADD for each product was extracted from the Swiss on-line database of pharmaceutical products [27]. For products with a range of recommended doses, the lowest value was used for orally administered antimicrobials. For antimicrobials administered by injection, the highest value was used. This protocol was based on previous studies demonstrating that oral antimicrobials are often administered at below the recommended dosage, and injections are more likely to be administered at above the recommended dosage [7, 21]. To estimate the number of days at risk, the median length of the fattening period was taken from the data collected by questionnaire. The kg weight of pigs was calculated as the total number of pigs produced in one year multiplied with the average weight at the beginning of fattening. Since weight was not available on all of the study farms, the average weight at the beginning of fattening (26.8 kg) in 2014 was obtained from one of the main Swiss pig marketers (personal communication M. Reich, Anicom, Switzerland).

All data were entered into NCSS 9 and checked for plausibility and counts per group. Continuous data, where a non-linear relationship with the outcome was expected, were grouped into several categories. Univariable screening of all potential risk factors was performed using chi-squared tests. For factors that contained less than 5 counts per group, fisher's exact tests were performed. Variables with p-values < 0.1 were considered for entry into the multivariable logistic regression model. All potential risk factors were screened for correlation among each other. If a high correlation between two

variables was observed (phi > 0.7), the biologically more meaningful variable was selected for the model. The multivariable logistic regression model was built with a stepwise forward selection procedure. Only variables significantly associated with being a case farm (p < 0.05) were retained in the model. Biologically meaningful interactions between the risk factors were tested, but none of them was significant.

Competing interests

The present study was initiated by SUISAG, a private company owned mainly by the Swiss federation of pig producers (Suisseporcs). The SUISAG divisions of veterinary Pig Health Service (SGD), breeding and reproduction deliver different services in the pig sector, for example veterinary consulting. The SUISAG has well established connections with various stakeholders, e.g. with authorities, farm veterinarians and marketers. The present study, which was part of the FitPig project (http://www.hafl.bfh.ch/fitpig), was funded by the Federal Food Safety and Veterinary Office (FSVO), Federal Office for Agriculture (FOAG), Federal Office for Public Health (FOPH) and the Suisseporcs. The researchers worked independently, and no influence on study design, analysis, interpretation or results was exerted by the funding bodies. The authors declare that they have no competing interests.

Authors' contributions

CA helped to draft questionnaires, recruited participants, performed farm visits, managed the data, performed the statistical analysis and wrote the manuscript. GS participated in designing the study, assisted with the statistical analysis and revised the manuscript. PH and JM helped to draft questionnaires and performed farm visits together with CA. XS, PSP and PSC helped to draft the questionnaires. JP initiated the study, contributed to the study design, and consulted on practical and scientific aspects of the study. MH participated in designing the study, extracted the list of possible participants from the database, coordinated the working processes, assisted with the statistical analysis, and helped to draft the manuscript. All authors read and approved the final manuscript.

Authors' information

CA, PH and JM are postgraduate veterinarians (doctoral students). GS is veterinarian and head of the Veterinary Public Health Institute of the Vetsuisse Faculty Bern. She holds a doctorate degree in theriogenology, a masters degree (M. Sc.) in epidemiology and is diplomate of the European College of Veterinary Public Health. PSC is a postdoctoral veterinarian and head of a regional SGD office. XS is the veterinary head and associate professor of his institution. PSP is agronomist and associate director of his institution. JP is veterinarian and lecturer for pig production at her institution. MH is the veterinary project coordinator at her institution, and she is diplomate of the European College of Veterinary Public Health.

Acknowledgments

This research, which was part of the FitPig project, was funded by the Federal Food Safety and Veterinary Office (FSVO), Federal Office for Agriculture (FOAG), Federal Office for Public Health (FOPH) and the Suisseporcs.
Karin Zbinden verified the drafts of the questionnaires as a social science expert. Merel Postma provided the questionnaires of the Minapig project for supporting the development of the questionnaires. The veterinarians of the SGD supported the recruitment by cross-checking the list of potential participants. The veterinarians of the Association of Pig Medicine reported potential participating farms. We would like to thank John Berezowski for language editing of the manuscript.
We thank all those who contributed to this study and especially the participating farmers.

Author details

[1]SUISAG, Division SGD, Sempach, Switzerland. [2]Veterinary Public Health Institute, Vetsuisse Faculty, University of Bern, Bern, Switzerland. [3]Department for Farm Animals, Division of Swine Medicine, Vetsuisse Faculty, University of Zurich, Zurich, Switzerland. [4]Berne University of Applied Sciences, HAFL - Agricultural Sciences, Zollikofen, Switzerland.

References

1. European Centre for Disease Prevention and Control, European Food Safety Authority, European Medicines Agency. ECDS/EFSA/EMA first joint report on the integrated analysis of the consumption of antimicrobial agents and occurrence of antimicrobial resistance in bacteria from human and food-producing animals. EFSA Journal. 2015;13(1):4006.

2. Federal Food Safety and Veterinary Office FSVO: 2013 ARCH-Vet Gesamtbericht: Antibiotika-Vertriebsstatistik und Resistenzüberwachung bei Nutztieren in der Schweiz. http://www.blv.admin.ch/dokumentation/04506/04518/index.html?lang=de (2014). Accessed 18 May 2015.

3. Carmo LP, Schüpbach G, Müntener C, Alban L, Nielsen LR, Magouras I. Quantification of antimicrobial use in Swiss pigs: comparison with other Swiss livestock species and with Danish pigs. Porto, Portugal: Proceedings of SafePork 2015 Conference; 2015. p. 135.

4. OIE World Animal Health Information Database: WAHID Interface. http://www.oie.int/wahis_2/public/wahid.php/Countryinformation/Animalsituation. Accessed 12 May 2015.

5. Grave K, Torren-Edo J, Mackay D. Comparison of the sales of veterinary antibacterial agents between 10 European countries. J Antimicrob Chemother. 2010;65:2037–40.

6. Rushton J, Pinto Ferreira J, Stärk KD. Antimicrobial Resistance: The Use of Antimicrobials in the Livestock Sector. OECD Food, Agriculture and Fisheries Papers, No. 68, OECD Publishing. 2014. http://dx.doi.org/10.1787/5jxvl3dwk3f0-en. Accessed 4 May 2015.

7. Timmerman T, Dewulf J, Catry B, Feyen B, Opsomer G, de Kruif A, et al. Quantification and evaluation of antimicrobial drug use in group treatments for fattening pigs in Belgium. Prev Vet Med. 2006;74:251–63.

8. Müntener CR, Stebler R, Horisberger U, Althaus FR, Gassner B. Berechnung der Therapieintensität bei Ferkeln und Mastschweinen beim Einsatz von Antibiotika in Fütterungsarzneimitteln. Schweiz Arch Tierheilkd. 2013;155(6):365–72.

9. Visschers VHM, Iten DM, Riklin A, Hartmann S, Sidler X, Siegrist M. Swiss pig farmers'perception and usage of antibiotics during the fattening period. Livest Sci. 2014;162:223–32.

10. Sidler X. Antibiotikum senken, aber wie?. In: Brauchen Nutztiere Antibiotika? 15 Jahre AML Verbot. Tagungsbericht. ETH-Zürich, Institut für Agrarwissenschaften. 6 May 2014. ISBN 978-3-906466-37-X. p. 24–26.

11. Alban L, Dahl J, Andreasen M, Petersen JV, Sandberg M. Possible impact of the "yellow card" antimicrobial scheme on meat inspection lesions in Danish finisher pigs. Prev Vet Med. 2013;108:334–41.

12. Federal Ministry of Food and Agriculture. Mehr Schutz vor Antibiotika-Resistenzen durch Regelung im Arzneimittelgesetz. http://www.bmel.de/DE/Tier/Tiergesundheit/Tierarzneimittel/_texte/Antibiotika-Dossier.html?nn=539690&notFirst=true&docId=2661834. Accessed 9 June 2015.

13. Bos MEH, Taverne FJ, van Geijlswijk IM, Mouton JW, Mevius DJ, Heederik DJJ, et al. Consumption of antimicrobials in pigs, veal calves, and broilers in The Netherlands: quantitative results of nationwide collection of data in 2011. PLoS One. 2013;8(10):e77525.

14. Speksnijder DC, Mevius DJ, Bruschke CJ, Wagenaar JA. Reduction of veterinary antimicrobial use in the Netherlands. The Dutch success model. Zoonoses Public Health. 2015;62 Suppl 1:79–87.

15. van der Fels-Klerx HJ, Puister-Jansen LF, van Asselt ED, Burgers SLGE. Farm factors associated with the use of antibiotics in pig production. J Anim SCI. 2011;89(6):1922–9.

16. Hybschmann GK, Ersbøll AK, Vigre H, Baadsgaard NP, Houe H. Herd-level risk factors for antimicrobial demanding gastrointestinal diseases in Danish herds with finisher pigs. A register-based study. Prev Vet Med. 2011;98:190–7.

17. Casal J, Mateu E, Mejía W, Martín M. Factors associated with routine mass antimicrobial usage in fattening pig units in a high pig-density area. Vet Res. 2007;38:481–92.

18. Regula G, Torriani K, Gassner B, Stucki F, Müntener CR. Prescription patterns of antimicrobials in veterinary practices in Switzerland. J Antimicrob Chemother. 2009;63:805–11.

19. DANMAP Danish Programme for Surveillance of antimicrobial consumption and resistance in bacteria from animals, food and humans. DANMAP 2013-Use of antimicrobial agents and occurrence of antimicrobial resistance in bacteria from food animals, food and humans in Denmark: http://www.danmap.org/~/media/Projekt%20sites/Danmap/DANMAP%20reports/DANMAP%202013/DANMAP%202013.ashx. Accessed 8 June 2015.

20. European Medicines Agency, European Surveillance of Veterinary Antimicrobial Consumption. 2013. Sales of veterinary antimicrobial agents in 25 EU/EEA countries in 2011. http://www.ema.europa.eu/docs/en_GB/document_library/Report/2013/10/WC500152311.pdf. Accessed 8 June 2015.

21. Callens B, Persoons D, Maes D, Laanen M, Postma M, Boyen F, et al. Prophylactic and metaphylactic antimicrobial use in Belgian fattening pig herds. Prev Vet Med. 2012;106:53–62.

22. Postma M, Maes D, Mijten E, De Bie S, Dewulf J. Preliminary results on reduction of antimicrobial usage on pig farms after management improvement interventions. In: Book of Abstracts of the 13th International Symposium on Veterinary Epidemiology and Economics. Belgium, Netherlands. Session 38 - Antimicrobial use in vet practice. Aug 2012. p. 99. http://orbit.dtu.dk/fedora/objects/orbit:123085/datastreams/file_85fd15d8-5f16-4fc5-a125-caddfb9009a9/content. Accessed 5 Mar 2015.

23. Postma M, Sjölund M, Collineau L, Lösken S, Stärk KDC, Dewulf J, et al. Assigning defined daily doses animal: a European multi-country experience for antimicrobial products authorized for usage in pigs. J Antimicrob Chemother. 2015;70:294–302.

24. Moreno MA. Survey of quantitative antimicrobial consumption per production stage in farrow-to-finish pig farms in Spain. Vet Rec Open. 2014; doi: 10.1136/vropen-2013-000002

25. Rubio-González A, Potes Y, Ilán-Rodriguez D, Vega-Naredo I, Sierra V, Caballero B, et al. Abstract: Effect of animal mixing as a stressor on biomarkers of autophagy and oxidative stress during pig muscle maturation. Animal. 2015;8:1–7.

26. Stevens KB, Gilbert J, Strachan WD, Robertson J, Johnston AM, Pfeiffer DU. Characteristics of commercial pig farms in Great Britain and their use of antimicrobials. Vet Rec. 2007;161:45–52.

27. Informationssystem Clinipharm/Clinitox: a computer-based drug and poison information system for veterinarians. www.clinipharm.ch. 2013. Accessed 30 April 2015.

7

Etiology of acute respiratory disease in fattening pigs

Minna Haimi-Hakala[1†], Outi Hälli[1*†], Tapio Laurila[1], Mirja Raunio-Saarnisto[2], Tiina Nokireki[3], Taina Laine[3], Suvi Nykäsenoja[3], Kirsti Pelkola[3], Joaquim Segales[4,5], Marina Sibila[4], Claudio Oliviero[1], Olli Peltoniemi[1], Sinikka Pelkonen[3] and Mari Heinonen[1]

Abstract

Background: The objective of our study was to clinically and etiologically investigate acute outbreaks of respiratory disease in Finland. Our study also aimed to evaluate the clinical use of various methods in diagnosing respiratory infections under field conditions and to describe the antimicrobial resistance profile of the main bacterial pathogen(s) found during the study.

Methods: A total of 20 case herds having finishing pigs showing acute respiratory symptoms and eight control herds showing no clinical signs suggesting of respiratory problems were enrolled in the study. Researchers visited each herd twice, examining and bleeding 20 pigs per herd. In addition, nasal swab samples were taken from 20 pigs and three pigs per case herd were necropsied during the first visit. Serology was used to detect *Actinobacillus pleuropneumoniae* (APP), swine influenza virus (SIV), porcine reproductive and respiratory syndrome virus (PRRSV), porcine respiratory coronavirus (PRCV) and *Mycoplasma hyopneumoniae* antibodies. Polymerase chain reaction (PCR) was used to investigate the presence of porcine circovirus type 2 (PCV2) in serum and SIV in the nasal and lung samples. Pathology and bacteriology, including antimicrobial resistance determination, were performed on lung samples obtained from the field necropsies.

Results: According to the pathology and bacteriology of the lung samples, APP and *Ascaris suum* were the main causes of respiratory outbreaks in 14 and three herds respectively, while the clinical signs in three other herds had a miscellaneous etiology. SIV, APP and PCV2 caused concurrent infections in certain herds but they were detected serologically or with PCR also in control herds, suggesting possible subclinical infections. APP was isolated from 16 (80%) case herds. Marked resistance was observed against tetracycline for APP, some resistance was detected against trimethoprim/sulfamethoxazole, ampicillin and penicillin, and no resistance against florfenicol, enrofloxacin, tulathromycin or tiamulin was found. Serology, even from paired serum samples, gave inconclusive results for acute APP infection diagnosis.

Conclusions: APP was the most common cause for acute respiratory outbreaks in our study. SIV, *A. suum*, PCV2 and certain opportunistic bacteria were also detected during the outbreaks; however, viral pathogens appeared less important than bacteria. Necropsies supplemented with microbiology were the most efficient diagnostic methods in characterizing the studied outbreaks.

Keywords: Pig, Respiratory, Pathogen, Actinobacillosis, Swine influenza, Ascaris, Necropsy, Acute, Outbreak

---

* Correspondence: outi.halli@helsinki.fi
†Equal contributors
[1]Department of Production Animal Medicine, University of Helsinki, Paroninkuja 20, 04920 Saarentaus, Finland
Full list of author information is available at the end of the article

Background

Porcine respiratory disease complex (PRDC) is a syndrome caused by mixed viral and bacterial pathogens together with environmental, managerial and genetic factors [1]. A combination of pathogens are involved, e.g. viruses such as porcine reproductive and respiratory syndrome virus (PRRSV), porcine circovirus type 2 (PCV2), swine influenza virus (SIV), porcine respiratory coronavirus (PRCV), and various bacteria e.g. *Actinobacillus pleuropneumoniae* (APP), *Mycoplasma hyopneumoniae* (MHyo), *Mycoplasma hyorhinis, Haemophilus parasuis (H.parasuis), Pasteurella multocida* and *Streptococcus suis* [1–6]. Often it remains unclear which the primary pathogen is and which one is acting as a predisposing agent for other infections or as a secondary infection [2, 6, 7]. Many of these pathogens can also be found in clinically healthy pigs, but they are detected more often in pigs with respiratory symptoms [8]. The pathogenesis of multifactorial PRDC is difficult to determine, because primary and opportunistic pathogens modify their impacts in different cases [2].

Pathogens involved in PRDC vary considerably in various countries, regions and herds over time. In Finland, the prevalence of porcine respiratory pathogens differs substantially from the situation in continental Europe. The country has been free of ADV, PRCV and PRRSV for decades. Also, Finland is nearly free of swine enzootic pneumonia. In 2015, MHyo was detected in only one Finnish pig herd [9], and most Finnish pig production (97%) is included in the national health programme [10] requiring the absence of this pathogen. On the contrary, APP is a common pathogen causing respiratory problems [9]. SIV is a newcomer in the country. Avian-like H1N1 swine influenza A virus was found in the Finnish pig population for the first time in 2008 and A(H1N1)pdm09 influenza virus in 2009 [11]. PCV2 is a pathogen commonly found in the Finnish pig population, and many herd owners control it by vaccination. However, its role in respiratory infections in Finland has not been studied earlier. Overall, assessing which respiratory pathogens are involved in acute respiratory disease outbreaks in a country lacking major viral pathogens is very important.

The objective of our study was to clinically and etiologically investigate acute outbreaks of respiratory disease in Finland. This field study also aimed to evaluate the clinical use of various methods in diagnosing the respiratory infections under field conditions and to describe the antimicrobial resistance profile of the main bacterial pathogen(s) found during our study.

Methods

Study population

This case-control study was carried out between May 2011 and January 2014 in finishing or farrow-to-finish pig herds in southern and southwestern Finland. Practicing herd veterinarians and herd owners in the area were asked to contact the research group when acute respiratory symptoms became apparent in finishing pigs. Veterinarians were informed of the study via several emails, letters and at veterinary meetings along with an announcement in the Finnish Veterinary Journal. Herd owners were informed at farmer meetings organized by the major slaughterhouses. Case herds were included in the study if they had at least one pig room with finishing pigs displaying a cough, fever and lowered appetite. A total of 20 case herds were enrolled in our study.

Control herds (*N* = 8) were selected from herds taking part in another study during the same time period. They were selected as case herds according to similar geographical location, herd size and type (fattening and/or farrow-to-finish). The control herds consisted of herds where local practicing veterinarians regularly clinically checked for signs of disease, at least every 3 months, and no acute respiratory signs were diagnosed in the finishers at the time of our study.

Exact data on vaccination schemes were not available regarding case or control herds.

Herd visits, clinical examination and sample taking

Researchers visited all the study herds on two occasions. The first visit to each case herd occurred within 3 days of farmers informing the research group about the respiratory symptom visible in their finishing pigs. On average, the visits occurred eight (standard deviation [SD] 6) days after the owner first observed the clinical signs and 26 (SD 13) days after the pigs had arrived to the fattening room. The second visit to case herds occurred 33 (SD 5) days after the first visit. The first visit to the control herds occurred 22 (SD 21) days after the feeder pigs arrived at the finishing rooms and the second visit was conducted 58 (SD 16) days later.

If a case herd had more than one room designated for finishers, the room exhibiting the most severe respiratory symptoms was selected for sampling. With the control herds, the room housing feeder pigs that had arrived 1–3 weeks earlier was selected. At the beginning of the first herd visit, each pig in the room was forced to stand up while researchers counted the number of coughing and sneezing episodes in the room for 5 min. A coughing/sneezing episode was defined as a single cough/sneeze or a set of continuous coughing/sneezing by a single pig. For the incidence ratio calculations, the number of sneezing and coughing episodes was related to the number of pigs in the room (number of episodes per 100 pigs for 5 min). In the case herds, farmers were also instructed to mark pigs displaying respiratory symptoms with colour markings before the herd visit. These pigs along with the ones observed coughing during the herd visit were selected for sampling. In both the case and control herds, 20 pigs were caught with a snout snare, their rectal temperature was measured and they were ear-tagged and blood-sampled for serological investigations of APP, SIV, MHyo, PRRSV and PRCV. In addition, nasal swabs were taken from 20 pigs in the case herds for SIV determination by PCR. Control herd pigs were clinically free from respiratory symptoms. They were examined for acute SIV infection only serologically, with paired serum samples, as SIV is known to be only found in nasal discharge during the acute phase of infection [12]. We estimated that with a prevalence of 15–20% and 15 samples, we would find at least one affected animal with 15 samples (95% confidence level). Similarly, with a prevalence of 20–25%, we would need 10 samples to find at least one affected animal. Based on these estimations, 15 paired serum samples were used for APP and SIV serology, 15 samples collected during first herd visit for PCV2 PCR analysis and 12 samples collected during second herd visit for PRRS and PRCV serology and 10 samples for MHyo serology.

In the case herds, three non-medicated pigs (13–14 weeks of age on average) with the most evident respiratory signs were euthanized and necropsied during the first herd visit. A lung and the heart of these pigs were sent to a laboratory for pathological, virological and bacteriological analyses, including antimicrobial susceptibility testing. No exact records of past usage of antimicrobial medication of case herds were available. No control herd pigs were available for necropsy.

The second visit to each herd included an interview with the owner, a count of the coughing and sneezing episodes of the pigs in the same room as during the first herd visit, and rectal temperature measurement and blood sampling of the ear-tagged pigs.

Transport of samples to laboratory

The nasal swabs were inserted in a transporting media (Copan Universal Transport Medium, UTM-R, Copan Diagnostics Inc., Murrieta, USA) and surrounded with chilling gel packs before transportation to a laboratory, where they were analysed the next day. All blood samples were cooled to 4 °C and centrifuged at 3000 rpm for 10 min within 24 h after sampling. The sera were stored frozen in –18 °C until analysis. The lungs and hearts of the euthanized pigs were chilled with icepacks, sent to a laboratory and examined the next day. PCV2 analyses were performed in the laboratory of CReSA, Spain. All other analyses were conducted in the laboratory of the Finnish Food Safety Authority (Evira).

Pathology

A total of 60 lung samples from euthanized pigs from 20 case herds were examined. Gross lesions in the lungs including consolidation, abscesses and fibrinous or fibrotic pleurisy and other findings were recorded. Tissue samples were taken from the affected areas in the lungs. The samples were fixed by immersion in 10% neutral formalin, embedded in paraffin, cut in 4-μm thick sections and stained with haematoxylin and eosin. Lung tissue samples were additionally taken, especially from pneumonic lesions, were submitted to bacteriological examination and a sample of the lung tissue was also submitted to be PCR-tested for SIV. These macroscopic lung lesions together with histological and bacteriological results were used to classify the herds.

Bacteriology

For aerobic pathogen detection, the lung tissue samples were cultivated on bovine blood agar and incubated at 37 °C. In addition, for possible APP biotype 1 and *Haemophilus parasuis* isolation, the samples were cultivated on bovine blood agar with a *Staphylococcus aureus* streak and incubated under a 5% CO_2 atmosphere at 37 °C. The small colonies showing enhanced growth around the *S. aureus* streak were isolated and confirmed by a positive Camp reaction. They were tested using multiplex PCR, which identified the species and APP serotypes 2, 5 and 6 [13]. The non-haemolytic NAD-dependent isolates with a negative CAMP reaction were further tested for *Haemophilus parasuis* using biochemical tests (oxidase, catalase, urease, fermentation of xylose, mannitol, inulin, trehalose and xylose supplemented with NAD and horse serum). All APP isolates obtained were tested for antimicrobial susceptibility.

The antimicrobial susceptibility of the APP isolates was determined using a broth microdilution method (penicillin, ampicillin, tetracycline, enrofloxacin, trimethoprim/sulfamethoxazole; VetMICTM, National Veterinary Institute SVA, Uppsala, Sweden) and a disk diffusion method (tiamulin 30 μg, tulathromycin 30 μg; Mast Diagnostics, Merseyside, UK) following the Clinical and Laboratory Standards Institute (CLSI) guidelines [14]. Susceptibility results were categorized as susceptible (S), intermediate (I) or resistant (R) using specific breakpoints for APP according to CLSI [15]. As no specific breakpoints have been determined for penicillin and trimethoprim/sulfamethoxazole, the interpretative criteria for the HACEK group were applied [16]. If the inhibition zone from the tulathromycin test showed a non-susceptible phenotype, susceptibility was further tested using the broth microdilution method (Sensititre®, Trek Diagnostics, East Grinstead, UK). APP ATCC 27090 was used as a quality control strain. If at least one APP strain was categorized as an I or an R in the antimicrobial susceptibility test, the entire herd was classified as either intermediate or resistant.

Virology

Swine influenza virus

SIV RNA was extracted from the lung ($N = 60$) and nasal swab ($N = 400$) suspensions using a QiaAmp ViralRNA Mini Kit (Qiagen, Hilden, Germany). All samples used for virus detection were subjected to influenza A M-gene-specific real-time RT-PCR [17] and A(H1N1) pdm09 -specific real-time RT-PCR [18]. Results were expressed as detected or not detected.

Porcine circovirus type 2

PCV2 was tested by PCR on serum samples of the first 15 pigs out of the 20 collected in the case and control herds during the first farm visit. DNA was extracted from 200 μL of serum using BioSprint® 96 DNA Blood kit (Qiagen, GmbH, D-40724 Hilden) on the Bio Sprint 96 system (Qiagen). Positive and negative extraction controls were added to each extraction plate. DNA samples were processed by means of a standard PCV2 PCR method [19]. Negative controls were added after every 10 samples in each PCR plate. PCR products were run by electrophoresis on a 2% agarose gel stained with ethidium bromide. Results were expressed as the percentage of PCR-positive samples per herd.

Herd classification based on microbiological and pathological outcome

The case herds were classified according to the pathology, bacteriology and virology of the three lung samples examined from each herd and the nasal swab samples examined for SIV.

A herd was considered to suffer from acute respiratory disease caused by APP (coded as CL-APP) when pigs examined pathologically exhibited either 1) typical pathological gross lesions for APP (various sizes of consolidated dark or grayish well-demarcated pneumonic areas or a consolidation with necrotic areas often together with local pleurisy) in at least two out of the three lung samples together with isolation of APP bacteria in two or three lung samples, or 2) characteristic pathological lesions in at least one lung sample and either a necrotic area indicative of APP infection or mild consolidated lesions in another lung sample combined with isolation of APP bacteria in all three lung samples.

A herd was considered to suffer from respiratory disease caused by an acute *Ascaris suum* (coded as CL-ASC) infestation when the following two criteria were fulfilled: 1) at least two out of the three pigs examined pathologically in these herds had compatible gross lesions (typically heavy, wet and mottled red lungs) compatible with an *A. suum* infestation, and 2) detection of gross ascarid larvae in the tracheal froth and/or in the histological sections of these lung samples. The lung samples defined as having lesions caused by an *A. suum* infestation had no other gross lesions characteristic of another specific respiratory pathogen.

A case herd was considered to suffer from acute swine influenza infection (coded as CL-SIV) if SIV was detected by PCR in at least one of the three examined lungs or in at least one of the 20 nasal swab samples.

Miscellaneous etiology (coded as CL-MISC) was considered if variable pneumonic lesions in the lung samples were observed and the abovementioned criteria were not fulfilled.

Serology

Actinobacillus pleuropneumoniae

In the laboratory, we analysed samples of the first 15 pigs out of the 20 collected with paired samples available from both herd visits. APP antibodies were measured using two commercial test kits: IDEXX APP-ApxIV ELISA (IDEXX, Liebefeld-Bern, Swizerland) to detect antibodies against ApxIV toxin, which is produced by all known APP serotypes (19), and IDvet ID Screen APP 2 indirect ELISA (IDvet, Grabels, France) to detect antibodies against lipopolysaccharides (LPS) specific to APP serotype 2 (APP2) with a sensitivity of 82.9% and a specificity of 99.6% for IDEXX APP ApxIV Elisa and a specificity of 99.68% for IDVet APP2 Elisa. Both tests were performed according to the manufacturer's instructions. The absorbance values (percentage of positive control) from the paired samples were compared. Seroconversion at the individual pig level was defined as an increase in absorbance. A herd was considered to suffer from an acute APP infection if at least one individual pig seroconverted based on at least one serologic test (ApxIV toxin or APP2 LPS) between the herd visits.

Swine influenza

The samples of the first 15 pigs out of the 20 collected with paired serum samples available from both herd visits available were analysed from each herd. All blood samples were tested with influenza A antibody ELISA (ID Screen® Influenza A Antibody Competition, IdVet, Grabels, France) according to manufacturer instructions. A sample was considered unclear when the competition percentage (S/N%) was 46–49% and positive when the competition percentage was ≤45%. If a herd had at least one unclear or positive blood sample (pig) in the ELISA test in either of the samplings (first or second), blood samples of that herd were further analysed using a hemagglutination inhibition (HI) test according to European Surveillance Network for Influenza in Pigs [20]. This was done with the antigens H1N1 (SW/Best/96), H1N2 (SW/Gent/7625/99) and H3N2 (SW/St. Oedenrode/96). All antigens were provided by GD Animal Health Service (Deventer, NL). A sample was considered HI positive if the HI titer was ≥1:20. Seroconversion at the individual pig level was defined as an increase in the HI titer between the first and second samples. A herd was considered to have an acute SIV infection if at least one individual pig seroconverted based on the HI test between herd visits.

Mycoplasma hyopneumoniae

Ten serum samples collected from the case herds during the second herd visit were examined for antibodies against MHyo. The antibodies were detected using a blocking ELISA commercial kit (MHyo ELISA, Oxoid, Basingstoke, UK), following manufacturer's instructions. Samples with an optical density value less than 50% of the OD buffer control were interpreted as positive. The sensitivity and specificity of the ELISA test was 100% and 98%, respectively.

Porcine reproductive and respiratory syndrome virus and porcine respiratory coronavirus

Serological screening for PRCV and PRRSV were carried out in 12 samples collected from each case herd during the second herd visit. A commercially available TGEV/PRCV ELISA test (SVANOVIR®, Boehringer Ingelheim Svanova, Uppsala, Sweden) with a sensitivity of 93% and specificity of 97% and PRRSV (PRRS Virus Antibody Test Kit, IDEXX Laboratories, Hoofddorp, NL) with a sensitivity of 98.8% and specificity of 99.9% were used according to the manufacturers' instructions. The PRCV test result was interpreted as negative when the percent inhibition was <45 and PRRSV test result negative when the S/P ratio was <0.4. A farm should be considered positive for PRRSV or PRCV if one or more samples were judged positive.

Statistical data analyses

All statistical data analyses were performed using Stata 14.0 (StataCorp LP, Texas, USA) and the statistical significance of p-value <0.05 was used.

Body temperature of the studied case and control herd animals was compared using unconditional linear regression. Prevalence of clinical signs (coughing and sneezing) during the first and second herd visits and in the case and control herds were modelled as count data (number of coughing/sneezing episodes per 5 min) using a Poisson or negative binomial model.

The percentages of PCR-positive samples in serum (PCV2) were compared between the case and control herds using the Wilcoxon rank sum test, because the proportion was not normally distributed.

The proportion of APP and SIV seroconverted animals were calculated for both tests in each herd and compared between the case and control herds using unconditional linear regression. Herd status (acute APP or SIV infection yes/no) based on the serological results was compared between the case and control herds using the chi square test.

Results
Farm characteristics and season

Out of the 20 case herds, 19 had fatteners only and one was a farrow-to-finish herd. Case herds had an average of 901 (SD 511) fatteners per herd and 234 (SD 101) pigs in each room. The control herds consisted of six fattening and two farrow-to-finish herds with an average of 1075 (SD 400) fattening pigs per herd and 265 (SD 167) pigs per room. In the case and control herds, the pigs originated from an average of 3.7 (SD 6.4) and 1.1 (SD 0.3) different piglet-producing herds, respectively. The season of the first herd visit was relatively similar in case and control herds: spring 20% of case vs. 0% of control herds, summer 20% vs 25%, autumn 25% vs. 50% and winter 35% vs. 25%. Most of the herd visits were done during the year 2012 (60% of case and 62% of control herds), because that was the time when farmers and practicing veterinarians were actively informed about the project.

Clinical signs

Average rectal temperatures of the pigs during the first herd visit were 39.7 °C (SD 0.3, N = 448) and 39.4 °C (SD 0.3, N = 160) in the case and control herds, respectively (p = 0.01). Corresponding figures for the second herd visit were 39.3 °C (SD 0.1, N = 427) and 39.3 °C (SD 0.2, N = 155) (p = 0.3) for the case and control farms, respectively.

An average 4.0 (SD 3.8, N = 17, case herds) and 0.2 (SD 0.3, N = 8, control herds) coughing episodes were counted per 100 pigs during the first herd visit. The incidence rate ratio (IRR) for coughing episodes (case vs. control herds) was 16.5 (p < 0.01) during the first herd visit. By the second visit the coughing episodes in the case herds decreased to the same level as in the control herds: 0.6 (SD 0.8) for the case rooms and 0.4 (SD 0.5) for the control rooms. No difference in IRR was observed for the coughing episodes during the second herd visit (IRR 1.5, p = 0.5).

During the first herd visit, case pigs averaged 12.2 sneezing episodes per 100 pigs (SD 11.1) and the control pigs averaged 5.5 (SD 5.3). The IRR for sneezing episodes (case vs. control herds) was 1.9 (p = 0.1) during the first herd visit. By the second visit, the sneezing episode count in the case herds had decreased down to the same frequency as in the control herds: 5.5 (SD 4.4) in the case herds and 3.9 episodes per 100 pigs in the control herds (SD 3.3; p = 0.2).

Classification of respiratory infection status in the herds

Fourteen (70%) out of 20 case herds were classified as having respiratory infection caused by APP (CL-APP) based on the pathological and bacteriological results. Three case herds were classified with a miscellaneous

(CL-MISC) respiratory infection unassociated with a specific pathogen and three other herds (15%) were diagnosed to suffer from acute *A. suum* infections (CL-ASC) based on the examination of lung samples. Two of the latter herds also had APP seroconverted pigs, and one of these two herds had gross lesions caused by APP in one lung sample.

Bacterial pathogens were isolated from the pig lungs of 18 (90%) case herds. Of these, 12 (66%) herds had APP only (11 of these herds were classified as CL-APP herds and one as a CL-ASC herd). Four herds (22%) had APP together with another bacteria (three of these herds were classified as CL-APP and one as CL-MISC herds) and two (11%) only had other pathogens (all classified as CL-MISC herds). No specific bacteria were detected in the pig lungs from two farms (10%). Other encountered bacteria included *Escherichia coli, P. multocida, S. aureus, Actinomyces* spp., *Streptococcus dysgalactiae subs. Equisimilis, S. suis* and *Streptococcus* spp. and gram- and CAMP-negative and NAD-dependent rodbacterium. The PCR testing showed all APP cultures to be APP serotype 2.

A herd-level summary containing relevant pathological, virological and serological results is presented in Table 1.

All lung and nasal swab samples were SIV negative. Thus, none of the case herds was diagnosed to suffer from acute SIV infection based on PCR even though some herds were serologically positive.

APP antimicrobial susceptibility
Forty-four APP isolates obtained from 16 case herds were tested for antimicrobial resistance. APP isolates from six herds (38%) were intermediately resistant and one herd (6%) tested resistant to tetracycline. Isolates from one herd (6%) were intermediately resistant while two herds (13%) had isolates resistant to trimethoprim/sulfamethoxazole. Isolates from two herds (13%) were resistant to ampicillin and penicillin. Altogether, five isolates resistant or intermediately resistant to at least two different antimicrobials were detected from three herds. No resistance to florfenicol, enrofloxacin, tiamulin or tulathromycin was found. Minimum inhibitory concentration (MIC) distribution is presented in Table 2 and growth inhibition zone distribution of APP strains in Table 3.

Serology
Actinobacillus pleuropneumoniae
Antibodies to ApxIV toxin were detected during the first sampling in 14 (70%) case and six (75%) control herds. Respectively, APP2 antibodies were found in six (30%) case and five (62.5%) control herds. Seroconversion to either ApxIV toxin or APP2 LPS was detected in at least one pig in 19 (95%) case herds and six (75%) control herds. These 19 case and six control herds were

classified to suffer from an ongoing acute APP infection based on the serology results. No difference was observed in the occurrence of acute APP infection between the case and control herds ($p = 0.1$). Seroconversion to ApxIV toxin was detected in 68.8% (SD 26.7) of the individual animals in the case herds and in 67.5% (SD 43.7) in the control herds. Seroconversion to APP2 LPS was detected in 38.3% (SD 27.9) of individual animals in the case herds and in 38.9% (SD 27.8) in the control herds. No difference was found in the proportion of seroconverted animals between the case and control herds (ApxIV toxin $p = 0.9$, APP2 $p = 0.9$).

Swine influenza virus
During the first sampling, SIV antibodies were found in pigs in eight (40%) case and three (37.5%) control herds. Three out of 20 case (15%) and two out of eight control (25%) herds were classified with an ongoing acute SIV infection at the time of the herd visits based on the seroconversion of at least one sampled pig. No difference was found in the number of acute SIV herds between the case and control herds ($p = 0.5$). On average, 5.9% (SD 9.1) of individual animals had seroconverted in the case herds and 8.5% (SD 12.8) in the control herds based on the HI test. No difference was found in the proportion of seroconverted animals between the case and control herds ($p = 0.7$).

Other pathogens
All samples tested were negative against PRRSV, Mhyo and PRCV antibodies.

Porcine circovirus type 2
Six out of 20 (30%) case herds and two out of eight (25%) control herds had at least one PCR-positive serum, respectively. A total of 29 PCV2 PCR-positive samples with mean percentage of positive samples per herd 9.7% (SD 18.2) were detected in the case herds and one positive (1.7%, SD 3.1) in each control herd. No difference was observed in the proportion of PCV2 PCR-positive samples between the case and control herds.

Discussion
Actinobacillus pleuropneumoniae was the most common cause of acute respiratory outbreaks in the studied finishing pig herds. However, SIV, *Ascaris suum*, PCV2 and certain opportunistic bacteria appeared to cause concurrent infections, potentially contributing to the respiratory disease outcome. SIV and PCV2 were detected also in control herds suggesting possible subclinical infections in these herds. Serology alone was not effective in determining the cause of a respiratory outbreak, but pathology and bacteriology were considered useful in reaching a complete diagnosis. In addition to

Table 1 Summary of diagnostic results of 20 case herds exhibiting a respiratory outbreak and of eight control herds with no respiratory symptoms in finishing pigs

Herd	Herd status	Herd classification[a]	Bacteriology	APP (serology)[b]	SIV (serology)[b]	SIV (detection)[c]	PCV2 (PCR)[d]
1	case	CL-APP	APP, Actinomyces sp.	Yes	Yes	No	3 (20%)
2	case	CL-ASC	No specific bacteria	No	No	No	0
3	case	CL-ASC	APP	Yes	No	No	0
4	case	CL-APP	APP	Yes	No	No	0
5	case	CL-APP	APP	Yes	No	No	0
6	case	CL-APP	APP	Yes	No	No	0
7	case	CL-MISC	gram-, CAMP-, NAD dependent rod-bacterium; S. aureus	Yes	Yes	No	0
8	case	CL-APP	APP	Yes	No	No	2 (13%)
9	case	CL-APP	APP	Yes	No	No	0
10	case	CL-APP	APP	Yes	No	No	0
11	case	CL-APP	APP	Yes	No	No	13 (67%)
12	case	CL-ASC	No specific bacteria	Yes	No	No	4 (27%)
13	case	CL-APP	APP, Str. dysgalactiae subsp. equisimilis, E.coli	Yes	No	No	0
14	case	CL-MISC	Str. suis, Streptococcus sp.	Yes	No	No	9 (47%)
15	case	CL-APP	APP, P. multocida	Yes	No	No	0
16	case	CL-APP	APP	Yes	Yes	No	0
17	case	CL-APP	APP	Yes	No	No	0
18	case	CL-APP	APP	Yes	No	No	2 (13%)
19	case	CL-APP	APP	Yes	No	No	1 (7%)
20	case	CL-MISC	APP, P. multocida	Yes	No	No	0
21	control	NA	NA	No	No	NA	1 (7%)
22	control	NA	NA	Yes	No	NA	0
23	control	NA	NA	Yes	Yes	NA	0
24	control	NA	NA	No	No	NA	0
25	control	NA	NA	Yes	No	NA	0
26	control	NA	NA	Yes	No	NA	1 (7%)
27	control	NA	NA	Yes	No	NA	0
28	control	NA	NA	Yes	Yes	NA	0

Abbreviations: CL-APP acute APP infection, CL-ASC acute Ascaris suum infection, CL-MISC acute infection of miscellaneous etiology, APP Actinobacillus pleuropneumoniaen, A. suum Ascaris suum, S. aureus Staphylococcus aureus, P. multocida Pasteurella multocida, E.coli Escherichia coli, Actinomyces sp. Actinomyces species, Haemophilus sp. Haemophilus species, Str. dysgalactiae subsp. equisimilis Streptococcus dysgalactiae subspecies equisimilis, Str. suis Streptococcus suis, SIV swine influenza virus, PCV2 porcine circovirus 2, NA not available
[a]Main necropsy diagnosis based on pathological and bacteriological results from three necropsied pigs
[b]Seroconversion in ≥1 out of 15 pigs sampled
[c]SIV detection with PCR from ≥1 nasal sample out of 20 pigs or from ≥1 lung sample of three necropsied pigs
[d]Number and percentage (in parentheses) of PCV2 positive samples per herd in PCR analysis

this, bacteriology together with antibiotic resistance determination was valuable in selecting the correct medication to be used, which is important in practice.

Clinical examination of the case herd pigs revealed respiratory signs including higher rectal temperature and coughing when compared to the control herd pigs. We were unfortunately unable to acquire exact data on the mortality in the rooms, because some animals in several herds were moved before or between herd visits to other rooms housing sick animals. However, the clinical signs

in the herds were quite mild compared to those reported in experimental studies [21]. During the first herd visit, the average rectal temperature of the case pigs was 39.7 °C and by the second herd visit it was at the same level as in the control herds. In a study by Loeffen et al. [22], pigs in 15 respiratory outbreaks, caused by similar pathogens as in our study, showed respiratory symptoms with fever rising to 40–42 °C, which is much higher than the body temperature measured in our study. We cannot rule out missing the peak body temperature in our study

Table 2 Minimum inhibitory concentrations (MIC) for six antimicrobial agents for the *Actinobacillus pleuropneumoniae* strains (*N* = 44) isolated from lung samples collected from 60 finishing pigs in 16 out of 20 case herds

Anti-microbial	No. of isolates with MIC (µg/ml)												%Res
	≤0.015	0.03	0.06	0.12	0.25	0.5	1	2	4	8	16	32	
PEN				8	16	17		1	2				7
AMP						41			3				7
TET						27	16				1		39
ENR			38	3	3								0
SXT[a]					38	2	2	2					9
FFN						44							0

MICs equal to or lower than the lowest concentration tested are given as the lowest concentration
Abbreviations: *PEN* penicillin, *AMP* ampicillin, *TET* tetracycline, *ENR* enrofloxacin, *SXT* trimethoprim/sulfamethoxazole, *FFN* florfenicol, *%Res* Percentage of intermediately resistant or resistant APP isolates out of all isolates
[a]concentration of trimethoprim given, in concentration ratio 1/19

pigs, as this might have happened earlier than our first herd visit. In addition to coughing, sneezing was very commonly heard in our study herds. However, sneezing was also diagnosed frequently in the control herds and its occurrence did not decrease by the second herd visit, indicating a persistent cause present in all herd types.

APP2 was the main causative agent for acute respiratory infections in Finnish finishing pigs. Previous Finnish studies screening the APP serotypes present in the country have revealed that APP2 is a common serotype together with several others [23, 24]. However, these older studies detected only antibody prevalence, but did not establish the connection between antibody prevalence and clinical disease. Our present study considered APP2 to be the main etiological agent of respiratory outbreak in the majority of herds (14 out of 20). In addition, APP2 was isolated from two other herds: one herd with miscellaneous etiology of its respiratory outbreak and one herd with lung lesions caused by *A. suum*.

It is difficult to compare the role of APP in respiratory infections in various countries, as study herds have usually not been selected and sampled in the same way as in our study. A study on clinical outbreaks carried out in the Netherlands in a manner similar to ours found APP to be the most likely cause in five out of 16 clinical outbreaks [22]. Other researchers have often used slaughterhouse data and/or serology, but pathological findings from samples taken during visible clinical symptoms have not been used. This is most likely due to the difficulty in carrying out such field studies. In France, a cross-sectional study on infectious agents in respiratory diseases was performed in 125 French swine herds without including any information concerning the clinical situation of the herds [25]. The researchers found that APP2 (serological diagnosis) was significantly associated with extensive pleuritis in the slaughterhouses, but not with pneumonia. In addition, an association between pneumonia or pleuritis in the slaughterhouses and seropositivity to APP was found in three other studies [26–28].

Serology has indeed been used in several studies examining APP causing respiratory infections in finishing pigs, but serological results have usually not been connected to clinical findings or acute outbreaks. Herds e.g. in Spain [27], Italy [28], Canada [29] and Belgium [30] have commonly been found positive for APP antibodies. In our study, antibodies against ApxIV toxin and APP2 LPS were found in both the case and control herds already during the first herd visit. Detectable antibody levels have been reported 1–3 weeks after experimental infection [31]. Pigs in our study may have been in contact with APP long enough to enable some of them to have seroconverted earlier than the first herd visit. We know that the herd owners waited for an average of 8 days before communicating about a respiratory outbreak, which is quite a long time. Estimating the role of subclinical infections is also difficult. Subclinical APP

Table 3 Growth inhibition zones for two antimicrobial agents for 44 Actinobacillus pleuropneumoniae strains isolated from lung samples collected from 60 finishing pigs in 16 out of 20 case herds

Antimicrobial	No. of isolates with GIZ (mm)																	%Res
	6	7	8	9	10	11	12	13	14	15	16	17	18	19	20	21	22	
TIA									9	10	15	4	1	2	2		1	0
TUL				1[a]	1	9	11	6	7	4	2	2		1				0

Abbreviations: *TIA* tiamulin, *TUL* tulathromycin, *GIZ* growth inhibition zone, *%Res* Percentage of intermediately resistant or resistant APP isolates out of all isolates
[a]The isolate was tested also with the broth microdilution method and was found susceptible to tulathromycin (MIC value 32 µg/ml)

infection is known to potentially cause seroconversion [29]. A subclinical APP infection was possibly ongoing in the control herds during the time of our study and the presence of an infection went unnoticed by the herd owner and the research personnel. Our study found that the use of serology in APP detection, in either single sampling or paired samples, for the diagnosis of acute respiratory disease in field conditions is of little value, because no exact information of the initiation time of the infection is available and because of subclinical infections. However, when the beginning of an infection is known, as is often the case in experimental studies, or when the course of the infection is followed [32], serology remains a valuable diagnostic tool [30].

Three out of 20 outbreaks had a miscellaneous etiology. The pathology and bacteriology of these herds revealed findings incompatible with the set criteria for acute APP or SIV infections and the presence of bacteria such as APP, *E. coli*, *P. multocida*, *S. aureus*, *Actinomyces* spp., *S. dysgalactiae subs. Equisimilis*, *S. suis* and *Streptococcus* spp. APP serology showed seroconversion in each of these herds. SIV seroconversion additionally happened in one herd. Other researchers have also found that reaching a proper diagnosis is not always easy under field conditions despite using several diagnostic methods. Researchers studying respiratory outbreaks in 16 herds in the Netherlands could not reach a definitive diagnosis in four herds [23]. They concluded that secondary bacteria might have played a role in the clinical outbreaks where no evident cause could be found. It is also possible the primary pathogen could not be identified in our study, despite the utilization of several diagnostic methods.

Ascaris suum infection was found to be the main cause of respiratory clinical signs in three case herds (15%). At least in Finland this pathogen has been considered a minor disease agent, especially in modern management systems with concrete floors and without outdoor access. It is widely known that *A. suum* can cause verminous pneumonia, as the larvae migrate through the lung tissue during their lifecycle [33]. Also, slaughterhouse statistics from Finnish yearly figures of approximately 2 million slaughter pigs confirm the importance of *A. suum* infestations (Finnish Food Safety Authority, personal communication). Liver condemnations due to milk spots caused by *A. suum* were recorded in an average 6.5% of the finishing pigs slaughtered during the years 2010–2015. Other, more specific diagnostic methods for ascarids, have shown the prevalence of this parasite to be high. For example, antibodies against *A. suum* were observed in 39% of the study herds in a Danish study on finishing pigs [34]. A higher prevalence was found in Serbia when using the flotation method, with approximately 50% of swine herds being *A. suum* positive [35]. Ascariasis is a clinically relevant disease, as it

can cause production losses [36] and impair the immunity achieved by vaccinations [37]. Also, proper diagnosis is of utmost importance. The administration of antimicrobial agents is useless as a treatment method against ascariasis.

Viral pathogens appeared to be less important as a cause of acute respiratory symptoms in finishing pigs in our study. The significance of SIV infection varies in other studies. For example, a clinical field study in the Netherlands showed SIV to be the most frequent main cause of a clinical outbreak in 16 herds [21]. In a recent study in Brazil, nearly 70% of the nasal swab samples taken from piglets expressing signs of respiratory disease were PCR-positive for SIV. Furthermore, SIV was the most common finding in the virological evaluations of diseased animals showing lung lesions [38]. However, studies also exist in which SIV is detected from pigs suffering from respiratory symptoms or slaughtered finishing pigs with lung lesions, but other pathogens are more frequently observed [6, 8, 39]. Typically for SIV, the virus is often detected in combination with other pathogens [6, 38]. In our present study, SIV was not found in the nasal swabs or lung samples and none of the case herds were therefore classified to suffer from an acute respiratory infection caused by SIV. However, results from the nasal swabs might be at least partly false-negative because our nasal swab sampling took place fairly late compared to optimal timing. Herds were visited approximately 8 days after clinical signs commenced and, therefore, it might be more correct to designate case herds as suffering from sub-acute respiratory disease instead of acute respiratory disease, especially in the case of SIV infection. Nasal swabs should be taken within 4 days after infection onset to attain the optimal detection of SIV [12]. Serology revealed that three case herds out of 20 appeared to have had a concurrent SIV infection. Two out of the eight control herds also had pigs that had seroconverted and possibly suffered from subclinical SIV infection. In addition, both the case and control herds had antibodies already during the first herd visit. SIV serology, similarly to APP serology, should be understood more as a monitoring tool rather than as a diagnostic one. Nowadays, a convenient diagnostic sample is oral fluid, since at a population level, the presence of a pathogen may be detected for a longer period [40].

PCV2 has been associated with several disease syndromes collectively named porcine circovirus diseases [41]. The role PCV2 plays in PRDC has been suggested to always involve interaction or synergism with other respiratory pathogens [42]. The proportion of PCV2-positive animals was similar in the case and control farms of our study. PCV2 is a ubiquitous virus and hence PCR-positive animals occurring on a farm is very likely irrespective of the farm's disease status. When blood sample analysis is based only on a standard PCR method (positive and negative, but no quantification of viral counts) without histopathology or detection of the virus in lymphoid tissues, the method is not sufficient for establishing the actual role of PCV2 in clinical disease. However, we did not see compatible PCV2 gross pathology during the field autopsies carried out on the case farms. Based on the lack of typical circovirus gross pathology and no difference in the proportion of PCR-positive animals between the case and control farms, we concluded that PCV2 probably did not play a major role in acute respiratory disease detected on the case farms despite the pathogen being present on farms. Vaccinating pigs against PCV2 infections is a very common preventive measure in Finland, and this has most likely contributed to the low occurrence of the pathogen.

According to our hypothesis, certain pathogens causing acute respiratory symptoms in pigs, namely Mhyo, PRRSV and PRCV, were not found in the studied Finnish herds. Especially Mhyo and PRRSV are important pathogens involved in respiratory infections in many pig-producing countries despite PRRSV not being detected in certain countries e.g. Finland [6, 8, 24, 43]. Certain PRCV strains can also contribute to respiratory disease [44]. The lack of these pathogens as causative agents of respiratory outbreaks in Finland makes the situation of finishing pig herds quite different and favourable compared to respiratory disease scenarios in several countries located across the world. The absence of these pathogens may have a significant impact on the prevalence of other respiratory pathogens. However, the similar disease situation is present also in specific pathogen free herds in other countries than Finland, and these farms and their veterinarians might benefit from obtained results.

The vaccination history of study animals may have had some influence on serological results. We do not know the exact vaccination scheme utilized for study animals. However, we know that at the time of the study, Finnish sow herds generally vaccinated all sows against erysipelas, parvovirus and colibacillosis and a vaccination of piglets against PCV2 is very common in the country. We also know that very few (most likely none of the herds in our study) herds vaccinated against APP or SIV. Based on that estimation, it is unlikely that vaccinations would have had any significant effect on APP serology.

In our present study, APP strains were susceptible to most of the tested antimicrobials. Only tetracycline resistance was detected in more than 10% of the isolates. Similar results have been found in other European countries. Thus, resistance to tetracycline among porcine APP is a growing problem. Other studies have occasionally observed resistance to penicillin, ampicillin and trimethoprim/sulfamethoxazole [45–49]. The Ministry of Agriculture and Forestry in Finland issued its first national recommendation for prudent antibiotic use in

animals as early as 1996 [50]. Currently, the first-choice antimicrobial agent recommended in APP infections is G-penicillin and the second choice is tiamulin or tetracycline. It is notable that a few isolates were found to be resistant also to penicillin, ampicillin and trimethoprim/sulfamethoxazole, which further emphasizes the need to investigate the resistance of APP strains when selecting the appropriate treatment.

From a practical standpoint, the field necropsies supplemented with microbiological analysis was the most valuable diagnostic tool combination for detecting the main cause of acute respiratory infections in our study. Field necropsies have several advantages: the technique is simple, inexpensive and not pathogen-specific, preliminary results are promptly available and antimicrobial susceptibility results can be obtained from bacteria isolated from lesions. However, field necropsies are disadvantageous, since if acute disease is not leading to mortality, euthanasia should be performed. In acute respiratory outbreaks, field necropsies, sample-taking and antimicrobial susceptibility testing are extremely important, because resistance to certain recommended antimicrobials does exist. Susceptibility testing is necessary not only from the field veterinarian's and single pig herd's point of view, but also from a national policymaker's perspective. Serology cannot be used alone in diagnosis, but offers detailed information about possible pathogens causing mainly subclinical infections. Also other diagnostic methods could be used. In addition to the already mentioned oral fluids, tracheobronchial swabs [51] or lavage [52] would be of help. Their disadvantage is the need for special equipment and/or sedation of the pig, which might limit this sampling method under field conditions.

Conclusions

APP serotype 2 was the most common cause for acute respiratory outbreaks in finishing pigs in Finland and *A. suum* or other opportunistic bacteria caused acute coughing episodes in some herds. Viral pathogens appeared to have a minor role in causing the clinical signs. Field necropsies supplemented with microbiological analysis were the most valuable diagnostic tool combination in detecting the main cause of the infections under field conditions. Bacterial isolation from the lungs was especially important in assessing antimicrobial susceptibility and for optimizing antimicrobial treatment, because some resistance, especially to tetracycline, was found among the APP strains causing disease. Serological diagnostics were not optimal in the diagnosis of the respiratory outbreaks of our study. Although several different diagnostic methods were used, the primary pathogen causing the outbreak remained questionable in some herds.

Acknowledgements
We wish to thank all the farmers who let us conduct herd visits to their herds and all the veterinarians who informed us of acute cases. We are grateful to the students of the University of Helsinki that attended the herd visits and helped us collect the samples.

Funding
This work was partly funded by the ESNIP3 Consortium (European Surveillance Network for Influenza in Pigs 3, grant #259949, FP7-Influenza-2010). Funding for this study was also obtained from the Ministry of Agriculture and Forestry of Finland (Makera-funding) and from major slaughterhouses (Atria, HK Scan and Snellman).

Authors' contributions
MHH and OH wrote the draft of the manuscript. MHH, OH, TL, CO and MH conducted the herd visits. The following persons conducted the laboratory analyses: MR-S (APP serology, MHyo), KP (bacteriology), TN (SIV, PRRS and PRCV), TL (pathological examinations), SN (antimicrobial susceptibility), JS and MS (PCV2). SP analysed the APP serological results. OH conducted the statistical analyses. All authors took an active part in planning the study and commenting on the data analysis and the manuscript. All authors read and approved the final manuscript.

Competing interests
The authors declare that they have no competing interests.

Author details
[1]Department of Production Animal Medicine, University of Helsinki, Paroninkuja 20, 04920 Saarentaus, Finland. [2]Finnish Food Safety Authority Evira, PO Box 198, 60101 Seinäjoki, Finland. [3]Finnish Food Safety Authority Evira, Mustialankatu 3, 00790 Helsinki, Finland. [4]Centre de Recerca en Sanitat Animal (CReSA, IRTA-UAB), Campus de la Universitat Autònoma de Barcelona, 08193 Bellaterra, Spain. [5]Departament de Sanitat i Anatomia Animals, Facultat de Veterinària, UAB, 08193 Bellaterra, Barcelona, Spain.

References
1. Brockmeier S, Halbur P, Thacker E. Porcine respiratory disease complex. In: Brogden K, Guthmiller J, editors. Polymicrobial diseases. Washington (DC): ASM Press; 2002. Chapter 13.
2. Thacker E, Halbur P, Ross R. Mycoplasma hyopneumoniae potentiation of porcine reproductive and respiratory syndrome virus-induced pneumonia. J Clin Microbiol. 1999;37:620–7.
3. Harms P, Halbur P, Sorden S. Three cases of porcine respiratory disease complex associated with porcine circovirus type 2 infection. J Swine Health Prod. 2002;1:27–30.
4. Choi Y, Goyal S, Soo JH. Retrospective analysis of etiologic agents associated with respiratory diseases in pigs. Can Vet J. 2003;44:735–7.
5. Kim J, Chung H-K, Chae C. Association of porcine circovirus 2 with porcine respiratory disease complex. Vet J. 2003;166:251–6.
6. Hansen MS, Pors SE, Jensen HE, Bille-Hansen V, Bisgaard M, Flachs EM, Nielsen OL. An investigation of the pathology and pathogens associated with porcine respiratory disease complex in Denmark. J Comp Pathol. 2010;143:120–31.
7. Fachingera V, Bischoff R, Jedidiab A, Elbersa K. The effect of vaccination against porcine circovirus type 2 in pigs suffering from porcine respiratory disease complex. Vaccine. 2008;26:1488–99.
8. Palzer A, Ritzmann M, Wolf G, Heinritzi K. Associations between pathogens in healthy pigs and pigs with pneumonia. Vet Rec. 2008;162:267–71.
9. Evira. Animal Diseases in Finland, year statistics, Evira publications 2015 (in Finnish).
10. Sikava, Stakeholders health and welfare register for swineherds in Finland. Animal Health ETT, Seinäjoki, Finland. https://www.sikava.fi/PublicContent/IntroductionInEnglish. Accessed 2 Apr 2016.
11. Nokireki T, Laine T, London L, Ikonen N, Huovilainen A. The first detection of influenza in the Finnish pig population: a retrospective study. Acta Vet Scand. 2013;55(69):1–7.
12. Brown I, Done S, Spencer Y, Cooley W, Harris P, Alexander D. Pathogenicity of a swine influenza H1N1 virus antigenically distinguishable from classical and European strains. Vet Rec. 1993;132(24):598–602.
13. Jessing S, Angen Ø, Inzana T. Evaluation of a multiplex PCR test for simultaneous identification and Serotyping of Actinobacillus pleuropneumoniae serotypes 2, 5, and 6. J Clin Microbiol. 2003;41:4095–100.
14. CLSI. Performance Standards for Antimicrobial Disk and Dilution Susceptibility Tests for Bacteria isolated from Animals; Approved Standard – Third Edition. CLSI Document M31-A3. Wayne: Clinical and Laboratory Standards Institute; 2008. p. 35–36,83.
15. CLSI. Methods for Antimicrobial Dilution and Disk Susceptibility Testing of Infrequently isolated or Fastidious Bacteria; Approved Guideline - Second Edition. CLSI Document M45-A2. Wayne: Clinical and Laboratory Standards Institute; 2010. p. 22–23.
16. CLSI. Performance Standards for Antimicrobial Disk and Dilution Susceptibility Tests for Bacteria Isolated from Animals; Second Informational Supplement. CLSI Document VET01-S2. Wayne: Clinical and Laboratory Standards Institute; 2013. p. 15–24.
17. Spackman E, Senne D, Myers T, Bulaga L, Garber L, Perdue M, Lohman K, Daum L, Suarez D. Development of a real time reverse transcriptase PCR assay for type a influenza virus and the avian H5 and H7 haemagglutination subtypes. J Clin Microbiol. 2002;40:3256–60.
18. Rönkkö E, Ikonen N, Kontio M, Haanpää M, Kallio-Kokko H, Mannonen L, Lappalainen M, Julkunen I, Ziegler T. Validation and diagnostic application of NS and HA gene-specific real-time reverse transcription-PCR assays for detection of 2009 pandemic influenza a (H1N1) viruses in clinical specimens. J Clin Microbiol 2011;49:2009–2011.
19. Quintana J, Balasch M, Segales J, Calsamiglia M, Rodriguez-Arrioja GM, Plana-Duran J, Domingo M. Experimental inoculation of porcine circoviruses type 1 (PCV1) and type 2 (PCV2) in rabbits and mice. Vet Res. 2002;33:229–37.
20. ESNIP. Haemagglutination inhibition (HI) assay. Standard protocols ESNIP. European Surveillance Network for Influenza in Pigs 2 http://www.esnip.ugent.be/page7/page7.html.
21. Hennig I, Teutenberg-Riedel B, Gerlach G-F. Downregulation of a protective Actinobacillus pleuropneumoniae antigen during the course of infection. Microb Pathog. 1999;26:53–63.
22. Loeffen WLA, Kamp EM, Stockhofe-Zurwieden N, APKMI v N, Bongers JH, Hunneman WA, AEW E, Baars J, Nell T, FG vZ. Survey of infectious agents involved in acute respiratory disease in finishing pigs. Vet Rec. 1999;145:123–9.
23. Levonen K, Seppänen J, Veijalainen P. Actinobacillus-pleuropneumoniae serotype-2 antibodies in Finnish pig health-scheme herds. J Veterinary Med Ser B. 1994;41:567–73.
24. Levonen K, Seppänen J, Veijalainen P. Antibodies against 12 serotypes of Actinobacillus pleuropneumoniae in Finnish slaughter sows. J Veterinary Med Ser B. 1996;8:489–95.
25. Fablet C, Marois-Crehan C, Simon G, Grasland B, Jestin A, Kobisch M, Madec F, Rose N. Infectious agents associated with respiratory diseases in 125 farrow-to-finish pig herds: a cross-sectional study. Vet Microbiol. 2012;157:152–63.
26. Meyns T, Van Steelant J, Rolly E, Dewulf J, Haesebrouk F, Maes D. A cross-sectional study of risk factors associated with pulmonary lesions in pigs at slaughter. The Vet J. 2011;187:388–92.
27. Fraile L, Alegre A, López-Jiménez R, Nofrasias M, Segalés J. Risk factors associated with pleuritis and cranio-ventral pulmonary consolidation in slaughter-aged pigs. Vet J. 2010;184:326–33.
28. Merialdi G, Dottori M, Bonilauri P, Luppi A, Gozio S, Pozzi P, Spaggiari B, Martelli P. Survey of pleuritis and pulmonary lesions in pigs at abattoir with a focus on the extent of the condition and herd risk factors. Vet J. 2012;193:234–9.
29. MacInnes JI, Gottschalk M, Lone AG, Mecalf DS, Ojha S, Rosendal T, Watson SB, Friendship RM. Prevalence of Actinobacillus pleuropneumoniae,

Actinobacillus suis, Haemophilus parasuis, Pasteurella multocida, and Streptococcus Suis in representative Ontario swine herds. Can J Vet Res. 2008;72:242–8.

30. Chiers K, Donne E, Van Overbeke I, Ducatelle R, Haesebrouck F. Actinobacillus pleuropneumoniae infections in closed swine herds: infection patterns and serological profiles. Vet Microbiol. 2002;85:343–52.

31. Costa G, Oliveira S, Torrison J, Dee S. Evaluation of Actinobacillus pleuropneumoniae diagnostic tests using samples derived from experimentally infected pigs. Vet Microbiol. 2011;148:246–51.

32. Andreasen M, Nielsen JP, Baekbo P, Willeberg P, Botner A. A longitudinal study of serological patterns of respiratory infections in nine infected Danish swine herds. Prev Vet Med. 2000;45:221–35.

33. Corwin RM, Stewart TB. Internal parasites. In: Straw BE, D'Allaire S, Mengeling WL, Taylor DJ, editors. Diseases of swine. Ames: Blackwell Science Ltd.; 1999. p. 713–30.

34. Ellegaard B, vandekerckhove E, Vlaminck J, Geldhof P, Haugegaard J. Investigation of the prevalence of Ascaris suum infections in Danish finishing herds using a new serological test. Proceedings of the 23th International Pig Veterinary Society Congress (IPVS). 2014, 629.

35. Ilíc T, Becskei Z, Tasi'c A, Dimitrijevi'c S. Follow-up study of prevalence and control of ascariasis in swine populations in Serbia. Acta Parasitol. 2013; 58(3):278–83.

36. Kipper M, Andretta I, Monteiro SG, Lovatto PA, Lehnen CR. Meta-analysi of the effects of endoparasites on pig performance. Vet Parasitol. 2011;181:316–20.

37. Steenhard NR, Jungersen G, Kokotovic B, Beshah E, Dawson HD, Urban JF Jr, Roepstorff A, Thamsborg SM. Ascaris suum infection negatively affects the response to a Mycoplasma hyopneumoniae vaccination and subsequent challenge infection in pigs. Vaccine. 2009;27(37):5161–9.

38. Schmidt C, Cibulski SP, Andrade CP, Teixeira TF, Varela AP, Scheffer CM, Franco AC, deAlmeida LL, Roehe PM. Swine influenza virus and association with the porcine respiratory disease complex in pig farms in southern Brazil. Zoonoses Public Health. 2016;63:234–40.

39. Nakharuthai C, Boonsoongnern A, Poolperm P, Wajjwalku W, Urairong K, Chumsing W, Lertwitcharasarakul P, Lekcharoensuk P. Occurence of swine influenza virus infection in swine with porcine respiratory disease complex. Southeast Asian J Trop Med Public Health. 2008;39:1045–53.

40. Decorte I, Stenseels M, Lambrecht B, Cay AB, De Regge N. Virus in spiked oral fluid and samples from individually housed, experimentally Infected pigs: Potential role of porcine oral fluid in active influenza A virus surveillance in swine. PLoS ONE. 2015;10(10):e0139586.

41. Gillespie J, Opriessing T, Meng XJ, Pelzer K, Buechener-Maxwell V. Porcine circovirus type 2 and porcine circovirus-associated disease. J Vet Intern Med. 2009;23:1151–63.

42. Chae C. A review of porcine circovirus 2-associated syndromes and diseases. Vet J. 2005;169:326–36.

43. Monger VR, Stegeman JA, Koop G, Dukpa K, Tenzin T, Loeffen WL. Seroprevalence and associated risk factors of important pig viral diseases in Bhutan. Prev Vet Med. 2014;117:222–32.

44. Saif L, Pensaert MB, Sestak C, Yeo S-G, Jung K. Coronaviruses. In: Diseases of Swine, 10th ed., 2012. Zimmermann JJ, Karriker LA, Ramirez A, Schwartz KJ, Stevenson GW, editors. Iowa: John Wiley et Sons, Inc.

45. Gutiérrez-Martín C, del Blanco N, Blanco M, Navas J, Rodríguez-Ferri E. Changes in antimicrobial susceptibility of Actinobacillus pleuropneumoniae isolated from pigs in Spain during the last decade. Vet Microbiol. 2006;115:218–22.

46. Kucerova Z, Hradecka H, Nechvatalova K, Nedbalcova K. Antimicrobial susceptibility of Actinobacillus pleuropneumoniae isolates from clinical outbreaks of porcine respiratory diseases. Vet Microbiol. 2011;150:203–6.

47. Vanni M, Merenda M, Barigazzi G, Garbarino C, Luppi A, Tognetti R, Intorre L. Antimicrobial resistance of Actinobacillus pleuropneumoniae isolated from swine. Vet Microbiol. 2012;156:172–7.

48. de Jong A, Thomas V, Simjee S, Moyaert H, El Garch F, Maher K, Morrissey I, Butty P, Klein U, Marion H, Rigaut D, Vallé M. Antimicrobial susceptibility monitoring of respiratory tract pathogens isolated from diseased cattle and pigs across Europe: the VetPath study. Vet Microbiol. 2014;172:202–15.

49. Wasteson Y, Roe DE, Falk K, Roberts MC. Characterization of tetracycline and erythromycin resistance in Actinobacillus pleuropneumoniae. Vet Microbiol. 1996;48:41–50.

50. Permanent work group on antimicrobials of the Ministry of Agriculture and Forestry. Recommendations for the Use of Antimicrobials against the Most Common Infectious Diseases of Animals. Evira publications 3/2009 (in Finnish).

51. Giacomini E, Ferrari N, Pitozzi A, Remistani M, Giardiello D, Maes D, Alborali GL. Dynamics of Mycoplasma hyopneumoniae seroconversion and infection in pigs in the three main production systems. Vet Res Commun. 2016;40:81–8.

52. Woolley LK, Fell S, Gonsalves JR, Walker MJ, Djordjevic SP, Jenkins C, Eamens GJ. Evaluation of clinical, histological and immunological changes and qPCR detection of Mycoplasma hyopneumoniae in tissues during the early stages of mycoplasmal pneumonia in pigs after experimental challenge with two field isolates. Vet Microbiol. 2012;161:186–95.

8

Feed additives decrease survival of delta coronavirus in nursery pig diets

Katie M. Cottingim[1], Harsha Verma[2], Pedro E. Urriola[1], Fernando Sampedro[2], Gerald C. Shurson[1] and Sagar M. Goyal[2]* (iD)

Abstract

Background: Feed contaminated with feces from infected pigs is believed to be a potential route of transmission of porcine delta coronavirus (PDCoV). The objective of this study was to determine if the addition of commercial feed additives (e.i., acids, salt and sugar) to swine feed can be an effective strategy to inactive PDCoV.

Results: Six commercial feed acids (UltraAcid P, Activate DA, KEMGEST, Acid Booster, Luprosil, and Amasil), salt, and sugar were evaluated. The acids were added at the recommended concentrations to 5 g aliquots of complete feed, which were also inoculated with 1 mL of PDCoV and incubated for 0, 7, 14, 21, 28, and 35 days. In another experiment, double the recommended concentrations of these additives were also added to the feed samples and incubated for 0, 1, 3, 7, and 10 days. All samples were stored at room temperature (~25 °C) followed by removal of aliquots at 0, 7, 14, 21, 28, and 35 days. Any surviving virus was eluted in a buffer solution and then titrated in swine testicular cells. Feed samples without any additive were used as controls. Both Weibull and log-linear kinetic models were used to analyze virus survival curves. The presence of a tail in the virus inactivation curves indicated deviations from the linear behavior and hence, the Weibull model was chosen for characterizing the inactivation responses due to the better fit. At recommended concentrations, delta values (days to decrease virus concentration by 1 log) ranged from 0.62–1.72 days, but there were no differences on virus survival among feed samples with or without additives at the manufacturers recommended concentrations. Doubling the concentration of the additives reduced the delta value to ≤ 0.28 days ($P < 0.05$) for all the additives except for Amasil (delta values of 0.86 vs. 4.95 days). Feed additives that contained phosphoric acid, citric acid, or fumaric acid were the most effective in reducing virus survival, although none of the additives completely inactivated the virus by 10- days post-inoculation.

Conclusions: Commercial feed additives (acidifiers and salt) may be utilized as a strategy to decrease risk of PDCoV in feed, specially, commercial feed acidifiers at double the recommended concentrations reduced PDCoV survival in complete feed during storage at room temperature. However, none of these additives completely inactivated the virus.

Keywords: Feed additives, Inactivation kinetics, Porcine delta coronavirus, Survival, Swine, Transmission, Virus

Background

There are three enteric coronaviruses that can cause gastrointestinal illness in young pigs e.g., transmissible gastroenteritis virus (TGEV), porcine epidemic diarrhea virus (PEDV), and porcine delta coronavirus (PDCoV) [1]. Transmissible gastroenteritis virus has been present in the United States since 1946, but PEDV and PDCoV were introduced more recently in 2013 and 2014, respectively. The spread of PEDV among swine herds was rapid; and strict biosecurity measures known to prevent transmission of other viruses such as porcine respiratory and reproductive syndrome virus were ineffective; later contaminated complete feed was demonstrated to be a route for PEDV transmission that has been overlooked in previous biosecurity protocols [2]. Therefore, for disease prevention purposes, it is essential to understand proper feed handling procedures that minimize risk of transmission, and to identify methods that can rapidly inactivate these viruses if present in feed.

Commercial swine feed is often fortified with various additives, including acidifiers such as organic and/or inorganic acids to control bacterial and mold growth in

* Correspondence: goyal001@umn.edu
[2]Department of Veterinary Population Medicine, University of Minnesota, St. Paul, MN 55108, USA
Full list of author information is available at the end of the article

feed, increase growth performance of animals, improve nutrient digestibility, and control harmful bacteria in the animal gut [3]. Acidifiers are often added to feed as an alternative to the use of antibiotics as growth promoters and to control pathogens such as *Salmonella* spp. [4, 5]. Nursery pigs are believed to obtain the greatest benefit from the addition of acidifiers, and the addition of acidifiers has been shown to increase growth rate by 12% [6]. Acidifiers are also effective in reducing diarrhea and mortality while maintaining adequate growth of nursery pigs [6]. This study was conducted to determine if the addition of commercially available feed additives (salt, sugar, and acidifiers), at recommended or double the recommended concentrations, is effective in reducing the survival of PDCoV in feed.

Methods
Virus propagation
The strain of PDCoV was obtained from the National Veterinary Services Laboratory (NVSL; Ames, IA). Stock virus was propagated in swine testicular cells. The cells were grown in Minimum Essential Medium with Earle's salts supplemented with L-glutamine (Mediatech, Herndon, VA), 8% fetal bovine serum (Hyclone, South Logan, UT), 50 µg/mL gentamicin (Mediatech), 150 µg/mL neomycin sulfate (Sigma, St. Louis, MO), 1.5 µg/mL fungizone (Sigma), and 455 µg/mL streptomycin (Sigma). The maintenance medium included 5 µg/mL of trypsin (Gibco, Life technologies, Grand Island, NY) and the same antibiotics as previously described. Cells inoculated with the virus were incubated at 37 °C under 5% CO_2 and were observed for the appearance of virus-induced cytopathic effects (CPE) for up to 6 days post-infection. The infected cells were subjected to 3 freeze-thaw cycles (−80 °C/25 °C) followed by centrifugation at 2500 × g for 15 min at 4 °C. The supernatant was collected, aliquoted, and stored at −80 °C until use.

Virus titration
Serial 10-fold dilutions of all samples were prepared in maintenance medium followed by inoculation in monolayers of swine testicular cells contained in 96-well microtiter plates (Nunc, NY, USA) using 100 µL/well and 3 wells per dilution. Inoculated cells were incubated at 37 °C under 5% CO_2 for up to 6 days and examined daily under an inverted microscope for the appearance of CPE. The highest dilution showing CPE was considered the end point. Virus titers were calculated as Tissue Culture Infectious Dose $TCID_{50}$/mL by the Karber method [7].

Feed matrix and laboratory analysis
The CGI Enhance ground commercial starter feed used in this experiment was obtained from VitaPlus (Madison, WI). This feed is designed for feeding pigs from 5–10 days

post-weaning and does not contain any animal derived by-products. The feed was confirmed to be negative for PDCoV by real time reverse transcription-polymerase chain reaction (RT-PCR). A sample of the feed was submitted to Minnesota Valley Testing Laboratories (New Elm, MN), where dry matter (DM; method 930.15), ether extract (method 2003.05), crude protein (CP; method 990.03), crude fiber (method 920.39), and ash (method 942.05) were analyzed following standard procedures [8]. The chemical analysis results of the feed were 91.43% DM, 4.47% EE, 24.2% CP, 2.02% crude fiber, and 9.45% ash on as is basis.

Feed additives
Six commercial feed acidifiers, UltraAcid P, (Nutriad, Dendermonde, Belgium), Activate DA (Novus International, St. Charles, MO), Acid Booster (Agri-Nutrition, DeForest, WI), Kemgest (Kemin Agrifoods, Des Moines, IA), Luprosil (BASF, Florham Park, NJ), and Amasil (BASF, Florham Park, NJ) were evaluated when added at their manufacturers' recommended concentrations (Table 1). In addition, the effect of sodium chloride and sucrose on virus survival was also evaluated. In a second experiment, PDCoV survival was evaluated by adding the double of the recommended amounts of these feed additives.

Virus inoculation procedure
Forty-eight aliquots of feed (5 g/aliquot) were placed in plastic scintillation vials and the recommended concentrations of each feed additive were added. There were a total of 8 observations at each of the 6-time point for each of the 9 dietary combinations (control and 8 additives). Another set of 40 aliquots of feed were used at double of the recommended concentrations of the additives, for a total of 8 replications per each of the 5-time points and 9 dietary combinations (Table 1). Subsequently, 1 mL of PDCoV (initial titer 3.2 × 10^5 $TCID_{50}$/mL) was added to all vials. The control treatment consisted of vials containing feed and virus but no feed additive. The samples were thoroughly mixed using a vortex mixer and stored at room temperature (~25 °C). An individual vial served as the experimental unit, and one vial from each set was removed at 0, 7, 14, 21, 28, and 35 days to determine the degree of virus inactivation. In the experiment involving double the recommended concentrations of additives, samples were removed and evaluated for virus inactivation at 0, 1, 3, 7, and 10 days. Different time points were selected to account for greater virus inactivation in the early stages of inoculation. To determine the amount of virus inactivation at each time point, the surviving virus in each vial was eluted by adding 10 mL of 3% beef extract-0.05 M glycine solution at pH 7.2. After thorough mixing by vortexing, the vials were centrifuged at 2500 × g for 15 min. Serial 10-fold dilutions of the supernatants (eluates) were

Table 1 Commercial name of feed additives, active ingredients, concentration when mixed with complete feed at the manufacturers' recommended doses (1×) and twice the manufacturers' recommended doses (2×) along with pH of the diet and additive mixture

Feed additive (Manufacturer); (Active ingredients)	Amount		pH[1]	
	1×	2×	1×	2×
Complete feed	0	0	$5.82^c \pm 0.02$	$5.82^c \pm 0.02$
UltraAcid P (Nutriad, Dendermonde, Belgium); (orthophosphoric, citric, fumaric, and malic acids)	150 mg	300 mg	$5.84^c \pm 0.03$	$5.78^c \pm 0.02$
Acid Booster (Agri-Nutrition, DeForest, WI); (phosphoric, citric, and lactic acids)	10 mg	20 mg	$5.84^c \pm 0.02$	$5.84^{cg} \pm 0.05$
KEMGEST (Kemin Agrifoods, Des Moines, IA); (phosphoric, fumaric, lactic, and citric acid)	10 mg	20 mg	$4.20^e \pm 0.03$	$3.98^e \pm 0.03$
Activate DA (Novus International, St. Charles, MO); (fumaric, benzoic, and 2-hydroxy-4-methylthiobutanoic acids)	20 mg	40 mg	$5.50^b \pm 0.03$	$5.11^b \pm 0.02$
Luprosil (Propionic acid, BASF, Florham Park, NJ); (99.5% propionic acid)	56 µl	112 µl	$5.74^d \pm 0.03$	$5.67^d \pm 0.03$
Amasil (Formic Acid, BASF, Florham Park, NJ); (61% formic acid, 20.5% sodium formate, 18.5% water)	46 µl	92 µl	$5.88^c \pm 0.03$	$5.88^{gh} \pm 0.01$
Sugar (Shoppers Value, Eden Prairie, MN); (sucrose)	20 mg	40 mg	$3.22^f \pm 0.04$	$2.93^f \pm 0.02$
Salt (Essential Every-day, Eden Prairie, MN); (sodium chloride)	20 mg	40 mg	$4.93^a \pm 0.05$	$4.39^a \pm 0.03$

[1]Results shown are means of three replications; different superscripts differ at ($P < 0.05$)

inoculated in swine testicular cells as previously described for virus titration. The amount of surviving virus was calculated and compared with that in control vials (no additive) and was expressed as $\log_{10}$ TCID$_{50}$/mL. All treatments were applied and analyzed in triplicate.

Measurement of pH
Fifty mL of distilled water was added to 5 g of feed contained in a 100 mL glass flask. The feed suspension was stirred at room temperature for 2 h using a magnetic stirrer. The pH was measured using a pH probe (Fisher Scientific, Waltham, MA) at 0, 15, 30, 60, and 120 min. The final pH value was calculated as the average of the values at different time intervals. The average pH for feed was 5.82 ± 0.02 and this value was used to compare the pH values after the addition of feed additives.

Mathematical models
Inactivation kinetics data (log TCID$_{50}$/mL) were analyzed by using GInaFIT software, a freeware add-on for Microsoft Excel (Microsoft, Redmond, WA) [9]. The traditional log-linear model developed by Bigelow and Esty (1920) was used to characterize the survival curves of PDCoV by using the following equation [10]:

$$\text{Log N} = \text{Log} N_0 - (k \times t) \tag{1}$$

where N is the amount of surviving virus after treatment, N_0 is the initial virus titer, k is the kinetic parameter (day^{-1}), and t is the treatment time (d). The kinetic parameter k is usually expressed as D, which is also known as 'decimal reduction time' (time required to

reduce initial virus titer by 90% or 1 log at a certain temperature) and was calculated as:

$$\text{D} = \frac{2.3}{k} \tag{2}$$

The Weibull distribution function has been used to describe non-linear inactivation patterns of different microorganisms after thermal and non-thermal processing. Assuming that the temperature resistance of the virus is governed by a Weibull distribution, Mafart et al. [11] developed the following equation [12]:

$$Log(N) = \log(N_0) - \left(\frac{t}{\delta}\right)^n \tag{3}$$

where N is the surviving virus titer after treatment, N_0 is the initial virus titer, δ is the time (min or days) of first logarithm decline in virus titer, and n is the shape parameter. The n value provides an indication of the shape of the response curve. If $n > 1$, the curve is convex (it forms a shoulder-shaped response), if $n < 1$, the curve is concave (it forms a tail-shaped response), and if $n = 1$, the curve is a straight line and can be described by a linear model.

Statistical analysis
Three replicates per treatment were used to determine how well the model fit the experimental data by calculating the Adj. R^2 defined as follows:

$$\text{Adj. } R^2 = \left[1 - \frac{(m-1)\left(1 - \frac{SSQregression}{SSQtotal}\right)}{m - j}\right] \tag{4}$$

where m is the number of observations, j is the number of model parameters, and SSQ is the sum of squares.

The effect of different additives on the kinetic parameters and survival of virus was assessed by using a mixed model (SAS, v9.3; SAS Inst. Inc., Cary, NC) that included the effect of additives and time as fixed effects and replicate/batch as random effects. Each vial was considered as the experimental unit. Data were analyzed for outliers and the presence of a normal distribution using the UNIVARIATE procedure of SAS that calls for calculations of sample moments, measurements of location and variability, standard deviation, test for normality, robust estimates on scale, missing values among others. The LSMEANS statement in SAS was used to calculate treatment means adjusted for model effects, while Tukey's test was used to determine differences among treatments. For this study, significance was considered when $P < 0.05$.

Results

Effect of additives on the survival of PDCoV in feed at their recommended concentrations

The goodness of model fit was analyzed by comparing the Adj. R^2 values from the log-linear and Weibull models. The Adj. R^2 values for the log-linear model (0.48–0.57) were less than those obtained for the Weibull model (0.86–0.93), indicating that the Weibull model provide a better fit of the experimental data (Table 2). This is explained mainly because the appearance of a resistant fraction of the virus that was able to survive longer than the length of the experiment (35 days). This residual survival produced long tails in the survival curves characterized by shape parameters (n) less than 1. This nonlinear behavior resulted in D-values that overestimated virus survival (14.13–15.52 days), while the delta values obtained with the Weibull model were between 0.86 and 1.72 days. Weibull prediction values showed much faster inactivation

kinetics and thus characterized better the virus survival curves.

In spite differences in virus inactivation kinetics, none of the additives appear to be effective in completely inactivating the virus. The total amount of virus inactivation over the sampling period of 35 days was 3 log reduction for the control sample and all the additives evaluated, indicating that none of the additives added at the manufacturers' recommend doses were effective in reducing PDCoV survival.

Effect of additives on the survival of PDCoV in feed at twice the recommended concentration

Doubling the concentrations of feed additives resulted in faster PDCoV inactivation kinetics (0.0004–0.28 days) for all additives, except for sucrose and formic acid (Table 3). UltraAcid P and KEMGEST provided faster initial virus inactivation kinetics than the other additives, and the delta values were estimated to be 35 s. However, most of the survival curves suggested that a large fraction of the virus remained resistant to the treatment with the appearance of tails (n values < 1) and a maximum inactivation degree achieved of 2 log after 10 days of storage. The addition of Luprosil (0.06 days), Acid Booster (0.28 days), and sodium chloride (0.09 days) resulted in the greatest virus inactivation with 2.3-3.0 log reduction after 10 days of storage at room temperature.

The pH of the complete feed without addition of acidifiers was greater than pH of the same complete feed with the addition of Luprosil, Activate DA, KEMGEST, Acid Booster, and Amasil. The pH of the complete feed with addition of UltraAcid P was not different from that of the complete feed. There was no correlation between the pH values of the diet with the addition of acidifiers and the inactivation kinetics of PDCoV (delta values; Fig. 1). Interestingly, the virus appeared to survive better at pH values lower than 3 and at pH 7 to 8.

Table 2 Kinetic parameters and correlation coefficients corresponding to the log-linear and Weibull models fitted to survival curves of Porcine Delta coronavirus (PDCoV) in complete feed and feed additives included at the manufacturers' recommended concentrations

Additive[1]	Log reduction (35 days)	Log-linear model		Weibull model		
		D-value	Adj R^2	Delta (days)	Shape parameter (n)	Adj R^2
Control	3.0	14.73 ± 1.04	0.55	0.86 ± 0.64	0.27	0.92
UltraAcid P	3.0	15.52 ± 2.09	0.48	0.62 ± 0.56	0.23	0.89
Acid Booster	3.0	14.41 ± 0.90	0.57	1.72 ± 1.85	0.32	0.86
KEMGEST	3.0	14.73 ± 1.04	0.55	0.86 ± 0.64	0.27	0.92
Activate DA	3.0	14.73 ± 1.04	0.55	0.86 ± 0.64	0.27	0.92
Luprosil	3.0	14.13 ± 0.90	0.55	1.00 ± 0.79	0.29	0.93
Formic Acid	3.0	14.73 ± 1.04	0.55	0.86 ± 0.64	0.27	0.92
Sugar	3.0	14.73 ± 1.04	0.55	0.86 ± 0.64	0.27	0.92
Salt	3.0	14.41 ± 0.90	0.57	1.70 ± 1.85	0.32	0.89

[1]UltraAcid P, (Nutriad, Dendermonde, Belgium), Activate DA (Novus International, St. Charles, MO), Acid Booster (Agri-Nutrition, DeForest, WI), Kemgest (Kemin Agrifoods, Des Moines, IA), Luprosil (BASF, Florham Park, NJ), and formic acid (BASF, Florham Park, NJ)

Table 3 Kinetic parameters and correlation coefficients corresponding to the Weibull model fitted to PDCoV survival curves in complete feed and feed additives that were added at twice the manufacturers recommended concentrations

Additive[1]	Log reduction (10 days)	Log-linear model		Weibull model		
		D-value[1]	Adj R^{2*}	Delta[2] (days)	Shape parameter (n)	Adj R^{2*}
Control	2.0	6.05 ± 0.00	0.46	0.35^{be} ± 0.00	0.23	0.86
UltraAcid P	2.0	7.42 ± 0.00	0.22	0.0004^{a} ± 0.00	0.05	0.99
Acid Booster	2.7	4.65 ± 1.24	0.59	0.28^{be} ± 0.18	0.27	0.93
KEMGEST	2.0	7.42 ± 0.00	0.22	0.0004^{a} ± 0.00	0.05	0.99
Activate DA	2.0	6.74 ± 0.60	0.18	0.12^{bd} ± 0.20	0.13	0.72
Luprosil	2.3	4.97 ± 2.40	0.27	0.06^{b} ± 0.03	0.13	0.69
Formic Acid	2.0	8.52 ± 0.00	0.08	4.95^{ac} ± 0.00	0.02	0.50
Sugar	2.0	10.00 ± 0.00	0.13	4.94^{ac} ± 0.00	0.07	0.17
Salt	3.0	4.41 ± 0.52	0.55	0.09^{bd} ± 0.02	0.22	0.91

[1]UltraAcid P, (Nutriad, Dendermonde, Belgium), Activate DA (Novus International, St. Charles, MO), Acid Booster (Agri-Nutrition, DeForest, WI), Kemgest (Kemin Agrifoods, Des Moines, IA), Luprosil (BASF, Florham Park, NJ), and formic acid (BASF, Florham Park, NJ)
[a, b, c, d]Means of 3 replications; different superscripts differ at ($P < 0.05$)
[e]Trend comparing 2× Acid Booster vs. control ($P < 0.1$)

Discussion

Organic, inorganic, or blends of acids are commonly added to swine feeds to control pathogens such as *Salmonella* spp. [13]. To our knowledge, this is the first study that has evaluated the impact of commercially available acids, sodium chloride, and sucrose on the survival of PDCoV in swine feed. When these commercial additives were added at the manufacturers' recommended doses, none of them were effective in decreasing survival of PDCoV, we had to add all acidifiers at twice the manufacturer recommended concentrations to observe inactivation of PDCoV in complete swine feed. In contrast, PEDV is inactivated by similar acidifiers at the manufacturers' recommended concentration; Activate DA (0.81 d) and KEMGEST (3.28 d) produced inactivation PEDV that was faster than inactivation in the control diet [14].

The current experiment focused on determining inactivation kinetics of commercial additives available to the United States feed industry, and did not focus on evaluating the specific active ingredients present in these additives that may inactivate PDCoV. However, based on the description and order of the active ingredients listed for each

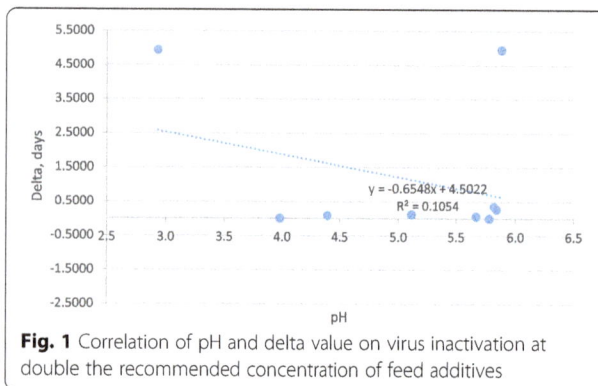

Fig. 1 Correlation of pH and delta value on virus inactivation at double the recommended concentration of feed additives

commercial additive, it appears that some form of phosphoric acid (pKa 6.9×10^{-3}) was present in UltraAcid P and KEMGEST, which suggests that this acid may be potentially responsible for inactivation of PDCoV. Phosphoric acid has been shown to inactivate pathogens such as *Salmonella* spp. on stainless steel surfaces, but there are no data available on inactivation of viruses in animal feed [15].

Inactivation of PDCoV was greater in the presence of KEMGEST than Acid Booster, but the active ingredients in these two feed additives are similar, with the exception of fumaric acid present in KEMGEST. Furthermore, fumaric acid was also present in UltraAcid P, which was also effective in rapidly inactivating PDCoV. Therefore, it is possible that fumaric acid in KEMGEST and UltraAcid P may be the primary component that causes PDCoV inactivation. Studies have shown that fumaric acid is an effective antimicrobial that reduces survivability of *E. coli* [16] and *Salmonella* spp. [17]. It is believed that changes in pH affect viruses by increasing sensitivity to deoxyriobonuclease [18] and by altering the virus capsid by the loss of structural proteins [18]. The RNA of RNA-containing viruses (such as PDCoV) is sensitive to ribonuclease at all pH levels tested (pH 3–9) [19]. At pH levels of 5 and 7, RNA was hydrolyzed and there was an absence of ribonuclease. There is no clear pattern or indication of a specific acid that inactivates PDCoV and more research is needed to depict the acid or combination of acid that can completely inactivate the virus.

Comparing data from this experiment with data on inactivation of PEDV, it appears that PDCoV is more labile than PEDV to environmental temperature and storage conditions because the delta values for PDCoV were, in general, much less (<2 d) than 17 days observed for PEDV [20]. Comparison of inactivation kinetics suggest that PEDV resists inactivation during feed storage to a greater extent than does PDCoV. There are limited data comparing the survival of enteric coronaviruses in the environment, but after the initial outbreak of each virus, PEDV infected more number of herds than PDCoV, this epidemiology and geographic distribution data suggest that PEDV survives longer than PDCoV and in agreement with observations of the current experiment [21, 22].

Addition of salt, but not sugar, to the control diet caused a decrease in delta values for inactivation of PDCoV. This observation is in agreement with inactivation of PEDV in complete swine feed, where adding both salt and sugar increased inactivation of PEDV [20]. Likewise, this observation is in agreement with results from an experiment that suggest that addition of phosphate supplemented salt mix to casting for sausage manufacturing increases inactivation of several viruses affecting swine such as Food and Mouth Disease Virus, Classical Swine Fever Virus, Swine Vesicular Disease Virus, and African Swine Fever Virus [23].

Conclusions

Using feed acidifiers could be an effective strategy to decrease the concentration of PDCoV in swine feed, but double the manufacturer's recommended concentration was required to observe an effect. Using feed acidifiers could be an effective strategy to decrease the concentration of PDCoV in swine feed, but double the manufacturer's recommended concentration was required to observe and effect. In spite the observed results on inactivation of PDCoV more experiments are needed to demonstrate the effectiveness of these treatments as means of preventing PDCoV transmission in feed on more applied settings. None of the treatments applied in this experiment were completely effective in inactivating PDCoV. Therefore, the strategy proposed in this research should be used in combination with other virus inactivation procedures within the processing and distribution steps for swine feed rather than a single kill step for virus inactivation.

Abbreviations
Adj. R^2: Adjusted coefficient of correlation; CP: Crude protein; DM: Dry matter; EE: Ether extract; PDCoV: Porcine delta coronavirus; PEDV: Porcine epidemic diarrhea virus; TCID: Tissue culture infectious dose

Acknowledgements
We thank Nhungoc Ti Luong for technical assistance in conducting this study.

Funding
We thank the National Pork Board for partial funding of this project and Cenex Harvest States for the fellowship provided to K.M. Cottingim.

Authors' contributions
KMC collected the data and wrote the manuscript, HV collected data and revised the manuscript, PEU designed the experiments, analyzed data and revised the manuscript, FS analyzed the data and revised the manuscript, GCS revised the manuscript, SMG designed the experiments, collected data, analyzed data, and revised the manuscript. All authors read and approved the manuscript.

Authors' information
SMG, HV, FS College of Veterinary Medicine, PEU, GCS, and KMC College of Food Agriculture, and Natural Resources Science at the University of Minnesota.

Competing interests
The authors declare that they have no competing interest.

Author details
[1]Department of Animal Science, University of Minnesota, St. Paul, MN 55108, USA. [2]Department of Veterinary Population Medicine, University of Minnesota, St. Paul, MN 55108, USA.

References
1. Saif LJ, Pensaert MB, Sestak K, Yeo S, Jung K. Coronaviruses. Diseases of Swine. Edited: Zimmerman JJ, Karriker LA, Ramirez A, Schwarts KJ, Stevenson GW. 2012, Wiley and Sons, Ames IA 501–524.
2. Dee S, Clement T, Schelkopf A, Nerem J, Knudsen D, Christopher-Hennings J, Nelson E. An evaluation of contaminated complete feed as a vehicle for porcine epidemic diarrhea virus infection of naive pigs following consumption via natural feeding behavior: proof of concept. BMC Vet Res. 2014;10:176.
3. Jacela JY, DeRouchey JM, Tokach MD, Goodband RD, Nelssen JL, Renter DG, Dritz SS. Peer r eviewed Practice t ip. Future. 2009;17:270–5.
4. Van Immerseel F, Cauwerts K, Devriese LA, Haesebrouck F, Ducatelle R. Feed additives to control Salmonella in poultry. Worlds Poult Sci J. 2002;58:501–13.
5. Koyuncu S, Andersson MG, Löfström C, Skandamis PN, Gounadaki A, Zentek J, Häggblom P. Organic acids for control of Salmonella in different feed materials. BMC Vet Res. 2013;9:81.
6. Tung CM, Pettigrew JE. Critical review of acidifiers. Rep NPB. 2008;5–169.
7. Karber G. 50% end-point calculation. Arch Exp Pathol Pharmak. 1931;162:480–3.
8. AOAC. Official Methods of Analysis of AOAC International. 2007.
9. Geeraerd AH, Valdramidis VP, Van Impe JF. GInaFiT, a freeware tool to assess non-log-linear microbial survivor curves. Int J Food Microbiol. 2005;102:95–105.
10. Bigelow WD. The logarithmic nature of thermal death time curves. J Infect Dis. 1921;528–536.
11. Mafart P, Couvert O, Gaillard S, Leguérinel I. On calculating sterility in thermal preservation methods: application of the Weibull frequency distribution model. Int J Food Microbiol. 2002;72(1):107–113.
12. Albert I, Mafart P. A modified Weibull model for bacterial inactivation. Int J Food Microbiol. 2005;100:197–211.
13. Juven BJ, Cox NA, Bailey JS, Thomson JE, Charles OW, Shutze JV. Survival of Salmonella in dry food and feed. J Food Prot. 1984;47:445–8.
14. Trudeau M, Verma H, Sampedro F, Urriola PE, Shurson GC, Goyal S. Survival and mitigation strategies of porcine epidemic diarrhea virus (PEDV) in complete feed. In: ADSA-ASAS 2015 Midwest Meeting. Asas. 2015.
15. Shen C, Luo Y, Nou X, Bauchan G, Zhou B, Wang Q, Millner P. Enhanced inactivation of Salmonella and Pseudomonas biofilms on stainless steel by use of T-128, a fresh-produce washing aid, in chlorinated wash solutions. Appl Environ Microbiol. 2012;78:6789–98.
16. Comes JE, Beelman RB. Addition of fumaric acid and sodium benzoate as an alternative method to achieve a 5-log reduction of Escherichia coli O157:H7 populations in apple cider. J Food Prot. 2002;65:476–83.
17. Kondo N, Murata M, Isshiki K. Efficiency of sodium hypochlorite, fumaric acid, and mild heat in killing native microflora and Escherichia coli O157: H7, Salmonella Typhimurium DT104, and Staphylococcus aureus attached to fresh-cut lettuce. J Food Prot. 2006;69:323–9.

18. Prage L, Pettersson U, Höglund S, Lonberg-Holm K, Philipson L. Structural proteins of adenoviruses: IV, Sequential degradation of the adenovirus type 2 virion. Virology. 1970;42:341–58.

19. Salo RJ, Cliver DO. Inactivation of enteroviruses by ascorbic acid and sodium bisulfite. Appl Environ Microbiol. 1978;36:68–75.

20. Trudeau MP, Verma H, Sampedro F, Urriola PE, Shurson GC, McKelvey J, Pillai SD, Goyal SM. Comparison of Thermal and Non-Thermal Processing of Swine Feed and the Use of Selected Feed Additives on Inactivation of Porcine Epidemic Diarrhea Virus (PEDV). PLoS One. 2016;11, e0158128.

21. USDA. Swine Enteric Coronavirus Disease (SECD) Situation Report - Oct 22. 2015. p. 1–18.

22. McCluskey BJ, Haley C, Rovira A, Main R, Zhang Y, Barder S. Retrospective testing and case series study of porcine delta coronavirus in U.S. swine herds. Prev Vet Med. 2016;123:185–91.

23. Wieringa-Jelsma T, Wijnker JJ, Zijlstra-Willems EM, Dekker A, Stockhofe-Zurwieden N, Maas R, Wisselink HJ. Virus inactivation by salt (NaCl) and phosphate supplemented salt in a 3D collagen matrix model for natural sausage casings. Int J Food Microbiol. 2011;148:128–34.

9

Surgical castration with pain relief affects the health and productive performance of pigs in the suckling period

Joaquin Morales[1]* , Andre Dereu[2], Alberto Manso[1], Laura de Frutos[1], Carlos Piñeiro[1], Edgar G. Manzanilla[3] and Niels Wuyts[2]

Abstract

Background: Surgical castration is still practiced in many EU countries to avoid undesirable aggressive behavior and boar taint in male pigs. However, evidence shows that castration is painful and has a detrimental influence on pig health. This study investigated the clinical and productive effects of surgical castration in the suckling period. A total of 3696 male pigs, 3 to 6 days old, comprising of 721 litters from two different farms were included in the study. Within each litter, half of the males were kept as intact males (IM) and half were surgically castrated (CM). Surgical castration was conducted by a trained farmer. Average daily gain (ADG), body weight at weaning (BWW), percentage of pre-weaning mortality (PWM) and antibiotic usage were measured. Pig major acute phase protein (PigMAP) serum concentrations were analyzed prior to castration, and on days 1 and 10 after castration. Productive performance data were analyzed using a linear mixed model. Mortality and percentage of pigs treated with antibiotics were analyzed using the Fisher's exact test.

Results: No overall differences in BWW and ADG were observed between the two groups. However, differences were observed when the same effects were analyzed in the 25% lightest, 50% medium and 25% heaviest pigs at birth. PWM was higher in CM than in IM groups (6.3% vs 3.6%; $p < 0.001$), especially in the light (12.2% vs 6.2%; $p = 0.02$) and in the medium (5.5% vs 2.7%; $p = 0.04$) weight groups. In the heaviest pigs group PWM was not affected by castration, but IM tended to show higher ADG ($p = 0.06$) and showed higher BWW (8.0 kg vs 7.8 kg; $p = 0.05$) than CM. There were no differences in percentage of pigs treated with antibiotics between the two groups (5.8% vs 5.8%; $p = 0.98$) in this study. Furthermore, PigMAP was increased in CM the day after castration (0.944 mg/ml vs 0.847 mg/ml; $p = 0.025$), but there was no difference between CM and IM groups at day 10.

Conclusions: Surgical castration has a negative impact on production in the suckling period because it causes an increase in PWM, especially in pigs in the three lower quartiles for body weight, and negatively affects the BWW in pigs born in the highest quartile for body weight.

Keywords: Boar breeding, Entire boars, Pre-weaning pig mortality, Stop castration, Suckling piglet, Surgical castration, Swine

* Correspondence: joaquin.morales@pigchamp-pro.com
[1]PigCHAMP Pro Europa S.L. c, Santa Catalina, 10, Segovia, Spain
Full list of author information is available at the end of the article

Background

Intact male pigs have better feed conversion and can have higher growth rates than surgically castrated pigs (barrows) [1]. However, in many countries, male pigs are routinely castrated to prevent boar taint that results from the presence of androstenone or skatole [2], and also to reduce undesirable aggressive and sexual behaviour following the onset of puberty [3, 4].

Current European legislation allows surgical castration up to an age of 7 days of age [5]. However, as castration of pigs is also a substantial animal welfare problem, European agreements specified that from 2012 onwards physical castration of pigs should be performed with prolonged analgesia and/or anesthesia and that it should be abandoned totally by 2018 [6]. Available evidence shows that castration is both painful and stressful for the animal during and for some time after the castration [7, 8]. Potential complications associated with surgical castration include hemorrhage, excessive swelling or edema and infection: these can reduce performance, compromise health and, in some cases, increase mortality. A meta-analysis of 15 studies in 2009 showed that male piglets that had been surgically castrated had significantly higher mortality rates than their intact littermates [9]. However, existing literature provides little consistent information about the effects of surgical castration on the timing and causes of mortality, the incidence of different disease problems and on how the growth rate of the castrated pigs is affected in the suckling period.

This study aims to evaluate the clinical and productive effects of surgical castration with pain relief in the suckling period and to describe the different causes of mortality associated with this surgical procedure.

Methods
Animals, facilities and experimental design

This research was carried out at two one-site commercial swine herd farms, located in Segovia, Spain. Both farms were farrow-to-finish farms and were located in the same geographical area, had the same genetic lines and feed provider and similar size (630 and 570 reproductive sows in Farm 1 and Farm 2, respectively). The experimental design was a randomized block design, including surgical castration as the main effect, resulting in two experimental treatment groups with surgically castrated males (CM) and male pigs kept as intact males (IM).

Any sows with a clinical history of high incidence of abortions, high percentage of stillborn or high percentage of pre-weaning mortality were excluded from the study. At day 107 of gestation sows were moved from the gestation barn to farrowing pens. In both farms, each farrowing pen had a partially slatted floor and a heat bulb for the piglets. A blank creep feed was offered from

day 14 of age to the piglets *ad libitum*. Following normal practice in both farms, teeth clipping and tail docking were performed on all piglets enrolled in this study before Study Day 0. Male pigs were individually identified by ear tagging, weighed and randomized on Study Day 0 (day 3 to 6 of life). Randomization was done within litter at individual animal level and based on body weight. A different randomization list was used for each litter. Directly after randomization piglets in CM group were surgically castrated. Cross-fostering was only allowed before Study Day 0. The study observations ended on weaning at 28 days of age of the piglets. Normal animal housing and management procedures usually employed on the farms were used throughout the experimental period and animals were managed in compliance with the European farm animal welfare regulations [5].

Surgical castration procedure

A non-steroidal anti-inflammatory drug (NSAID) (meloxicam; 0.4 mg meloxicam/kg body weight, Contacera®: Zoetis) was administered 30 min before castration to mitigate pain, following recommendations proposed by O'Connor *et al.* [10]. The use of NSAIDs was not a common practice in the two farms selected, but the study aimed to represent the 'best practice' as it should be applied according to the 2012 European agreement [6]. Farm workers, previously trained by a veterinarian in order to standardise the procedure between farms, performed the castration according to normal farm practice between days 3 and 6 of life. In brief, piglets were restrained by the farmer workers. Two vertical incisions were made in the scrotum and the testes were removed after tearing off the spermatic cord. After castration, a topical antibiotic was administered on the injury area (oxytetracycline; Tenicol spray: MSD) for 5 s. Routine use of an antibiotic spray was used in this study in order to ensure optimal post-surgical recovering in the castrated group.

Observations and measurements

A general physical examination was performed for all enrolled pigs on Study Day 0. Body weight was measured from all piglets on Study Day 0 (3–6 days of age) and at weaning (28 days of age), and average daily gain (ADG) in the study period was calculated. Daily general health observations were carried out by the farm workers and ill or injured piglets were promptly examined and treated by the veterinarian. For all treatments the following information was recorded: animal identification, date, product used, dose, frequency, as well as reason for treatment (the routine use of the post castration antibiotic spray was not recorded or analysed as a treatment in the study observation period). In addition, for any piglet found dead or euthanized on welfare grounds during the study, a necropsy was conducted and the reason for death was recorded. Piglets in very poor health were removed from the study and placed with a nurse sow to give them a chance to recover. All adverse health observations were recorded. The different reasons for mortality or removals were listed as deaths associated to complications following the surgical castration procedure, meningitis, diarrhoea, runt piglets and other causes that could be related to post-castration complications. Meningitis was assigned to piglets that showed nervous signs (leaning head, pedaling and convulsions) before death or sudden deaths. Diarrhoea was assigned to piglets showing liquid faeces, dehydration, and poor body condition before death. Runt piglets were piglets which showed poor body condition and cachexia as the only clinical signs before death. All other minor causes of death or removal (e.g. dermatitis) were classified as 'other'.

Different reasons for antibiotic treatment interventions were classified as diarrhoea, dermatitis, runt piglets, meningitis, respiratory signs (coughing, rapid breathing, discharges from the eyes-conjunctivitis, sneezes, etc) and lameness (arthritis).

An acute phase-protein, PigMAP (Major Acute Phase-protein of Pigs), was used as an unspecific biomarker to quantify inflammation and/or stress. Fifty litters from Farm 1 and 40 litters from Farm 2 were randomly selected using a random number table for blood sampling. In each of these 90 litters, two piglets (1 CM and 1 IM) were also randomly selected (180 piglets in total; 100 in Farm 1 and 80 in Farm 2) and were blood sampled by venopunction of the vena cava on day 0 (before castration), day 1 (the day after castration) and day 10. Serum was immediately removed after centrifugation at 3500 g for 5 min, and kept frozen (–20 °C) until their analysis. PigMAP concentration in serum was measured by sandwich ELISA with two monoclonal antibodies, using a commercial kit (pigMAP kit ELISA, Acuvet biotech, Zaragoza, Spain) as described earlier [11].

Statistical analysis

All treatment differences were assessed at the 2-sided 0.05 alpha level of significance and trends were reported for alpha = 0.10. In all cases of an interaction with $p < 0.10$, the interaction was studied. Multiple comparisons were adjusted using Tukey's correction.

Piglets were classified based on their weight at day 0 in quartiles: light (25% lightest pigs), medium and heavy (25% heaviest pigs). The primary variables average weight at weaning and ADG were analyzed using a general linear model (proc GLM) including treatment, parity, farm and body weight group (light, medium, heavy) and all their second degree interactions as fixed factors.

PigMAP serum concentrations were analyzed using a linear mixed model (proc MIXED) with the fixed effects of treatment, parity, farm and second degree interactions effect.

Data on casualties and medication was analyzed using generalized linear models (proc GLIMMIX) including treatment, parity, farm, body weight group and all their second level interactions as fixed factors. When the frequency of events (casualties or medication) observed was 0 in any level of the independent variables (treatment, BW group or their interaction), the model did not converge, and the analysis was done using Fisher's exact test.

All statistical analyses were carried out using SAS version 9.4.

Results

A total of 3696 crossbred (Large White & Landrace x Pietrain) male pigs from 721 litters were included in the study. In Farm 1, a total of 1950 piglets from 363 litters and in Farm 2, 1746 piglets from 358 litters were included in the study. A total of 1848 piglets were assigned to each treatment group (IM, CM).

Productive performance (Table 1) showed an interaction between surgical castration and weight group (body weight at weaning, $p = 0.084$). Castration did not affect performance of light or medium piglets but heavy CM animals tended to have a lower ADG ($p = 0.059$) and had a lower body weight at weaning ($p = 0.05$). Pre-weaning mortality (Table 2) also showed an interaction between surgical castration and weight group ($p = 0.063$). Mortality was almost double for light ($p = 0.017$) and medium ($p = 0.041$) weight CM piglets but was not different for heavy CM animals ($p = 0.327$). No other variable or interaction affected productive performance or pre-weaning mortality.

The percentages for different causes of death are presented in Fig. 1. Percentage of mortality associated with the procedure of castration, with meningitis and losses of runt piglets were higher in CM than in IM group. In total 17 CM piglets died due to castration: 4 of them had a non-detected testicular hernia and died during the surgical procedure; 3 piglets died within 1 h after the surgical procedure showing an haemorrhage in the wound area and the other 10 died within 5 days after the procedure of castration showing an infection in the surgical area. No differences between CM and IM were observed in the other reasons of mortality or removal. Odds ratios for mortality were 2.3 (1.1, 4.8) for meningitis and 2.8 (1.3, 6.0) for runt pigs, when surgical castration was applied. Body weight group affected mortality associated to castration (0.75, 0.54 and 0.00% for light, medium and heavy piglets respectively; $p = 0.021$),

Table 1 Effect of surgical castration on growth rate in the suckling period by initial body weight group[a]

Item	Intact Males	Castrated Males	SEM[b]	P value[3]
Light pigs				
Initial number of pigs	476	459		
Body weight, day 0 (kg)	1.43	1.42	0.008	0.528
Body weight, day 28 (kg)	5.69	5.77	0.062	0.367
Average daily gain (g/day)	182.3	185.5	2.648	0.379
Medium pigs				
Initial number of pigs	921	931		
Body weight, day 0 (kg)	1.96	1.97	0.006	0.226
Body weight, day 28 (kg)	6.83	6.79	0.041	0.540
Average daily gain (g/day)	210.0	208.5	1.768	0.535
Heavy pigs				
Initial number of pigs	451	458		
Body weight, day 0 (kg)	2.55	2.57	0.012	0.388
Body weight, day 28 (kg)	7.97	7.81	0.063	0.050
Average daily gain (g/day)	237.4	230.4	2.615	0.059

[a]Pigs were split in three groups according to their initial body weight: light pigs (25% pigs with the lightest initial body weight), medium pigs (50% pigs with medium initial body weight) and heavy pigs (25% pigs with the heaviest initial body weight)
[b]Standard Error of Mean
[3]P-value for surgical castration treatment effect (Intact vs. Castrated male pigs) obtained by multiple comparisons using Tukey's correction

crushing (2.78, 1.03 and 0.77%; $p = 0.002$), and meningitis (1.60, 0.76, 0.33%; $p = 0.012$).

No differences in antibiotic treatment due to castration were observed in this study. Highest frequency of antibiotic treatment was to treat diarrhoea (4.20%) followed by treatment of meningitis (0.98%). Body weight group affected antibiotic treatment for meningitis (2.99, 1.46 and 0.66% for light, medium and heavy piglets respectively; $p = 0.002$).

PigMAP serum concentration was significantly higher in CM than in IM groups the day after castration, and these differences disappeared by day 10 (Table 3).

Discussion

Castration is a surgical procedure commonly performed in non-optimal hygiene conditions on 3–6 days-old piglets and results in open wounds. Until now, very little research quantifying the health and performance impact of castration on male piglets, especially in the suckling period, has been published.

In the present study, castration was conducted under commercial conditions by two experienced farmers. In brief, meloxicam was administered about 30 min prior to castration in male pigs in CM group, and a topical antibiotic was applied on the injury wounds after castration. No other manipulations were imposed, to replicate commercial situations as much as possible. Under these conditions, surgical castration almost doubled the percentage of pre-weaning mortality, mainly associated with runting of affected piglets, with fatal meningitis, and with the intra- and the post-surgery mortality. Most studies evaluating the consequences of castration rarely mention pre-weaning mortality [12], suggesting that there is no effect. However, analysis of data from commercial herds shows that poor hygiene at castration could promote the occurrence of arthritis, which itself may result in death of piglets [13]. In another study, a lower antibody response to an immune challenge in castrated piglets compared to entire piglets was observed [14], probably attributable to the stress reaction, which

Table 2 Effect of surgical castration on percentage of mortality in the suckling period by initial body weight group[a]

Item	Intact Males (%)	Castrated Males (%)	Odds ratio[b] (95% CI)	P value[3]
Light	6.3	12.2	2.2 (1.09, 4.25)	0.017
Medium	2.7	5.5	2.1 (1.02, 4.22)	0.041
Heavy	2.4	1.5	0.6 (0.15, 2.51)	0.327

[a]Pigs were split in three groups according to their initial body weight: light pigs (25% pigs with the lightest initial body weight), medium pigs (50% pigs with medium initial body weight) and heavy pigs (25% pigs with the heaviest initial body weight)
[b]Odds ratio of death
[3]P-value for surgical castration treatment effect (Intact vs. Castrated male pigs) obtained by multiple comparisons and using Tukey's correction

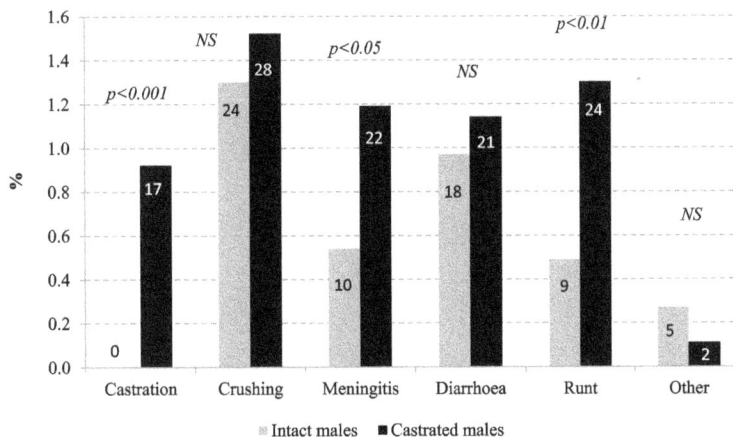

Fig. 1 Different reasons of losses in intact and in castrated male pigs during the suckling period in percent. Number of cases is detailed in each column

could explain the higher mortality. In our study, Pig-MAP serum concentration was significantly higher in CM than in IM the day after castration, confirming that physical castration causes tissue damage, inflammation and stress. This result is in accordance with a previous study [15], where a significant increase of haptoglobin serum concentration, another acute phase protein, 24 h after physical castration was also observed, likely associated with stress or with an inflammatory process. Since in this study most antibiotic interventions were not specific to castration, it was not possible to make an assessment about antibiotic usage as a result of castration or non-castration. Furthermore, it should be noted that all piglets in the CM group received a topical antibiotic (spray) as a post-surgery prophylactic measure.

Castration reduces undesirable aggressive and sexual behaviors, but it also stimulates fat deposition and has a negative effect on feed conversion [12]. In another study, a decrease in the growth rate of piglets was observed only in the days following surgery when it was carried out shortly after birth (3 days) [16]. These differences in weight gain had disappeared by weaning, as was also observed in the present study, prompting the conclusion that castration does not have long-term implications in

the suckling period. However, taking into account our observation that the mortality rate was almost double in CM group compared to the IM group, an alternative explanation is more likely: i.e. that there is a disproportional impact on weakest pigs (those with lowest bodyweight) in the CM group with higher mortality whilst in the IM group the survival rate of these low weight piglets was higher. The mean growth performance picture in the whole group obscures the effect of these opposite interactions.

Reduced health recovery may be related to less time nursing and more time lying down of castrated pigs [17]. Adequate colostrum intake and regular consumption of milk are required for control of gastro-intestinal diseases, hypoglycemia, starvation, and crushing of the pre-weaned pig [18]. In addition, lightweight pigs are most susceptible to diseases [19, 20], which was confirmed by the results of the present study. This observation is especially important in the current status of the swine industry, where selection for maximum prolificacy has resulted in an increase in litter size and more piglets weaned per litter. This rapid increase in litter size has resulted in an increase of light-birth-weight piglets [21], thus exacerbating the (negative) effects of castration as a critical management parameter. Moreover, in the group of pigs with the heaviest birth weight, even if surgical castration did not result in higher mortality, it compromised growth rates to weaning. This observation could be associated with stress and discomfort promoted by the castration procedure, affecting milk consumption. As a consequence of both higher mortality rate in the light pigs and poorer growth performance in the heavy pigs, surgical castration applied in 3 to 6 days of age male piglets has a negative impact on health, performance and economic production cost in the suckling period.

Table 3 Effect of surgical castration on PigMAP[a] serum concentration (mg/ml) at three different study days

Item	Intact Males	Castrated Males	SEM[b]	P value
Day 0	0.903	0.841	0.032	0.167
Day 1	0.847	0.944	0.030	0.025
Day 10	0.990	0.902	0.073	0.392

[a]Pig major acute phase protein
[b]Standard Error of Mean
Day 0 = sampling before castration, day 1 = 1 day after castration, and day 10 = 10 days after castration in castrated males. In intact male piglets, the days correspond to the intervention in their litter mates

Conclusions

Surgical castration promotes productive losses in the suckling period by causing an increase in pre-weaning mortality in pigs born with the lowest body weights, and negatively affects growth rate and weaning body weight in pigs born with highest body weights. Main causes of mortality related to surgical castration were runt pigs, meningitis and the surgical and post-surgical complications of the castration procedure.

Abbreviations

ADG: Average daily gain; BWW: Body weight at weaning; CM: Surgically castrated male pigs; IM: Intact male pigs; PigMAP: Pig major acute phase protein; PWM: Pre-weaning mortality

Acknowledgements

The farmers and their stockmen are greatly acknowledged for agreeing to engage in the trial and for working in good cooperation with the investigation team.

Funding

Zoetis Inc. funded the study.

Authors' contributions

JM was investigator of the study and wrote the manuscript; AD monitored the study and participated in the experimental design of the study; AM was Clinical Research Manager; LF participated in animal manipulations and data collection; CP participated in the experimental design and in the discussion of results; EM performed the statistical study and reviewed the manuscript; NW participated in the experimental design, reviewed the manuscript and wrote the conclusion. All authors read and approved the final manuscript.

Competing interests

AD and NW are employees from the company sponsor.

Author details

[1]PigCHAMP Pro Europa S.L. c, Santa Catalina, 10, Segovia, Spain. [2]Zoetis Inc, Hoge Wei 10, 1930 Zaventem, Belgium. [3]Teagasc, Pig Development Department, Moorepark, Fermoy, Co Cork, Ireland.

References

1. Bonneau M. Use of entire males for pig meat in the European Union. Meat Sci. 1998;49:S257–72.
2. Zamaratskaia G, Squires EJ. Biochemical, nutritional and genetic effects on boar taint in entire male pigs. Animal. 2009;3:1508–21.
3. Cronin GM, Dunshea FR, Butler KL, McCauly I, Barnett JL, Hemsworth PH. The effects of immune- and surgical castration on the behaviour and consequently growth of group-housed, male finisher pigs. Appl Anim Behav Sci. 2010;81:111–26.
4. Rydhmer L, Lundström K, Andersson K. Inmunocastration reduces aggressive and sexual behaviour in male pigs. Animal. 2010;4:965–72.
5. European Union. Council Directive 2008/120/EC of 18 December 2008 laying down minimum standards for the protection of pigs. OJ L 47, 18.2.2009.
6. European Commission. European Declaration on alternatives to surgical castration of pigs. https://ec.europa.eu/food/sites/food/files/animals/docs/aw_prac_farm_pigs_cast-alt_declaration_en.pdf. Accessed 19 May 2017.
7. Hay M, Vulin A, Genin S, Sales P, Prunier A. Assessment of pain induced by castration in piglets: behavioral and physiological responses over the subsequent 5 days. Appl Anim Behav Sci. 2003;82:201–18.
8. Kluivers-Poodt M, Houx BB, Robben SRM, Koop G, Lambooij E, Hellebrekers LJ. Effects of a local anaesthetic and NSAID in castration of piglets, on the acute pain responses, growth and mortality. Animal. 2012;6:1469–75.
9. Allison J, Pearce M, Brock F, Crane JA. 2010. A comparison of mortality (animal withdrawal) rates in male fattening pigs reared using either physical castration or vaccination with Improvac® as the method to reduce boar taint. Proc. 21st IPVS Congress, Vancouver, Canada. July 18-21. 2010, p. 1139.
10. O'Connor A, Anthony R, Bergamasco L, Coetzee J, Gould S, Johnson AK, Karriker LA, Marchant-Forde JN, Martineau GS, McKean J, Millman ST, Niekamp S, Pajor EA, Rutherford K, Sprague M, Sutherland M, von Borell E, Dzikamunhenga RS. Pain management in the neonatal piglet during routine management procedures. Part 2: Grading the quality of evidence and the strength of recommendations. Anim Health Res Rev. 2014;15:39–62.
11. Piñeiro M, Lampreave F, Alava MA. Development and validation of an ELISA for the quantification of pig major acute phase protein (Pig-MAP). Vet Immunol Immunop. 2009;127:228–34.
12. Prunier A, Bonneau M, von Borell EH, Cinotti S, Gunn M, Fredriksen B, Giersing M, Morton DB, Tuyttens FAM, Velarde A. A review of the welfare consequences of surgical castration in piglets and the evaluation of non-surgical methods. Anim Welf. 2006;15:277–89.
13. Strom I. Arthritis in piglets. Dansk Veterinaertidsskrift. 1996;79:575–7.
14. Lessard M, Taylor AA, Braithwaite L, Weary DM. Humoral and cellular immune responses of piglets after castration at different ages. Can J Anim Sci. 2002;82:519–26.
15. Lackner A, Goller K, Ritzmann M, Heinritzi K. 2002. Acute phase proteins in castration of piglets. Proc. 17th IPVS Congress, Ames, IA, USA. June 2-5. 2002, Vol 2 p. 253.
16. Kielly J, Dewey CE, Cochran M. Castration at 3 days of age temporarily slows growth of pigs. Swine Health Prod. 1999;7:151–3.
17. McGlone JJ, Nicholson RI, Hellman JM, Herzog DN. The development of pain in young pigs associated with castration and attempts to prevent castration: Induced behavioral changes. J Anim Sci. 1993;71:1441–6.
18. Roy B, Kumar A, Lakhani GP, Jain A. Causes of pre-weaning mortality in India. Schol J Agric Sci. 2014;4:485–93.
19. Beaulieu AD, Aalhus JL, Williams N, Patience JF. Impact of piglet birth weight, birth order, and litter size on subsequent growth performance, carcass quality, muscle composition, and eating quality of pork. J Anim Sci. 2010;88:2767–78.
20. Fix JS, Cassady JP, Holl JW, Herring WO, Cusbertson MS, See MT. Effect of piglets birth weight on survival and quality of commercial market swine. Livest Sci. 2010;132:98–106.
21. Bérard J, Kreuzer M, Bee G. Effect of litter size and birth weight on growth, carcass and pork quality, and their relationship to postmortem proteolysis. J Anim Sci. 2008;86:2357–68.

10

Production results from piglets vaccinated in a field study in Spain with a Type 1 Porcine Respiratory and Reproductive virus modified live vaccine

Guillermo Cano[1*], Marcia Oliveira Cavalcanti[2], Francois-Xavier Orveillon[3], Jeremy Kroll[4], Oliver Gomez-Duran[3], Alberto Morillo[1] and Christian Kraft[2]

Abstract

Background: PRRS is a viral disease of pigs and sows that is one of the most costly to the pig industry worldwide. The disease can be controlled by focusing on different aspects. One of them is the vaccination of piglets, which is more controversial and difficult to manage than the vaccination of sows. However, pig producers could consider a piglet vaccination strategy if it reduces the negative clinical disease and improves zootechnical performance, decreases the probability to be infected and/or reduces the spread of the virus once the vaccinated piglet is infected. The efficacy of a novel PRRS modified live vaccine (Ingelvac PRRSFLEX® EU) was studied in a blinded, side-by-side placebo controlled field study of piglet vaccination including piglets weaned for three consecutive weeks (week groups 1, 2 and 3).

Results: This study established that PRRS piglet vaccination resulted in significantly better weight gain, seen as early as 4 weeks after vaccination, in naturally challenged pigs. Vaccine efficacy was supported by statistically significant increases in Average Daily Weight Gain (ADWG) among week group 3 vaccinated pigs from vaccination to the end of the study and statistically significant increases in bodyweight and ADWG from inclusion to 10 weeks of age in week group 2 vaccinated piglets. However, no differences were noted in week group 1 presumably because more than 30 % of the vaccinated pigs were viremic at the time of vaccination. Furthermore, the proportion of pigs showing any abnormal clinical sign at least once at any of the examination time points was lower in vaccinated pigs than in control pigs. Based on the viremia results (qPCR), early onset of PRRS was detected in this herd. Viremia occurred at the time of vaccination in week group 1 and shortly after vaccination in week groups 2 and 3. Peak wild type PRRSV infection was assumed at 4 weeks post vaccination in all groups based on the number of PRRS positive pigs in the control groups.

Conclusion: This study establishes that vaccination of piglets with Ingelvac PRRSFLEX® EU at 4 weeks of age improves weight gain and reduces the appearance of clinical sings during the growing period, even when the piglets are infected shortly after vaccination.

Keywords: PRRSV, Piglets, Vaccination, Average daily weight gain

* Correspondence: gcano@testsandtrial.com
[1]Tests and Trials S.L., Monzon, Spain
Full list of author information is available at the end of the article

Background

Porcine Reproductive and Respiratory Syndrome (PRRS) is a viral disease of pigs and sows that is one of the most costly to the pig industry worldwide. Nieuwenhuis et al. [1] have calculated a decrease of 1.7 pigs sold per sow during the outbreak period in The Netherlands while in North America 1.44 weaned pigs per sow/year were lost to PRRS [2]. Increasing costs of PRRS between 2005 and 2010 were estimated between 3 and 109 € per sow in Europe [1] and at 2.36$ per pig weaned in US [2].

The disease can be controlled by focusing on different management aspects. Different strategies must be taken into account by veterinarians once a herd has become infected and often include: the fast and reliable diagnosis of an outbreak, internal and external biosecurity measures, control of secondary infections and immunization.

Nowadays, live attenuated and inactivated vaccines are available globally. Also strategies of injections with serum containing live PRRS virus (PRRSV), so called Live Virus Inoculation (LVI) have been used to consistently expose the sow herd [3] but neither of them, vaccines or LVI inoculation are considered to have a high efficacy specially when applied to piglets [4, 5]. Due to the high genetic variability of the virus [6, 7] almost all the infections in the field can be considered as heterologous to existing vaccines [8].

The vaccination of piglets is more controversial among European Veterinarians and difficult to manage (timing and compliance) than the vaccination of sows due to the fact that i) if naïve piglets are infected with genotype 1 PRRSV, the clinical signs of the respiratory disease are not always evident [9], ii) because there is frequent interaction with other pathogens which affects the clinical expression of the symptoms [10] and iii) if the proportion of viremic piglets after weaning is high, the time needed to generate an effective immunity is probably longer than the infection time [11].

Piglet vaccination strategies could be taken into account by the producers if i) the vaccination of piglets decreases the probability to be infected and/or ii) if the vaccination of piglets reduces the spread of the virus once the vaccinated piglet is infected.

Average daily gain and mortality are the performance variables most affected by PRRSV status of piglets [2]. Neither feed conversion rate nor the percentage of pigs sold to the primary market are commonly affected by the PRRSV status of piglets in outbreaks with type 1 virus [2] even though in some cases differences in feed conversion rate has been found [12].

The present study was designed to investigate the efficacy of Ingelvac PRRSFLEX® EU vaccine in 4 week old piglets under field conditions to prevent the productive and clinical effects caused by PRRSV. Primary parameters of vaccine efficacy were the productive performance based on the Bodyweight (BW) and the Average Daily Weight Gain (ADWG). Secondary parameters investigated were viremia, serological response, mortality, clinical signs and concomitant treatments.

Methods
Animals and experimental design

The study was performed under normal husbandry field conditions according to Good Clinical Practice (GCP VICH GL9) in two treatment groups. The trial was designed as a randomized, blinded and included an unvaccinated negative control group of piglets. The treatment group received a single intramuscular administration of Ingelvac PRRSFLEX® EU vaccine (PRRS 94881 Modified Live Virus (MLV; vaccinated group) at the minimum titer level indicated for use, while the other group received 1 mL of Phosphate Buffered Saline (PBS) intramuscularly as a negative control group (unvaccinated group). The primary efficacy parameter was weight gain and was compared between vaccinated and unvaccinated pigs. Secondary parameters of the study were mortality, viremia, serology and clinical signs.

A total of 1364 commercial crossbreed pigs (healthy by clinical observation) were included in the study at 4 weeks of age and were distributed to two treatment groups: 690 pigs were administered Ingelvac PRRSFLEX® EU (vaccinated pigs) and 674 pigs a PBS solution (unvaccinated pigs). Three replicates of vaccinated and unvaccinated pigs were included in the study in consecutive weeks: 224, 230 and 236 vaccinated pigs were included in the first Week Group (WG 1), the second Week Group (WG 2) and the third Week Group (WG 3), respectively, and 214, 226 and 234 unvaccinated pigs in WG 1, WG 2 and WG 3, respectively. Study pigs were weaned at 3 weeks of age from the same sow farm. Treatment groups were balanced by sex and initial bodyweight within each replication group. The animal phase finished at the end of the fattening period that was considered when the first pig from each replicate group was ready to go to slaughter.

The selected farm had a previous history of PRRS infection with clinical signs in grower-finisher pigs and was confirmed in a herd pre-screening with PRRSV serology and quantitative Polymerase Chain Reaction (qPCR). Positive qPCR samples were sequenced (Open Reading Frame (ORF) 5) to ensure a heterologous field challenge. In addition, animals were tested for *Actinobacillus pleuropneumoniae* (APP), Swine Influenza Virus (SIV) and Porcines Circovirus Type 2 (PCV2). Sows from the breeding herd were vaccinated with a commercial live attenuated PRRSV vaccine; therefore, seropositive pigs born from vaccinated sows were included in the study. Pigs were fed a commercial ration appropriate for their age and weight. Feed and water were available ad libitum.

All study pigs were housed in barns appropriate for their breed and age, and were kept under similar conditions of climate, air quality, ventilation, temperature, air humidity and light. In the post-weaning facilities, pigs from the week groups were distributed in different rooms. WG 1 in rooms 1, 2, 7 and 8; WG 2 in rooms 3, 4, 5 and 6 and WG 3 in rooms 1, 2, 9 and 10 (see Fig. 1). Piglets of different WG in the same room were kept in separate pens. Vaccinated pigs were housed separately from the unvaccinated pigs until entry into fattening. Due to the different sizes of rooms, the randomization of the rooms to the treatment groups was done considering the room effect. Cross-contamination was prevented by strict biosecurity rules implemented on the farm for the duration of the study. In the fattening facilities, vaccinated and unvaccinated pigs were commingled and distributed in three buildings.

Pigs were individually weighed at four time points: at vaccination prior to administration of Ingelvac PRRSFLEX® EU or PBS, at 4 weeks post-vaccination, at the beginning of fattening (10 weeks post-vaccination) and at the end of the study. For WG1 and WG2, the end of the study was at 17 weeks post-vaccination and for WG 3 at 16 weeks post-vaccination. ADWG for the intervals between weighing at vaccination and weighing at 4, 10 and 16–17 weeks post-vaccination were calculated for each pig individually. Homogeneity of the BW at the end of the study was calculated from Coefficient of Variation (1-CV) for every group and within week group.

Mortality was recorded throughout the study for calculation of the mortality rate. Furthermore, study pigs were clinically examined at weeks 4, 10, 14 and 16 or 17 post-vaccination. Special attention was given to the respiratory signs (dyspnea, cough) and apathy, but skin alterations (petechiae, crust, anemia or icterus), joint disorders and diarrhea were also recorded. Collective and individual treatments were also recorded throughout the study.

Collection and processing of samples
Blood samples were collected from 73 vaccinated (24, 23 and 26 in WG 1, WG 2 and WG 3, respectively) pigs and 69 unvaccinated pigs (22, 24 and 23 in WG 1, WG 2 and WG 3, respectively). In each pen, at least one pig of middle weight was chosen to be bled at vaccination time. Blood samples were drawn prior to administration

of Ingelvac PRRSFLEX® EU or PBS. Additional blood samples were collected from the same pigs at 4, 10, 14 and 16 or 17 weeks after vaccination. Blood samples were collected by jugular *venipuncture using 4 mL dry vacuum tubes* and were processed within 24 h after collection in order to obtain serum by centrifugation at 3000 rpm during 10 min. Serum samples were stored frozen at –80 °C until the end of the study. Then, the serum samples were sent to Boehringer Ingelheim Veterinary Research Center GmbH & Co. KG to be tested for PRRS antibodies by ELISA (HerdChek PRRS X3 Antibody Test Kit,IDEXX Laboratories, Inc.), and detection of PRRSV-EU specific RNA via real-time reverse transcription PCR. Proportions of positive animals were calculated per time point of examination.

Vaccine and placebo product description
Piglets were vaccinated intramuscularly in the neck with one dose (1 ml) of Ingelvac PRRSFLEX® EU vaccine with a minimum titer as indicated on the vaccine label instructions at 4-weeks of age. Control animals were administered one dose of vaccine corresponding solvent (PBS) without vaccine content. No other vaccinations or treatments were administered to the animals on at least 3 days before and after the PRRS vaccine treatment.

Data analysis
Statistical analysis was performed with R software [13]. All tests were designed as two-sided tests and differences were considered as statistically significant if $p \leq 0.05$ For BW and ADWG, differences between treatment groups were tested using analysis of variance and subsequent t-tests. Treatment group (PRRS 94881 MLV or PBS), week group (WG 1, WG 2 or WG 3), their interaction (Group*WG) and sex (male or female) were included as factors in the statistical model. The initial weight (BW at vaccination time) was used as covariate for all post-treatment time points and for all periods. Least squares means of the groups and differences between least squares means with 95 % Confidence Intervals (95 % CI) were calculated from the analysis of variance. Homogeneity at final BW was tested comparing variances of BW at the end of the study using a Fisher's test. Differences in proportions (qPCR positive, ELISA positive, mortality rate, clinical observations and concomitant treatments) between the treatment groups were tested by Fisher's

Unvaccinated pigs	Vaccinated pigs	Unvaccinated pigs	Unvaccinated pigs	Vaccinated pigs	Vaccinated pigs	Vaccinated pigs	Unvaccinated pigs	Unvaccinated pigs	Vaccinated pigs
Room 1	Room 2	Room 3	Room 4	Room 5	Room 6	Room 7	Room 8	Room 9	Room 10
WG1 WG3	WG1 WG3	WG 2	WG 2	WG 2	WG 2	WG 1	WG 1	WG 3	WG 3

Fig. 1 Layout of the pigs at weaning

exact test. Wilson's confidence interval for a single proportion was also calculated for every proportion.

Results

The farm showed a high degree of PRRSV positive animals in a pre-screening before the study started. Positive qPCR samples were sequenced (ORF 5, see Additional file 1) and results showed identities of 88.94, 88.45 and 92.74 % to Lelystad virus (GenBank Accession Number: M96262), Porcilis® PRRS (the PRRSV isolate of the commercial live attenuated PRRS virus vaccine used in sows; GenBank Accession Number: KJ127878) and Ingelvac PRRSFLEX® EU (GenBank Accession Number: KT988004), respectively. Moreover, the pre-screening revealed pigs were positive for APP, SIV and PCV2 antibodies.

BW and ADWG from vaccinated and unvaccinated pigs are shown in Table 1. Vaccinated pigs showed better growth parameters than unvaccinated pigs at 10 weeks after vaccination. Nevertheless, looking at the 3 week groups separately, there were differences ($p < 0.05$) between vaccinated and unvaccinated pigs in WG 2 and WG 3 but not in WG 1 (Table 1).

The BW of vaccinated pigs from WG 2 at 4 and 10 weeks after vaccination was higher ($p < 0.05$) than unvaccinated pigs within the same WG. ADGW increased from vaccination to 4 and 10 weeks after vaccination ($p < 0.05$; Table 1).

The BW in WG 3 of vaccinated pigs was higher ($p < 0.05$) at week 16 after vaccination and ADWG increased from vaccination to 16 weeks after vaccination ($p < 0.05$; Table 1).

The BW uniformity at the end of fattening was better in vaccinated pigs than in unvaccinated ($p < 0.05$; Table 1). Taking into account week groups separately, the BW uniformity of vaccinated pigs improved only in WG 3 ($p < 0.05$; Table 1) and there were not differences between groups ($p > 0.05$) in WG 1 and WG 2.

Percentage of PRRSV RNA positive pigs by qPCR throughout the study is shown in Figs. 2 and 3 for vaccinated and unvaccinated pigs. Peak of viremia with 80 % (68–88; 95 % CI) of vaccinated pigs and 83 % (72–91 %; 95 % CI) of unvaccinated pigs tested positive was at 4 weeks after vaccination. For all the time points, no differences were observed in the prevalence of viremic animals between vaccinated and unvaccinated pigs. For pigs in WG1, the PRRSV field infection was on-going at vaccination time with 38 % (19–59 %; 95 % CI) of vaccinated pigs and 27 % (11–50 %; 95 % CI) of unvaccinated

Table 1 Bodyweight (BW) and average daily weight gain (ADWG) at different observation periods. Least square mean ± standard error

Parameter	Week Group 1 + 2 + 3		Week Group 1		Week Group 2		Week Group 3	
	Unvaccinated pigs	Vaccinated pigs	Unvaccinated pigs	Vaccinated pigs	Unvaccinated pigs	Vaccinated pigs	Unvaccinated pigs	Vaccinated pigs
Number of animals	674	690	214	224	226	230	234	236
BW (kg) at								
Vaccination	5.8 ± 0.05	5.8 ± 0.05	5.8 ± 0.09	5.7 ± 0.09	5.7 ± 0.09	5.7 ± 0.09	6.1 ± 0.09	6.1 ± 0.09
4 weeks post-vaccination	14.6 ± 0.10	14.7 ± 0.10	14.4 ± 0.17	14.1 ± 0.17	15.1[a] ± 0.17	15.6[b] ± 0.17	14.2 ± 0.17	14.3 ± 0.16
10 weeks post-vaccination	40.9[a] ± 0.23	41.5[b] ± 0.23	40.0 ± 0.41	39.4 ± 0.40	43.3[a] ± 0.42	44.9[b] ± 0.41	39.3 ± 0.40	40.4 ± 0.40
16–17 weeks post-vaccination†	76.6 ± 0.37	76.9 ± 0.37	77.1 ± 0.65	76.4 ± 0.64	81.3 ± 0.66	80.9 ± 0.64	71.3[a] ± 0.64	73.4[b] ± 0.63
ADWG (g/d) from vaccination to								
4 weeks post-vaccination	310 ± 3.5	314 ± 3.4	306 ± 6.1	295 ± 6.0	328[a] ± 6.1	347[b] ± 6.0	296 ± 5.9	300 ± 5.9
10 weeks post-vaccination	486[a] ± 3.3	495[b] ± 3.2	474 ± 5.7	465 ± 5.6	519[a] ± 5.8	542[b] ± 5.7	465 ± 5.5	479 ± 5.5
16–17 weeks post-vaccination†	602 ± 3.2	605 ± 3.1	597 ± 5.6	591 ± 5.5	638 ± 5.6	635 ± 5.5	573[a] ± 5.4	590[b] ± 5.4
BW homogeneity‡ (%) at								
16–17 weeks post-vaccination†	85[a]	86[b]	86	86	87	87	82[a]	85[b]

BW Bodyweight, *ADWG* Average Daily Weight Gain

† The end of the study was at 17 weeks post-vaccination in week groups 1 and 2, and at 16 weeks post-vaccination in week group 3

‡ BW homogeneity was calculated from coefficient of variation (1-CV). It was tested comparing variances of BW using an F test

[a, b] Within week group, different letter in the same row indicates statistically significant difference ($p < 0.05$). Differences between treatment groups were tested using analysis of variance and subsequent t-tests

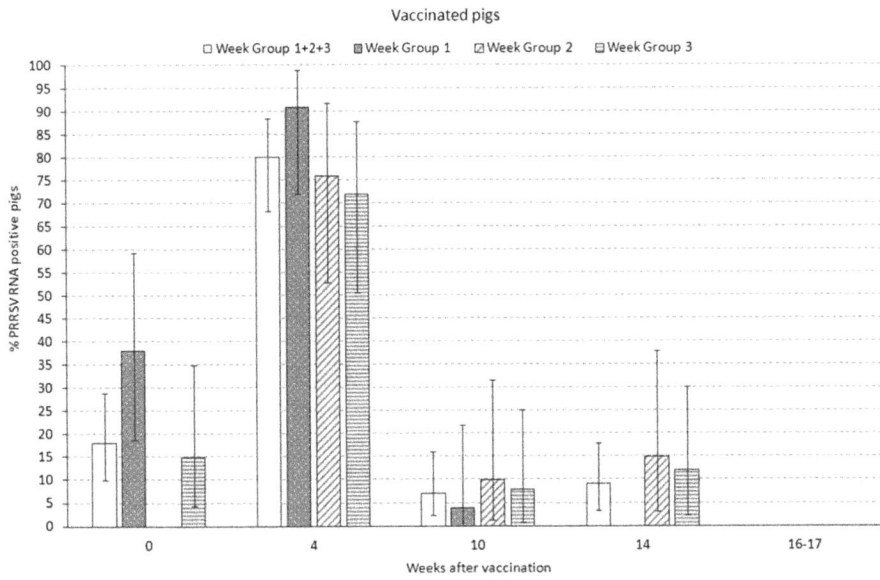

Fig. 2 Viremia in % positive pigs (qualitative) by qPCR at the different sampling times in 73 vaccinated pigs (24, 23 and 26 in week groups 1, 2 and 3, respectively). Percentage of positive pigs and confidence interval 95 %

pigs tested positive (see Figs. 2 and 3 at week 0). Notably, none of the vaccinated animals tested positive by PRRSV qPCR at the end of fattening while 3 % of the unvaccinated animals were still viremic at the end of fattening.

Percentages of pigs detected serologically positive by ELISA were determined in vaccinated and unvaccinated pigs. It was observed that 67 % (55–77 %; 95 % CI) of vaccinated pigs and 75 % (63–85 %; 95 % CI) of unvaccinated pigs were seropositive at vaccination, and that

99 % (92–100 %; 95 % CI) of vaccinated pigs and 92 % (83–98 %; 95 % CI) of unvaccinated pigs were already seropositive at 4 weeks post-vaccination. For all time points within this study, there was not statistical difference in the seroconversion rate between vaccinated and control pigs.

Since the wild type PRRSV infection took place very early during (WG 1) or after (WG 2 and WG 3) vaccination, it was not possible to determine the source of viremia in vaccinated animals.

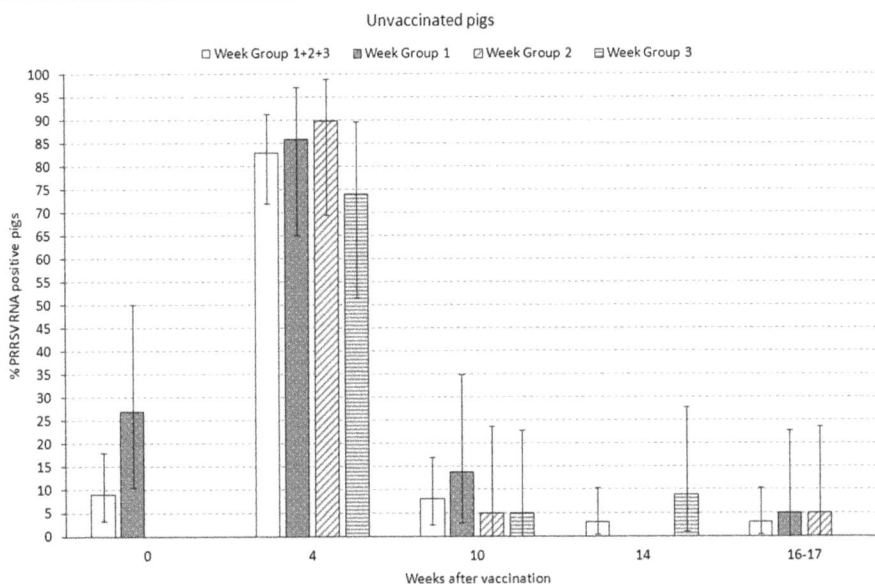

Fig. 3 Viremia in % positive pigs (qualitative) by qPCR at the different sampling times in 69 unvaccinated pigs (22, 24 and 23 in weeks groups 1, 2 and 3, respectively). Percentage of positive pigs and confidence interval 95 %

Table 2 summarizes the mortality, clinical signs and concomitant treatments throughout the study. Proportion of pigs showing any abnormal clinical sign at least once at any of the examination time points was lower ($p < 0.05$) in vaccinated pigs than in unvaccinated pigs, being the highest difference in WG 3 pigs. The most frequent signs were respiratory and skin alterations, being in both instance the proportion of affected pigs lower ($p < 0.05$) in vaccinated pigs than in unvaccinated ($p < 0.05$). Prevalence of joint disorders and diarrhea was generally low (1 % or lower).

Regarding concomitant treatments (Table 2), the proportion of vaccinated pigs treated individually at least once with a parenteral treatment was lower than in unvaccinated pigs ($p < 0.05$). The highest difference between vaccinated and unvaccinated pigs was in WG 2. About 98 % of the individual treatments administered were with injectable Enrofloxacin due to respiratory signs and in some cases due to diarrhea. Although collective treatments were restricted, a treatment with Doxycycline in water was administered to all piglets for 6 days once. The whole population was medicated including vaccinates and controls but as pigs of different ages were treated this occurred at a different time point in relation to the day of vaccination. Medication was at 4, 3 and 2 weeks postvaccination in WG 1, WG 2 and WG 3, respectively. This treatment was administered due to respiratory signs (sneezing and coughing), but also rough haircoat and thinness observed affecting all nursery rooms on the farm.

While numerically lower, there was no difference in mortality rate between vaccinated and unvaccinated pigs neither in the overall study nor within replicate groups (Table 2). None of the dead pigs examined in both treatment groups revealed PRRS related gross necropsy findings. The incidence of the findings recorded did not provide indications of a treatment-related pattern.

Discussion

This large field study was performed to investigate the efficacy of a novel PRRS MLV vaccine in terms of zootechnical parameters (BW and ADGW), in piglets of 4 weeks of age that originated from a vaccinated sow farm undergoing an active infection with a wild type PRRSV.

Vaccinated pigs showed better growth parameters than unvaccinated pigs at 10 weeks after vaccination. This performance improvement was observed in the critical period of virus circulation supporting the efficacy of the vaccine. When analyzing the data by separate cohorts it is clear that there were different responses to vaccination. Statistically significant differences for BW and ADWG at the end of the study were observed only in WG 3 pigs. Very few well controlled PRRS field trials have been conducted in Europe. The differences in BW and in ADWG observed among treatment groups in this study were not as remarkable as in previous reports [14–17]. Probably, this is due to the short time between the vaccination and the occurrence of the natural infection, which did not allow for better performance in vaccinated animals. In particular, the improvement in BW and ADWG could not be demonstrated in WG 1 probably because of a PRRSV wild type infection at the time of vaccination. This was confirmed through qPCR testing of pig sera at study day −1 before vaccination which showed 33 % PRRSV RNA pigs. In addition most of

Table 2 Percentage of mortality, pigs with clinical signs and pigs received concomitant treatments throughout the study (95 % CI)

Parameter	Week Group 1 + 2 + 3		Week Group 1		Week Group 2		Week Group 3	
	Unvaccinated pigs	Vaccinated pigs	Unvaccinated pigs	Vaccinated pigs	Unvaccinated pigs	Vaccinated pigs	Unvaccinated pigs	Vaccinated pigs
Number of animals	674	690	214	224	226	230	234	236
Mortality (%)	6.1	4.9	5.1	3.6	5.8	4.8	7.3	6.4
	(4.5–8.2)	(3.6–6.8)	(2.9–9.0)	(1.8–6.9)	(3.4–9.6)	(2.7–8.4)	(4.6–11.3)	(3.9–10.2)
Any clinical sign (%)†	8.3[a]	4.2[b]	7.0	3.6	6.2	3.0	11.5[a]	5.9[b]
	(6.5–10.6)	(2.9–6.0)	(4.3–11.2)	(1.8–6.9)	(3.7–10.1)	(1.5–6.2)	(8.1–16.3)	(3.6–9.7)
Respiratory signs (%)	4.7[a]	2.3[b]	3.3	1.8	3.1	1.3	7.7	3.8‡
	(3.4–6.6)	(1.4–3.7)	(1.6–6.6)	(0.7–4.5)	(1.5–6.3)	(0.4–3.8)	(4.9–11.8)	(2.0–7.1)
Skin alterations (%)	2.4[a]	0.7[b]	2.3	0.9	1.3	0.4	3.4	0.8
	(1.5–3.8)	(0.3–1.7)	(1.0–5.4)	(0.3–3.2)	(0.5–3.8)	(0.8–2.4)	(1.7–6.6)	(0.2–3.0)
Concomitant treatments (%)	23.0[a]	18.6[b]	15.5	15.6	21.2[a]	12.2[b]	32.5	27.5
	(20.0–26.3)	(15.8–21.6)	(10.4–19.8)	(11.5–21.0)	(16.4–27.0)	(8.6–17.0)	(26.8–38.7)	(22.2–33.6)

95 % CI: Wilson's Confidence Interval 95 % for a single proportion
† Respiratory signs and/or skin alterations and/or joint disorders and/or diarrhoea. Prevalence of joint disorders and diarrhoea was 1 % or lower
a, b Within week group, different letter in the same row indicates statistically significant difference ($p < 0.05$). Differences between the treatment groups were tested by Fisher's exact test

those previous studies were conducted in PRRS genotype 2 outbreaks under US conditions.

Proper vaccination against PRRSV or any MLV vaccines involves immunization of healthy pigs and proper timing of the vaccination event in relationship to onset of disease pressure on the farm. Under field conditions, the onset of immunity could be adversely affected by the presence of confounding factors, including the presence of other pathogens and vaccination in the face of an ongoing active PRRSV infection [14].

The interpretation of these results has to be done considering these circumstances; however, it seems that the vaccine protection even in the face of an existing infection was able to result in differences in BW and ADGW at 10 weeks of age. As the end of the study was set as the time when the first batch of pigs was sent to the slaughterhouse, we do not know if these differences carry over to batch closeout, where the entire economic impact is assessed by the producers.

Respiratory clinical signs, skin alterations and concomitant treatments were all found to be significantly reduced in vaccinated animals compared to unvaccinated animals suggesting a beneficial effect of vaccination on secondary infections and the general health status of the animals. Mortality was not statistically different between vaccinated and control pigs. This and other clinical parameters could be affected by the medication with Doxycycline to the population.

None of the necropsies performed during the study showed macroscopic signs of PRRSV infection, but detailed diagnostics of each case were not performed. While mortality was somewhat elevated at 4.9 and 6.1 % (vaccinated vs. control, respectively) it was lower than in other field studies that demonstrated statistical differences in reduction of mortality after vaccination [15]. We can assess that mortality was caused mainly by secondary infections in this trial (data not shown) as has been the case of other studies [18]. A more detailed diagnostic investigation of the deaths in this trial could help explain the lack of statistical reduction in mortality.

At inclusion in the study at 4 weeks of age most animals were serologically positive. This might be due to maternally derived antibodies from vaccinated dams or already signals the ongoing field infection that started during the suckling period. As vaccination is recommended from 17 days of life onwards, maternally derived antibodies should not have interfered with vaccination and were not likely providing protection as many were also positive for viral RNA. A limitation of this field study, since the wild type PRRSV infection took place very soon after vaccination or even before vaccination, was that it was not possible to determine the source of viremia in these animals. qPCR positive serum samples could be due to vaccine virus, the field virus (being viremic at vaccination time) or both as reported in other studies [11]. Sequencing of all positive samples may have provided further data to clarify this issue. Early PRRSV infection in this trial highlights the importance of ensuring breeding herd stability, defined by consistently weaning PRRSV negative piglets, to maximize the benefit of piglet vaccination [4, 17]. Other studies from North America have demonstrated that the direct benefits of PRRS vaccination in terms of efficacy depend on vaccination ahead of infection with field virus [14].

The PRRS field virus in this trial can be considered heterologous to the vaccine virus (92.74 % homology in ORF5). Murtaugh [19] indicates that a homology less or equal than 97–98 % can be considered as a different strain of the PRRSV, although the scientific community has not agreed on a defined cut off. Even though significant genetic differences were found between the strain circulating before vaccination and the vaccine strain, the vaccine provided partial clinical protection. However, to better understand the dynamics of the infection and the protection of the vaccine it would be advisable in future studies to perform such type of analyses.

Conclusions

This study establishes that vaccination of piglets with Ingelvac PRRSFLEX® EU at 4 weeks of age improves weight gain and reduces the appearance of clinical sings during the growing period, even when the piglets are infected shortly after vaccination. Evidence of vaccine benefits under field conditions was provided by improved performance in the period during the onset and peak viremia of wild-type PRRSV.

Abbreviations
ADWG, average daily weight gain; AEMPS, Agencia Española de Medicamentos y Productos Sanitarios; APP, Actinobacillus pleuropneumoniae; BW, bodyweight; CI, confidence interval; CV, coefficient of variation; LVI, live virus inoculation; MLV, modified live vaccine; ORF, open reading frame; PBS, phosphate buffered saline; PCV2, Porcines Circovirus Type 2; PRRS, Porcine Reproductive and Respiratory Syndrome; PRRSV, PRRS virus; qPCR, quantitative Polymerase Chain Reaction; RNA, ribonucleic acid; SIV, Swine Influenza Virus; WG, weight group.

Acknowledgements
Not applicable.

Funding
This study was totally financed by Boehringer Ingelheim Animal Health.

Authors' contributions
GC was the investigator of the study, wrote results section, performed the statistical study and reviewed the manuscript. AM wrote the introduction, the discussion and reviewed the results and the statistical study. MCO and CK developed the study design, monitored the study and reviewed the manuscript, FXO, OGD and JK wrote and reviewed the manuscript. All authors read and approved the final manuscript.

Competing interest
The authors declare that they have no competing interests.

Author details
[1]Tests and Trials S.L., Monzon, Spain. [2]Boehringer Ingelheim Veterinary Research Center GmbH & Co. KG, Hannover, Germany. [3]Boehringer Ingelheim Animal Health GmbH, Ingelheim, Germany. [4]Boehringer Ingelheim Vetmedica Inc., Ames, IA, USA.

References

1. Nieuwenhuis N, Duinhof TF, van Nes A. Economic analysis of outbreaks of porcine reproductive and respiratory syndrome virus in nine sow herds. Vet Rec. 2012;170(9):225.
2. Holtkamp DJ, Kliebenstein JB, Neumann EJ, Zimmerman JJ, Rotto HF, Yoder TK, et al. Assessment of the economic impact of porcine reproductive and respiratory syndrome virus on United States pork producers. J Swine Health Prod. 2013;21(2):72–84.
3. Fano E, Olea L, Pijoan C. Eradication of porcine reproductive and respiratory syndrome virus by serum inoculation of naive gilts. Can J Vet Res. 2005;69(1):71.
4. Kimman TG, Cornelissen LA, Moormann RJ, Rebel JMJ, Stockhofe-Zurwieden N. Challenges for porcine reproductive and respiratory syndrome virus (PRRSV) vaccinology. Vaccine. 2009;27(28):3704–18.
5. Linhares DCL, Cano JP, Torremorell M, Morrison RB. Comparison of time to PRRSV-stability and production losses between two exposure programs to control PRRSV in sow herds. Prev Vet Med. 2014;116(1–2):111–9.
6. Mateu E, Martín M, Vidal D. Genetic diversity and phylogenetic analysis of glycoprotein 5 of European-type porcine reproductive and respiratory virus strains in Spain. J Gen Virol. 2003;84(3):529–34.
7. Murtaugh MP, Stadejek T, Abrahante JE, Lam TTY, Leung FC-C. The ever-expanding diversity of porcine reproductive and respiratory syndrome virus. Virus Res. 2010;154(1–2):18–30.
8. Pileri E, Gibert E, Soldevila F, García-Saenz A, Pujols J, Diaz I, et al. Vaccination with a genotype 1 modified live vaccine against porcine reproductive and respiratory syndrome virus significantly reduces viremia, viral shedding and transmission of the virus in a quasi-natural experimental model. Vet Microbiol. 2015;175(1):7–16.
9. Martínez-Lobo FJ, Díez-Fuertes F, Segalés J, García-Artiga C, Simarro I, Castro JM, et al. Comparative pathogenicity of type 1 and type 2 isolates of porcine reproductive and respiratory syndrome virus (PRRSV) in a young pig infection model. Vet Microbiol. 2011;154(1–2):58–68.
10. Van Gucht S, Labarque G, Van Reeth K. The combination of PRRS virus and bacterial endotoxin as a model for multifactorial respiratory disease in pigs. Vet Immunol Immunopathol. 2004;102(3):165–78.
11. Labrecque MP, Cardinal F. Impact of PRRS vaccination timing in pigs with different maternal immunity levels. In: Proceedings of the 44th Annual Meeting of the American Association of Swine Veterinarians,San Diego, CA, USA. 2013. p. 327.
12. Kritas SK, Alexopoulos C, Kyriakis CS, Tzika E, Kyriakis SC. Performance of fattening pigs in a farm infected with both porcine reproductive and respiratory syndrome (PRRS) virus and porcine circovirus type 2 following sow and piglet vaccination with an attenuated PRRS vaccine. J Vet Med Ser Physiol Pathol Clin Med. 2007;54(6):287–91.
13. R Core Team. R: A language and environment for statistical computing Vienna, Austria. [Internet]. Vienna, Austria: R Foundation or Statistical Computing; 2014. Available from: http://www.R-project.org/
14. Philips RC, Edler RA, Holck JT. Vaccination with MLV vaccine to control PRRS in growing pigs. In: Proceedings of the 19th International Pig Veterinary Society Congress, Copenhagen, Denmark. 2006. p. 242.
15. Polson D, Baker RB, Philips RC, Hotze B. Improved growing pig performance in a large production system applying intensive management and vaccination protocol. In: Proceedings of the 20th International Pig Veterinary Society Congress, Durban, South Africa. 2008.
16. Angulo J, Philips RC, Cano JP. Growth peformance improvement and mortality reduction derived from a PRRS large scale control project in the US. In: Proceedings of the 21st International Pig Veterinary Society Congress, Vancouver, Canada. 2010. p. 973.
17. Robbins R, Harms P, Angulo J, Scheidt A, Philips RC, Kolb J. PRRSV control in finisher pigs, a large scale barn study in high dense area in USA. In: Proceedings of the 44th Annual Meeting of the American Association of Swine Veterinarians, San Diego, CA, USA. 2013. p. 255–7.
18. Trus I, Bonckaert C, van der Meulen K, Nauwynck HJ. Efficacy of an attenuated European subtype 1 porcine reproductive and respiratory syndrome virus (PRRSV) vaccine in pigs upon challenge with the East European subtype 3 PRRSV strain Lena. Vaccine. 2014;32(25):2995–3003.
19. Murtaugh M. Use and interpretation of sequencing in PRRSV control programs. In: Proceedings of the 2012 Allen D. Leman Swine Conference, St Paul, MN, USA. 2012. p. 49–55.

11

Lameness in piglets – should pain killers be included at treatment?

Mate Zoric[1,2]* ⓘ, Ulla Schmidt[3], Anna Wallenbeck[3] and Per Wallgren[1,2]

Abstract

Background: Joint swelling and lameness are the most obvious and persistent clinical signs of infectious arthritis in piglets. For a positive treatment effect of piglets with arthritis, early initiated treatments with antibiotics are desired. Hitherto pain-reducing drugs have rarely been used within veterinary medicine, but the potential of non steroid anti-inflammatory drugs (NSAID) are interesting from an animal welfare perspective. Therefore, the aim of this study was to compare the long term efficiency of treating lameness with and without pain relief. Further, the incidences of affected joints in lame piglets were analysed.

Results: In total 415 of the 6,787 liveborn piglets included in the study were diagnosed with lameness (6.1 %). Around 86 % of these diagnoses took place during the first 3 weeks of life. There was no difference in the incidence of lameness between the sexes, but lameness was most commonly diagnosed in the offspring to old sows (>4 parturitions). Lameness was diagnosed in about every second litter and on average about two pigs were diagnosed in the affected litters. The incidence of affected litters as well as affected piglets increased with ageing of the sows.

Treatments with antibiotics solely and in combination with NSAID improved ($P < 0.01$ to 0.001) the clinical status from day to day, but the clinical response did not differ between the two treatment groups.

Piglets that remained healthy were 1.1 and 1.7 kg heavier ($P < 0.001$) than piglets diagnosed with lameness at 5 and 9 weeks of age, respectively. There were no differences in piglet body weights between the treatment strategies at any time.

Conclusions: The clinical response to penicillin was good. It was neither improved nor reduced by a concurrent administration of NSAIDs. Nevertheless NSAIDs may improve the animal welfare due to pain relief. An important finding of this study was that decreasing pain due to lameness not was negative in a long term perspective, *i.e.* reducing pain did not lead to overstrain of affected joints and no clinical signs of adverse effects were noted. Therefore the use of NSAIDs ought to be considered to improve the animal welfare, at least in severe cases.

Keywords: Piglets, Lameness, Treatment, Penicillin, Non Steroidal Anti-Inflammatory Drugs, NSAID

Background

Abrasions, wounds and necrosis in the skin or on the hooves and accessory digits, are very common in newborn piglets [1]. Risk factors include floor type, nutrition and genetics [2, 3]. Skin lesions in piglets are presumably mainly a result of contact with the floor, especially during suckling [4–8]. The lesions are generally bilateral and most commonly observed as abrasions over the carpal joints [9, 10]. Such lesions are present already on day 3, they increase in magnitude until day 10 and thereafter decline [6, 8, 11]. Foot and skin lesions can contribute to lameness in two ways, either due to pain induced by the injury itself or by acting as an entrance for infections that spread to joints through bacteraemia and thereby induce arthritis and pain [2, 12]. Infectious arthritis are dominated by hemolytic streptococci, but also staphylococci and *E. coli* are frequently demonstrated [6, 8, 12, 13]. The streptococci domination suggests the sow to be a significant source of infection to the piglets [13, 14]. Lameness in suckling piglets is observed in about every

* Correspondence: mate.zoric@sva.se
[1]Department of Animal Health and Antimicrobial Strategies, National Veterinary Institute, SE-751 89 Uppsala, Sweden
[2]Department of Clinical Sciences, Faculty of Veterinary Medicine and Animal Sciences, Swedish University of Agricultural Sciences, Box 7054SE-750 07 Uppsala, Sweden
Full list of author information is available at the end of the article

second litter and around 75 % of the treatments against lameness are effectuated in piglets less than 3 week of age [12, 15, 16]. Apart from animal suffering, lameness contributes to losses in terms of dead piglets, decreased growth an increased use of manual labour and of antibiotics [16, 17].

Pain may of course be transient, but if the recovery period is prolonged the animal will be less competitive, e.g. at group feedings situations. If the pain cannot be effectively treated, culling may be the only practical option in pig farming [18]. Thus, the therapy of lame piglets ought to include measures aimed to decrease pain and thereby also minimize any adverse effect on feed intake [19].

Historically, little emphasis has been paid on pain management in veterinary medicine [20]. Pain has been regarded as a tool to keep animals tranquil to allow any injury to heal faster. Knowledge of pain management has been limited, both among veterinarians in the academic environment and in clinical practice [21]. However, supporting therapy with analgesic drugs (NSAIDs = Non Steroidal Anti-Inflammatory Drugs) has increased considerably in recent years [22], explained by a greater awareness and understanding of pain and painful conditions [23]. NSAIDs have anti-inflammatory, analgesic and antipyretic effects [24]. They have mainly a peripheral analgesic activity and acts by inhibiting the synthesis of prostaglandins, which in turn sensitivities nocisceptores (peripheral sensory nerve endings that react strong to tissue thermal, mechanical and chemical stimuli). Ketoprofen (2-(phenyl 3-benzoyl) propionic acid) is a NSAID of the 2-arylpropionic acid group (generically known as profens) with analgesic, anti-inflammatory and antipyretic properties [18].

To reduce pain in piglets, NSAIDs is at present the only realistic alternative since drugs of this class are the only long-acting analgesics with maximum residue limits (MRL) established for pigs in Europe [18]. However, as the analgesic is administered by intramuscular injection, treatment of large numbers of piglets have been concluded to be time consuming and potentially costly [25]. Further, if analgesic treatment of lame piglets leads to an increased mobility with the risk for over-load of affected joints with side effects in the future cannot be excluded. Therefore, the aim of this study was to investigate the clinical effects of concurrent treatment of lame piglets with NSAID-drugs and antibiotics to that of using antibiotics solely.

Results
Relationship to lameness and age of piglets
In total 415 out of 6,787 liveborn piglets were diagnosed with lameness (6.1 %) during the two and half years studied. Around 86 % of these diagnoses took place

during the first 3 weeks of life and the risk incidence of lameness decreased from 2.4 % during the first week of life to 0.3 % during the fifth week of life. There was no difference in the incidence of lameness between the sexes (Table 1).

Relationship with lameness and parity of sow
Overall, lameness was diagnosed in about every second litter, but the range of lame piglets varied from one to nine in affected litters (Table 2). The incidence of lameness was lowest in the litters of first and second parity sows and then increased with the age of the sows, both with respect to affected litters and to affected piglets within litter.

Clinical effect of treatments
Both treatment strategies, with penicillin solely or with penicillin in combination with NSAIDs, improved ($P < 0.01$ to 0.001) the clinical status (i.e. improved lameness score) from day to day but the treatment efficacy did not differ between the groups. Approximately 75 % of the piglets diagnosed with lameness was scored with severe signs of lameness (score 3) at the onset of treatment while 50 % were scored healthy or almost healthy (score 0 or 1) day 5 of treatment. The treatment efficacy is illustrated in Fig. 1, showing the day to day prevalence of piglets within the different diagnose codes.

Relationship to lameness and weight
The weights recorded at birth, 5 and 9 weeks of age are shown in Table 3. Piglets that remained healthy were 1.1 and 1.7 kg heavier than piglets attended with lameness at 5 and 9 weeks of age, respectively. Piglets attended for lameness performed equal regardless of treatments strategy (Fig. 1), but piglets that remained free from lameness grew 9 % faster ($P < 0.001$) than piglets diagnosed with lameness.

Distributions of the affected joints
A total of 454 joints were associated with lameness in 415 affected piglets. One clinically affected joint was recorded in 380 piglets (91.5 %), two joints in 31 piglets (7.5 %) and three joints in 4 piglets (1 %).

The distribution of the affected joints is shown in Fig. 2. It was evenly distributed between front and hind legs with 52.5 % in the front legs (Elbows 19.3 %; Carpus 9.9 %; Front Metacarpal joints 6.7 %; Front Hoofs 16.6 %) and 56.9 % in the hind legs (Hocks 16.1 %; Back Metacarpal joints 6.3 %; Back Hoofs 34.5 %).

In total, 56.8 % ($n = 258$) of the lesions were recorded on the left side of the piglets and 43.2 % ($n = 196$) on the right side.

Table 1 The mean incidence risk for being diagnosed for lameness with respect to week of age in 6,787 live born piglets

Age (Weeks)	Piglets medically treated for lameness (n)	Incidence risk of lameness (%)
1	166	2.4
2	119	1.8
3	72	1.1
4	35	0.5
5	23	0.3
In total	415 of 6,787	6.1
Whereof males	215 of 3,553	6.1
Whereof females	200 of 3,234	6.2

Necropsies, bacteria and antimicrobial resistance

Three lame piglets were culled before medical treatment and subjected to necropsy, including histopathological and microbiological examinations. One of the three pigs suffered from acute purulent arthritis, the other two of chronic arthritis, and all of the piglets were affected in more than one joint. Bacterial cultivations of three joints per animal demonstrated microbial growth in all piglets. The findings were *Streptococcus dysgalactiae* subsp. *equisimilis* in one piglet and *Staphylococcus hyicus* subsp. *hyicus* in two piglets. They were all sensitive to all antibiotics included in the in the [VetMIC™ GP-mo-A (version 2), National Veterinary Institute, NVI].

Discussion

This study was conducted at a research station with experienced staff that had good recording systems and written instructions for diagnosing diseases. Lameness was defined as lameness and/or swollen joint(s), thereby not differentiating lameness due to infections from lameness due to other causes. However, in a previous study where lame piglets were euthanized instead of medically treated, the diagnose arthritis was always made at necropsy [6, 8, 12], as also was the case with the three piglets sacrificed in this study. Thereby it is believed that most lame piglets actually suffered from arthritis, but as no etiological diagnose was made in the other piglets we prefer to use the term lameness.

During the two and half years studied, 415 of the 6,787 piglets born had been treated for lameness before the age of 5 weeks (6.1 %), whereof 86 % were diagnosed within 3 weeks from birth. Skin cuts have been discussed as an entry for infections, and castration may therefore predispose for lameness. However, as no difference in the incidence of lameness between the sexes were recorded, the results obtained concur previous reports [16, 26, 27], suggesting that castration in itself appear not to predispose to development of lameness - provided that it is effectuated skilfully and under aseptic conditions. Instead there was a correlation to the age of the sow, lameness was most commonly diagnosed in piglets born by old sows (>4 parturitions).

Lameness in piglets is of concern for both animal welfare and economic reasons. In intensive pig production the weight of the weaned piglet has a significant influence on lifetime performance. Low weight at weaning implies a loss of income for the farmer and might also influence the welfare of the affected animals negatively. Lameness, as well as other diseases [28], reduce the growth rate of the piglets and the piglets that were treated for lameness in this study grew 9 % slower than those not diagnosed with lameness. In a Danish study, piglets treated for lameness, diarrhoea or other infections were identified as main contributors to a decreased weight gain during the suckling period, with 38, 8 and 21 g per day, respectively [29].

Table 2 Prevalence of litters with lameness diagnosed in piglets by sow parity. Total prevalence, mean number and range of lame pigs in the affected litters, as well as the percentages of litters with one, two, three or more than three affected piglets

	Litters	Litters with lameness		Number of lame piglets in affected litters					
Parity	Total	n	%	Mean	Range	1 lame[A]	2 lame	3 lame	>3 lame
1	146	46	31.5 [A]	1.52	1-9	76 %[A]	15 %[A]	4 %[A]	4 %[A]
2	103	39	37.9 [AB]	1.51	1-6	74 %[AB]	18 %[A]	5 %[A]	5 %[A]
3	97	40	41.2 [AB]	1.74	1-6	55 %[BC]	28 %[A]	8 %[A]	8 %[AB]
4	62	33	53.2 [B]	2.15	1-6	48 %[C]	51 %[B]	15 %[AB]	15 %[AB]
>4	73	52	71.2 [C]	2.18	1-7	54%[C]	29%[A]	27%[B]	19%[B]

Different superscript letters within columns indicate significant pairwise differences with P < 0.05

Clinical score following treatment

Clinical score following treatment

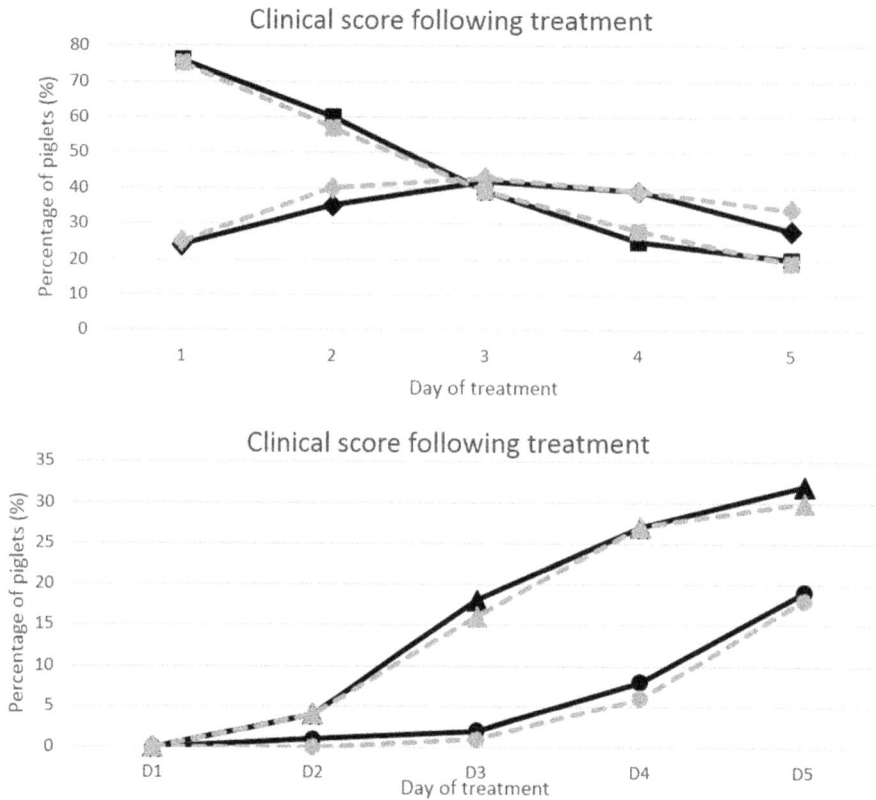

Fig. 1 The clinical score of lame piglets following treatment initiated on day 1. The clinical score of lame piglets treated with penicillin solely (grey dotted lines) compared to pigs treated with penicillin and NSAID (black lines). The decreasing prevalence of lame pigs with severe signs (diagnose code 3; squares) initially increased the prevalence of pigs with major clinical sigs (diagnose code 2; diamonds) from 25 to 40 %, but at day 5 also the prevalence of this diagnose had ceased somewhat (top). As a consequence, increasing levels of almost healthy (diagnose code 1; triangles) or healthy piglets (diagnose code 0; circles) were denoted (bottom). Note the different scales on the y-angles

Lame piglets are also believed to suffer from pain and stress, which is reported to have a negative influence on production [3]. Pain is defined as an unpleasant sensory and emotional experience that is associated with actual or potential tissue damage [30]. However, pain is subjective and therefore difficult to quantify, and there are no specific parameters for measuring pain [31]. Nevertheless, it is widely accepted that piglets may react to pain in three ways: trough vocalization, physiologically, and behaviorally [32, 33]. Thereby pain killers appear attractive in improving welfare for lame pigs. However, if analgesic treatment of lame piglets leads to an increased mobility during the acute lameness there might be a risk for overexertion of affected joints which in turn might induce long term negative side effects. Therefore it is important to note that no difference in weight gain between the two treated groups were recorded in this study. NSAID –treated piglets did not grew faster than non-NSAID-treated piglets, but neither did they grew slower which would have been expected if long term

Table 3 Mean weights of piglets treated for lameness during the first 9 weeks of life compared to piglets not attended with lameness. Every second lame piglet was treated with penicillin and NSAID and every second piglet was treated with penicillin solely. Least Square Means ± Standard Error

	Unaffected	Treated for arthritis		Treated with	Treated with	
		All		Penicillin + NSAID	Penicillin	
	(kg)	(kg)	P	(kg)	(kg)	P
Birth	1.5 ± 0.01 (n = 6373)	1.6 ± 0.02 (n = 412)	n.s.	1.5 ± 0.03 (n = 207)	1.6 ± 0.03 (n = 205)	n.s.
5 weeks	10.6 ± 0.11 (n = 4804)	9.5 ± 0.14 (n = 372)	<0.001	9.0 ± 0.20 (n = 184)	9.1 ± 0.20 (n = 188)	n.s.
9 weeks	24.3 ± 0.19 (n = 4161)	22.6 ± 0.26 (n = 354)	<0.001	21.7 ± 0.37 (n = 182)	22.4 ± 0.37 (n = 172)	n.s.

n.s. = not significant, P > 0.05

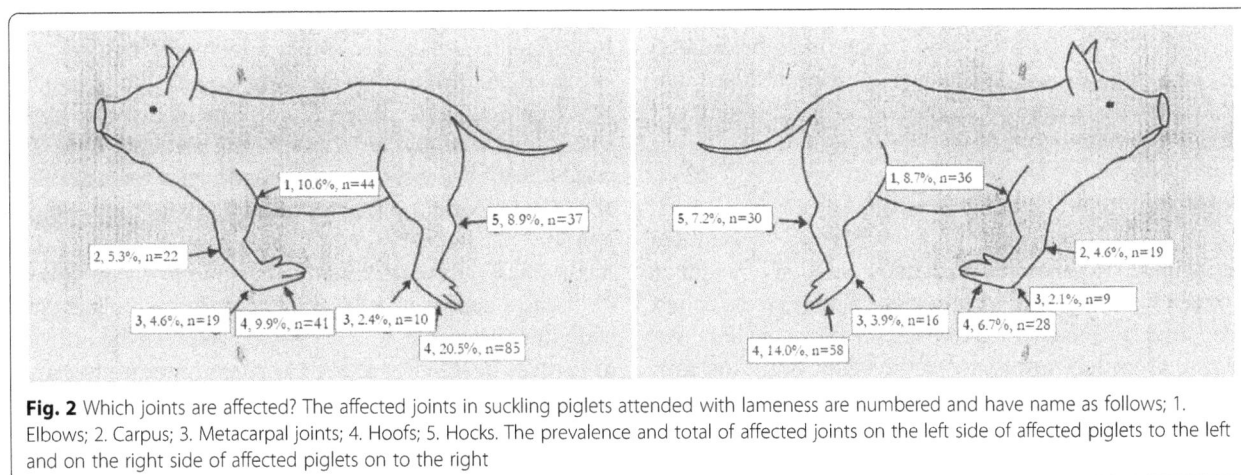

Fig. 2 Which joints are affected? The affected joints in suckling piglets attended with lameness are numbered and have name as follows; 1. Elbows; 2. Carpus; 3. Metacarpal joints; 4. Hoofs; 5. Hocks. The prevalence and total of affected joints on the left side of affected piglets to the left and on the right side of affected piglets on to the right

negative side effects would have been at hand. Use of NSAIDs in combination with antibiotics as treatment for lameness in piglets ought to therefore be considered for animal welfare issues, at least at severe cases of lameness.

In this study the clinical response of treatment penicillin was good, regardless of a similar treatment with NSAID or not. In both groups no piglet were given diagnose codes 0 or 1 (healthy or almost healthy) when initiating treatment, but 50 % of them were scored with 0 or 1 after 5 days of treatment. Yet it must be remembered that every 4th piglet diagnosed with severe lameness (diagnose code 3) when treatment was initiated still had that clinical score day 5, and that piglets diagnosed with lameness had a reduced weight gain. Since an early initiated treatment is concluded to be essential for a good treatment prognosis [16, 34], persisting clinical score might mirror the time for initiation of treatment in relation to the true onset of infection. It should also be emphasized that reducing pain pharmacologically in lame piglets not can replace the management routines, floor quality and good care.

Although lameness most commonly was observed in back hoofs, followed by elbows, front hoofs and hocks, lameness was fairly evenly distributed between joints. This indicated a septicemial spread of the infections associated with lameness, as previously also indicated by the association to abrasions [26]. We have no explanation for the diverging distribution between the left (56.8 %) and the right (43.2 %) side of the pig, but similar observations have previously been reported from 264 preweaning piglets in England where 42 % had abrasions on the left limbs and 38 % on the right limbs [35].

The microbial cause of lameness in piglets may vary and treatment of lame pigs leads to a permanent use of antibiotics in piglet production, which in turn may lead to antimicrobial resistance. Therefore, a causative diagnose, including defining of minimum inhibitory concentration (MIC) values, ought to regularly be made from joints of lame piglets in pig herds. In this herd, bacterial cultivations revealed *Streptococcus dysgalactiae* subsp. *equisimilis* and *Staphylococcus hyicus* subsp. *hyicus* as the cause of infectious arthritis, which concur with several other reports [6, 8], that were sensitive to all antibiotics included in the antimicrobial panels used.

Prompt treatment with antibiotics of piglets that limp due to infection is required to achieve a positive treatment effect [1, 36] and in agreement with the results obtained in this study many studies recommend penicillin as first choice of antibiotics [34, 37, 38]. It could be argued that the statement on immediate treatment of lame piglets would increase use of antibiotics, but it should be remembered that no "just-to-be-sure strategic disease preventing antimicrobial treatment" whatsoever take place in any Swedish herd. This is a responsible way to ensure a low use of antimicrobials, based on the fact that healthy pigs do not need antibiotics.

Conclusions

Piglets diagnosed with lameness had a reduced weight gain. Lameness was fairly evenly distributed between joints, which indicate a septicemic spread of the infections associated with lameness, as previously also indicated by the association to abrasions. The clinical response of penicillin was good, and it was neither improved nor reduced by a concurrent administration of NSAIDs. A significant finding of this study was that decreasing pain due to lameness not was negative in a long term perspective, *i.e.* reducing pain did not lead to overstrain of affected joints and no clinical signs of adverse effects were noted. Therefore the use of NSAIDs ought to be considered to improve the animal welfare, at least in severe cases.

Despite the generally good effect of penicillin, it was notable that around every 4th piglet diagnosed with severe lameness still scored so 4 days after initiating treatment. Since inserting treatment during the early cause of joint diseases has been suggested to be important for a good prognosis this may have been dependant on the onset of treatment in relation to the true onset of infection.

Methods
The study has been approved by the Ethical Committee for Animal Experiments, Uppsala, Sweden (reference number C 135/9). All lame piglets in the study would have been subjected to treatments with penicillin as a routine procedure regardless of the study, but none with NSAIDs.

Animals and management routines
The study was carried out at research station at Funbo-Lövsta, Swedish University of Agricultural Sciences. The farrow-to-finish herd comprised 110 sows (mainly purebred Yorkshire) and had been established for 30 years. The herd was free from diseases according to the "A List" of the Office International des Epizooties, and also from Aujeszky's disease, atrophic rhinitis, *Brachyspira* (*Serpuliana*) species, porcine epidemic diarrhoea, porcine reproductive and respiratory syndrome, *Salmonella* species and transmissible gastroenteritis.

Pregnant sows were housed in a deep-litter system in groups of about 16, but with individual feeding. Two weeks before farrowing, sows were transferred to a cleaned farrowing unit with 16 pens, each 8.4 m^2 in area and bedded with straw. Each piglet was weighed and given an identity (tattoo) at the day of birth. Navels were disinfected, canine teeth were filed when judged necessary and, canvas was glued to carpal joints to prevent abrasions. The piglets were also weighed when they were 5 weeks (at weaning) and 9 weeks old.

All 6,787 piglets born alive during a period of two and a half years were included in the study. The male piglets were castrated at 2, 3 or 4 days of age, and at the same time all the piglets received an intramuscular injection of 200 mg iron as iron dextran (Pigeron; Leo Pharmaceutical). The piglets were given a second iron injection when they were 14 days old, and they were offered commercial creep feed without antibiotics from 3 weeks of age; it contained 15.5 % crude protein, 1.0 % lysine, and 12.2 MJ metabolisable energy (ME)/kg (Växfor; Lantmännen, Svalöv, Sweden). No routine strategical treatment with antimicrobials whatsoever were made in the herd. Only pigs diagnosed with a disease were medically treated.

Lameness, treatment, necropsies, culture of bacteria, antimicrobial resistance
The herd veterinarian had made a written instruction to the staff. According to that instruction, lame piglets or piglets with visibly swollen joints were defined to suffer from lameness and should be parenterally treated with antimicrobials immediately. Benzyl penicillin (Penovet vet., Boehringer Ingelheim Vetmedica) was intramuscularly administered at a dose of 20 mg per kg bodyweight once a day for 5 days. Every second piglet was additionally injected with 3 mg ketoprofen (Romefen vet., Merial Norden) per kg bodyweight once a day for 3 days. Every medically treated piglet was colour-marked, and records of diseases and treatments were kept for each piglet. The staff was instructed to treat piglets affected by arthritis as early as possible to attain a fair treatment prognosis.

Three randomly selected lame piglets were culled instead of medically treated. At necropsy, samples for bacteriology were collected with sterile cotton swabs from up to 3 joints diagnosed with arthritis and from a normal joint from each pig. The samples were spread directly to blood agar (blood agar base No. 2; LabM, Salford, England + 5 % horse blood) and bromcresol purple-lactose agar (NVI art No.341200). The plates were incubated at 37 °C and read after 18 and 48 h. Isolates of staphylococci and streptococci were typed with methods used at the Bacteriological diagnostic laboratory at the National Veterinary Institute (NVI).

Isolates of staphylococci and streptococci were tested with respect to antimicrobial resistance towards penicillin, cephalothin, oxacillin +2 % NaCl, erythromycin, chloramphenicol, clindamycin, tetracycline, fusidic acid, gentamicin, kanamycin, ciprofloxacin, trimethoprim [VetMIC™ GP-mo-A (version 2), NVI].

Clinical examinations and evaluation of therapeutic efficacy
The occurrence of lameness was registered from birth until the age of 5 weeks and the clinical efficacies of treatment were assessed daily. When diagnosed lame, pigs were given a clinical score based on lameness swollen joints and general health status; 0 = healthy; 1 = almost healthy; 2 = manifest lameness; 3 severe lameness.

The occurrence of lameness and affected joints (Elbow, Carpus, Hock, Metacarpal joint, Hoof) in one or more legs were registered from birth until the age of 5 weeks.

Statistical analysis
Statistical analyses were performed using the Statistical Analysis Systems; SAS 9.2 (SAS, 2014). Data from the 6,787 liveborn piglets were included in the statistical analyses. Only the first incidence of arthritis in each piglet was taken into account and only complete recordings was included in the analyses. Differences in arthritis prevalence between sexes (male or female) and sow parities (1, 2, 3, 4, >4), as well as differences in clinical lameness status between treatments and change in clinical lameness status day to day

was analysed in bivariate two-by-two chi square tests using PROC FREQ. This procedure enabled pairwise competitions of prevalences between all classes (e.g. between specific parities). Differences in weight between pigs treated for arthritis and unaffected pigs were analysed with MODEL 1 and 2 and between lame pigs given the two different treatments with MODEL 3 and 4 using PROC MIXED.

MODEL 1: Birth weight = Lameness (yes or no) + Sex (Male or Female) + Parity (1, 2, 3, 4 or >4) + Sow + Sow*-Parity + e

MODEL 2: Weight at 5 weeks or Weight at 9 weeks = Lameness (yes or no) + Sex (Male or Female) + Parity (1, 2, 3, 4 or >4) + Sow + Sow*Parity + Birth weight + e

MODEL 3: Birth weight = Treatment (Penicillin + NSAID or Penicillin) + Sex (Male or Female) + Parity (1, 2, 3, 4 or >4) + Sow + Sow*Parity + e

MODEL 4: Weight at 5 weeks or Weight at 9 weeks = Treatment (Penicillin + NSAID or Penicillin) + Sex (Male or Female) + Parity (1, 2, 3, 4 or >4) + Sow + Sow*Parity + Birth weight + e

Where Lameness, Treatment, Sex and Parity were included as fixed effects, Sow and Sow*Parity were included as random effects and Birth weight was included as a continuous covariate.

Competing interests
The authors declare that they have no competing interests.

Authors' contributions
MZ, US, AW and PW initiated the study and designed it in cooperation. MZ was the main investigator and head writer of the manuscript with assistance from the other authors. All authors have read and approved the final manuscript.

Authors' information
MZ and PW are veterinarians working at the Department of Animal Health and Antimicrobial Strategies at the National Veterinary Institute and at the Department of Clinical Sciences at the Swedish University of Agricultural Sciences in Uppsala, Sweden. Both hold Swedish expert competence in porcine diseases, and PW is also an ECPHM-diplomat as well as professor in pig diseases at both the National Veterinary Institute and the Swedish University of Agricultural Sciences. MZ completed his PhD which focused on lameness in piglets in 2008 with PW as main supervisor. US work as a supervisor at the research station. AW is researcher and teacher at Department of Animal Breeding and Genetics and Department of Animal Environment and health at the Swedish University of Agricultural Sciences in Uppsala, Sweden. This work was initiated with a project aimed to analyse the incidence of lameness in piglets and to determine its influence on productivity, and has thereafter focused on risks for development of lameness in different housing system and treatment strategy.

Acknowledgements
This study was financed by grants from Foundation Mary Francke-Gustafson's fund and Foundation Carl-Fredrik von-Horn's fund at The Royal Swedish Academy of Agriculture and Forestry and the National Veterinary Institute.

Author details
[1]Department of Animal Health and Antimicrobial Strategies, National Veterinary Institute, SE-751 89 Uppsala, Sweden. [2]Department of Clinical Sciences, Faculty of Veterinary Medicine and Animal Sciences, Swedish University of Agricultural Sciences, Box 7054SE-750 07 Uppsala, Sweden. [3]Department of Animal Breeding and Genetics, Swedish University of Agricultural Sciences, Box 7023SE-750 07 Uppsala, Sweden.

References
1. Dewey CE. Diseases of the nervous and locomotor systems. In: Straw BE, Zimmerman JJ, D'Allaire S, Taylor DJ, editors. Diseases of swine. 9th ed. Ames, Iowa, USA: Blackwell Publishing Professional; 2006. p. 87–111.
2. Penny RHC, Edwards MJ, Mulley R. Clinical observations of necrosis of the skin of suckling piglets. Aust Vet J. 1971; doi: 10.1111/j.1751-0813.1971.tb02047.x.
3. Le HT, Nilsson K, Norberg E, Lundeheim N. Genetic association between leg conformation in young pigs and sow reproduction. Livest Sci. 2015; doi:10.1016/j.livsci.2015.05.025.
4. Mouttotou N, Green LE. Incidence of foot and skin lesions in nursing piglets and their association with behavioural activities. Vet Rec. 1999; doi:10.1136/vr.145.6.160.
5. Westin R, Algers B. Effects of farrowing pen design on health and behavior of the sow and piglets at farrowing and lactation. Sv Vet Tidn. 2006;8-9:21–7.
6. Zoric M, Nilsson E, Mattsson S, Lundeheim N, Wallgren P. Abrasions and lameness in piglets born in different farrowing systems with different types of floor. Acta Vet Scand. 2008; doi:10.1186/1751-0147-50-37.
7. Zoric M. Lameness in piglets. Dissertation. Faculty of Veterinary Medicine and Animal Science, Swedish University of Agricultural Sciences. Acta Universitatis Agriculturae Sueciae; 2008. http://pub.epsilon.slu.se/1862/ Accessed 01 Feb 2016.
8. Zoric M, Nilsson E, Lundeheim N, Wallgren P. Incidence of lameness and abrasions in piglets in identical farrowing pens with four different types of floor. Acta Vet Scand. 2009; doi:10.1186/1751-0147-51-23.
9. Gardner IA, Hird DW. Risk factors for development of foot abscess in neonatal pigs. J Am Vet Med Assoc. 1994;204:1062–7.
10. Persson S, Ehlorsson CJ, Håkansson U, Nilsson C. Golvytor i grisstallar. In: Jordbruksinformation 3. Jordbruksverket. 2006. http://webbutiken.jordbruksverket.se/sv/artiklar/golvytor-i-grisstallar.html Accessed 01 Feb 2016.
11. Zoric M. Lameness in piglets. Pig J. 2010;63:1–11.
12. Zoric M, Sjölund M, Persson M, Nilsson E, Lundeheim N, Wallgren P. Lameness in piglets. Abrasions in nursing piglets and transfer of protection towards infections with Streptococci from sow to offspring. J Vet Med B. 2004; doi: 10.1111/j.1439-0450.2004.00777.x.
13. Higgins R, Gottschalk M. Streptococcal diseases. In: Straw BE, Zimmerman JJ, D'Allaire S, Taylor DJ, editors. Diseases of swine. 9th ed. Ames, Iowa, USA: Blackwell Publishing Professional; 2006. p. 769–83.
14. Windsor RS. Streptococcal infections in young pigs. Vet Annu. 1978;18:134–43.
15. Egeli AK, Framsted T, Sunde M, Waage S. Lameness in piglets. Nor Vet Tidsskr. 2001;113:615–25.
16. Zoric M, Stern S, Lundeheim N, Wallgren P. Four-year study of lameness in piglets at a research station. Vet Rec. 2003; doi:10.1136/vr.153.11.323.
17. Zoric M, Sjölund M, Wallgren P. Financial impact of disease on pig production: V. Lameness. In: University of Parma (Italy), editor. Proceedings of the 6th European Symposium of Porcine Health Management, 7 – 9 May 2014, Sorrento, Italy. 2014. p. 191.
18. Fosse TK, Toutain PL, Spadavecchia C, Haga HA, Horsberg TE, Ranheim B. Ketoprofen in piglets: enantioselective pharmacokinetics, pharmacodynamics and PK / PD modelling. J Vet Pharmacol Therap. 2010; doi:10.1111/j.1365-2885.2010.01236.x.
19. Friton GM, Philipp H, Schneider T, Kleemann R. Investigation on the clinical efficacy and safety of meloxicam (Metacam*) in the treatment of non-infectious locomotor disorders in pigs. Berl Münch Tierärztl Wschr. 2003;116: 421–6.
20. Hewson CJ, Dohoo IR, Lemke KA, Barkema HW. Canadian veterinarians' use of analgesics in cattle, pigs, and horses in 2004 and 2005. Can Vet J. 2007; 48:155–64.
21. Information från Läkemedelsverket Supplement 1:2005. Smärtbehandling hos hund och katt – Behandlingsrekommendation. Läkemedelsverket, Medical Products Agency, Sweden. 2005. https://lakemedelsverket.se/upload/nyheter/2005/smarta_rek.pdf Accessed 01 Feb 2016.
22. Barz A, Breitinger I, Langhoff R, Zöls S, Ritzmann M, Heinritzi K. Examination of different options for combined administration of Metacam* and iron to piglets. In: IPVS 2008 Scientific Committee, editor. Proceedings of the 20th International Pig Veterinary Society Congress, 22 – 26 June 2008, Durban, South Africa, vol. 2. 2008. p. 472.
23. Breitinger I, Barz A, Langhoff R, Zöls S, Ritzmann M, Heinritzi K. Effects of Mederantil* premedication on castration-induced stress in male piglets. In: IPVS 2008 Scientific Committee, editor. Proceedings of the 20th International

Pig Veterinary Society Congress, 22 – 26 June 2008, Durban, South Africa, vol. 2. 2008. p. 585.

24. Rang HP, Dale MM, Ritter JM. Pharmacology. 4th ed, vol. 229. Edinburgh: Churchill Livingstone; 1999. p. 416–23.

25. Friendship R, Charbonneau G. Pain Control. In: Smith JH, editor. 13th London Swine Conference Proceedings. London, Ontario, Canada: Managing for production; 2013. p. 27–8.

26. Done S, Williamson SM, Strugnell BW. Nervous and Locomotor Systems. In: Zimmerman JJ, Karriker LA, Ramirez A, Schwartz KJ, Stevenson GW, editors. Diseases of swine. 10th ed. Ames, Iowa, USA: Wiley and Sons; 2012. p. 294–328.

27. Lameness in Pigs in Farrowing Houses. The Merck Veterinary Manual. http://www.merckvetmanual.com/mvm/musculoskeletal_system/lameness_in_pigs/lameness_in_pigs_in_farrowing_houses.html Accessed 01 Feb 2016.

28. Wallgren P. Ethical, ecological and economical considerations of diseases among pigs in Sweden. Sv Vet Tidn. 2000;13:685–94.

29. Johansen M, Alban L, Kjærsgård HD, Bækbo P. Factors associated with suckling piglet average daily gain. Prev Vet Med. 2004; doi:10.1016/j.prevetmed.2004.01.011.

30. Lemke KA. Understanding the pathophysiology of perioperative pain. Can Vet J. 2004;45:405–13.

31. White RG, DeShazer JA, Tressler CJ, Borcher GM, Davey S, Waninge A, et al. Vocalization and physiological response of pigs during castration with or without a local anesthetic. J Anim Sci. 1995;73:381–6.

32. Kluivers-Poodt M, Hopster H, Spoolder HAM. Castration under anaesthesia and/or analgesia in commercial pig production. Report 2007, 85, Animal Sciences Group Wageningen UR.

33. Hansson M, Lundeheim N, Nyman G, Johansson G. Effect of local anaesthesia and/or analgesia on pain responses induced by piglet castration. Acta Vet Scand. 2011; doi:10.1186/1751-0147-53-34.

34. Gottschalk M. Streptococcosis. In: Zimmerman JJ, Karriker LA, Ramirez A, Schwartz KJ, Stevenson GW, editors. Diseases of swine. 10th ed. Ames, Iowa, USA: Wiley and Sons; 2012. p. 841–55.

35. Mouttotou N, Hatchell FM, Green LE. The prevalence and risk factors associated with forelimb skin abrasions and sole bruising in preweaning piglets. Prev Vet Med. 1999; doi:10.1016/S0167-5877(99)00006-9.

36. Frohm H, Jacobson M, Zoric M. Clinical effects of NSAID treatment in piglets with arthritis. In: D'Allaire S, Friendship R, editors. Proceedings of the 21st International Pig Veterinary Society Congress, 18 – 21 July 2010, Vancouver, Canada, vol. 2. 2010. p. 1152.

37. Henry SC, Apley M. Therapeutics. In: Straw BE, D'Allaire S, Mengeling WL, Taylor DJ, editors. Diseases of swine. 8th ed. Ames, Iowa, USA: Iowa State University Press; 1999. p. 1155–62.

38. Swedres-Svarm 2014. Consumption of antibiotics and occurrence of antibiotic resistance in Sweden. Solna/Uppsala; 2014. http://www.sva.se/en/antibiotika/svarm-reports Accessed 01 Feb 2016.

12

A field efficacy and safety trial in the Netherlands in pigs vaccinated at 3 weeks of age with a ready-to-use porcine circovirus type 2 and *Mycoplasma hyopneumoniae* combined vaccine

Luuk Kaalberg[1], Victor Geurts[2] ⓘD and Rika Jolie[3*]

Abstract

Background: Respiratory diseases impair the health and welfare of growing pigs and impacts farmers' gains worldwide. Their control through a preventative medical approach has to be tailored according to the pathogens identified at farm level. In the Netherlands, several studies have emphasized the prominent role of *Mycoplasma hyopneumoniae*, Porcine Circovirus type 2 and Porcine Reproductive and Respiratory Syndrome Virus in such respiratory conditions. Further to the arrival on the Dutch market of the first commercially available bivalent vaccine against PCV2 and *M. hyopneumoniae*, Porcilis® PCV M. Hyo, a trial was designed to evaluate its safety and efficacy under local field conditions.

Material and methods: In a conventional farrow-to-finish 170-sow farm with a history of respiratory diseases and demonstrated circulation of both *M. hyopneumoniae* and PCV2, 812 piglets were randomised and included at weaning in either of the three following groups: PCVM (vaccinated with Porcilis® PCV M. Hyo), FLEX (vaccinated with CircoFLEX® and MycoFLEX®) or NC (negative control, injected with placebo). Piglets were vaccinated at 3 weeks of age (day 0) and a subset was bled and weighed at regular intervals up to slaughter. Lung slaughter checks were only performed on 64% of the pigs included on day 0.

Results and implication: No side effect of injection was observed in any of the three groups. Average daily weight gain was improved in both vaccinated groups as compared to the NC group, over the finishing period as well as from wean-to-finish. The PCVM group had a significantly lower PCV2 viremia area under the curve than the two other groups, and a significant reduction in the severity of the pneumonia-like lesions was observed at slaughter in the pigs of the PCVM group. A conservative estimate of the economic benefit of that vaccine was 2.84 € per finisher. This trial confirms that the vaccine is efficacious against the health and growth effects of PCV2 and *M. hyopneumoniae*, of practical advantage (single injection of a bivalent product) and well tolerated.

Keywords: PCV2, *Mycoplasma hyopneumoniae*, Bivalent vaccine, Randomised controlled field trial

* Correspondence: rika.jolie@merck.com
[3]Merck Animal Health, 2 Giralda Farms, Madison, NJ 07940, USA
Full list of author information is available at the end of the article

Background and regional context

Porcine Circovirus type 2 (PCV2) and *Mycoplasma hyopneumoniae* are two of the dominating pathogens in the global industry of fattening pigs. PCV2 infection can produce overt clinical diseases as well as subclinical growth retardation, the latter being considered as the most common form of PCV2 infection worldwide [1]. *M. hyopneumoniae* induces a chronic lung infection which impacts growth [2]. Both pathogens have developed immune evasion strategies that are still only partially understood [3, 4]. In growing pigs, these two pathogens, through their ability to interfere with effectors of both the innate [5, 6] and adaptive immune response [5, 7], tend to foster infections with other pathogens. Being both slow growers [5, 8] and immunity-wise discrete invaders [5, 9], PCV2 and *M. hyopneumoniae* have proven difficult to control by vaccination so far [10, 11].

In Europe, extensive epidemiological studies have been published on infectious risk factors of respiratory diseases. In France, it was shown that PCV2 seems to be of lesser importance in these disorders than *Mycoplasma hyopneumoniae* [12]. In Belgium, a recent cross-sectional study explored several infectious factors potentially associated with lung lesions at slaughter, but failed to include PCV2 among them, showing that it was not considered a relevant respiratory pathogen [13]. In the Netherlands on the other hand, PCV2, *Pasteurella multocida*, *Mycoplasma hyopneumoniae*, and swine influenza viruses (SIVs) were all found in a significantly higher frequency in herds having an elevated proportion of lung lesions (pneumonia) at slaughter, but with no clinical signs of post-weaning multisystemic wasting syndrome (PMWS) [14]. More recently, two reports added to this knowledge: i. in 27 Dutch farms with respiratory clinical signs, between November 2013 and October 2015, oral fluid sampling allowed to observe that finishers (pigs of 19–24 weeks of age) were positive for the genome of *M. hyopneumoniae* (> 75% of farms), PRRSV (35%), PCV2 and *Actinobacillus pleuropneumoniae* (100%)[1]; ii. in respiratory diseases outbreaks on 412 Benelux farms over a 4-year period, diagnostic test results confirmed the dominance of *M. hyopneumoniae*, PRRSV and PCV2 in fattening pigs, without seasonal variation.[2] Another study conducted in Germany also evidenced that PCV2 is a major component of respiratory diseases in that region [15]. However, the role of PCV2 in pneumonic lesions is rarely evoked in the field, where lung slaughter checks are exclusively considered as a monitoring tool to assess the prevalence of enzootic pneumonia; of note is that all lung lesion scoring systems are positively and significantly correlated [16]. Also, respiratory pathogens have been shown to interact with each other [17], e.g. *M. hyopneumoniae* as well as PRRSV have been shown to potentiate PCV2-associated lesions. One may also interfere with vaccination

against the other. Under experimental conditions, in pigs dually infected with *M. hyopneumoniae* and PCV2, the single vaccination against either pathogen has not been found to have an impact on the lung lesions induced by the other one. Conversely, piglet vaccination against *M. hyopneumoniae* was found to reduce PRRSV replication in co-infected piglets (as compared to non-vaccinated ones) (see [18] for a review). More lately, bivalent and combined vaccines against PCV2 and *M. hyopneumoniae* have become commercially available. While the practical interest of such products is obvious in terms of labour (a single injection as opposed to 2 injections for the monovalent vaccines), their preventative efficacy is regularly questioned in the field — partly because the epidemiology of respiratory diseases may vary locally. Comparative field data on the two single-shot 2-valence vaccines are scarcely available to the European prescribers. The present study's aim is providing such data, particularly adding to the European Medicines Agency's public assessment report on Porcilis® PCV M. Hyo, the first ready-to-use bivalent vaccine against PCV2 and *Mycoplasma hyopneumoniae*[3].

Case farm and trial setting

In the fall of 2014, a conventional 170-sow Dutch farrow-to-finish swine farm managed in a 2-week batch system with a history of PCV2-subclinical infection and of enzootic pneumonia was selected for a field trial. The former condition was characterized by a decreased average daily weight gain (ADWG) in the finishing phase over year 2014, as defined by [1]. Also, pre-trial investigations identified a PCV2 serological profile presenting an increase in antibody titers starting around 10 weeks of age; 16–22 week old pigs were also PCV2 PCR-positive in oral fluids, showing together an early and prolonged PCV2 circulation in the herd. The *M. hyopneumoniae* condition was evidenced by an elevated lung lesion score (LLS) assessed at slaughter (Madec scoring system [19]), which was above the average LLS of the slaughterhouse. Also, *M. hyopneumoniae* serology was partially positive in 16 week-old pigs, and completely positive in 22 week-old pigs; furthermore, the saliva samples of 16 week-old finishers were PCR-positive for *M. hyopneumoniae*. These results demonstrate that a herd infection took place during finishing. On that farm, sows, nursery and finisher pigs were housed in separate stables, although in a single site.

On the day of inclusion in the trial (d0), piglets of on average 21 days of age (16–26 days) were individually weighed and identified with their unique numbered ear tags (piglets appearing unhealthy were not identified, hence discarded). Within each litter, piglets were assigned to either of the three study groups.

Group 1 (PCVM, n = 269): vaccination with Porcilis® PCV M Hyo (MSD Animal Health, Boxmeer, the Netherlands), according to the product SPC[4]: 2 ml via the intramuscular (IM) route, in the neck.

Group 2 (FLEX, n = 267): vaccination with a single injection of CircoFLEX® and MycoFLEX® (Boehringer Ingelheim, Ingelheim, Germany), according to the product SPC[5]: 2 ml (2 × 1 ml dose) via the IM route, in the neck.

Group 3 (NC, n = 276): injection of saline, 2 ml via the IM route in the neck. Group 3 is the negative control group.

Because of the farm's 2-week batch production management, 6 batches of piglets were included in the trial, between Dec. 18, 2014 and March 5, 2015 (72 litters and 812 piglets in total). In half of these batches (#1, #3 and #5), around 10 piglets from each treatment group were randomly selected to be blood sampled on regular intervals (at 3, 10, 18 and 22 weeks of age). All trial piglets were also individually weighed on these dates. On d0, piglets selected for blood sampling received a red-paint dot on their ear-tag; blood sampling was performed after group allocation but before vaccination. There was no statistically significant difference between groups for age, and weight at inclusion, and sex (see Table 1).

Pigs from different groups were commingled throughout the study, according to the current farm practices.

Assessment of vaccine safety and efficacy

Although safety was not the primary objective for this study, the piglets were monitored for both local and systemic reactions immediately and 1 h after injections. No side effect was recorded in any of the three groups.

To assess the efficacy of the vaccines in the farms' context, three primary parameters were used: PCV2 viremia (genomic serum load) for protection towards infection; lung lesion score at slaughter for prevalence and severity of enzootic pneumonia; and average daily weight gain (ADWG) in the finishing period for the control of both pathogens (PCV2 and *M. hyopneumoniae*). Mortality was recorded as a secondary parameter; this allowed, together with primary parameters and slaughterhouse information, to estimate the economic impact of the vaccines.

The PCV2 viral load was determined by the Boxmeer MSD R&D Service Laboratory by a PCV2-specific real-time polymerase chain reaction [20].

All sampled control animals became PCV2 viraemic during the study (see Table 2). In the FLEX group 67% became viraemic and 43% in the PCVM group. The PCV2 viraemia, expressed as area under the curve (AUC), in the PCVM group was significantly lower than in the control group (ANOVA: $p < 0.0001$) and in the FLEX group (ANOVA: $p = 0.0022$). The FLEX group

Table 1 Overview of the number of animals, age at inclusion, sex and weight at vaccination or injection, per treatment group

	Control (N = 276)	FLEX (N = 267)	PCVM (N = 269)	Overall (N = 812)
Age (days)				
16	3 (1.1%)	3 (1.1%)	2 (0.7%)	8 (1.0%)
17	39 (14.1%)	35 (13.1%)	40 (14.9%)	114 (14.0%)
18	44 (15.9%)	42 (15.7%)	43 (16.0%)	129 (15.9%)
19	28 (10.1%)	27 (10.1%)	28 (10.4%)	83 (10.2%)
20	3 (1.1%)	3 (1.1%)	3 (1.1%)	9 (1.1%)
21	15 (5.4%)	16 (6.0%)	14 (5.2%)	45 (5.5%)
22	26 (9.4%)	25 (9.4%)	27 (10.0%)	78 (9.6%)
23	61 (22.1%)	58 (21.7%)	60 (22.3%)	179 (22.0%)
24	32 (11.6%)	33 (12.4%)	27 (10.0%)	92 (11.3%)
25	22 (8.0%)	22 (8.2%)	22 (8.2%)	66 (8.1%)
26	3 (1.1%)	3 (1.1%)	3 (1.1%)	9 (1.1%)
Gender				
Female	144 (52.2%)	136 (50.9%)	122 (45.4%)	402 (49.5%)
Male	132 (47.8%)	131 (49.1%)	147 (54.6%)	410 (50.5%)
Weight (kg)				
N	276	267	269	812
Mean	5.6	5.6	5.7	5.6
Standard deviation	1.54	1.56	1.57	1.56
Minimum	1.6	1.7	1.9	1.6
Maximum	10.2	10.2	10.0	10.2

Table 2 Mean PCV2 viraemia (expressed in log10 copies/µl DNA extract) by sampling time after admission and AUC, by trial group

	PCVM group	FLEX group	Negative control group
Admission	0.00 ± 0.00	0.00 ± 0.00	0.00 ± 0.00
Week 7	0.21 ± 0.52	0.75 ± 1.25	2.62 ± 2.02
Week 15	0.23 ± 0.69	0.92 ± 1.31	1.93 ± 1.12
Week 19	0.04 ± 0.12	0.29 ± 0.75	1.38 ± 1.29
AUC[a]	2.99/ 0.00[a]	12.11/ 3.90[b]	33.99/ 36.64[c]

Values with different superscript letters within the same row are statistically significantly different (ANOVA, [ab] $p = 0.0022$; [ac] $p < 0.0001$; [bc] $p < 0.0001$)
[a]Mean/Median

also had a statistically significant ($p < 0.0001$) lower viraemia compared with the control group. Two pigs (both from the FLEX group) were viraemic at vaccination and were not included in this analysis.

During the trial, wasting piglets were observed on the farm (contemporary batches), suggesting that PCV2 viral pressure was still present, although limited (overall mortality was low).

Lung lesion score was evaluated according to the Madec system, and a mixed ANOVA model was used to analyze these scores. Equivalent Goodwin scores [21] were calculated from the Madec scores and statistical analysis was performed on the log10-transformed total lung lesion scores[6]. The sample size of 300 pigs per group had a power above 80% to detect a difference of 0.15 in log10-transformed LLS (Goodwin system). This size was not achieved, since lungs from only 64% of pigs included on d0 were checked ($n = 518$); the rest of them were not scored for several reasons (death, loss of the ear tag or missed in the slaughter line). LLS can be interpreted however, since the proportion of pigs lost over the trial duration was comparable in each group (96 [36%] in the PCVM group, 104 [39%] in the FLEX group and 94 [34%]

in the NC group), mortality rate among each group was not statistically different: 36 pigs died or were culled during the study (3.3% (9/269) in the PCVM group, 4.5% (12/267) in the FLEX group and 5.4% (15/276) in the NC group) and the numerical difference in total LLS (Goodwin) between groups exceeds 0.15. There were differences in the proportion of lungs with enzootic pneumonia-like lung lesions between groups, with a proportion that was nearly double in the NC group compared with both vaccinated group (see Table 3). Also, average total LLS was higher in the NC group (0.4 ± 1.4) compared to both vaccinated groups (PCVM: 0.1 ± 0.6; FLEX: 0.2 ± 1.0). The difference between both vaccinated groups was not significant (mixed model ANOVA, $p = 0.4781$), but the difference in total LLS was significant between the PCVM and the NC groups ($p = 0.0163$). Finally, the severity of these lesions was significantly lower in the PCVM group as compared to the NC group (NC-PCVM = 0.14; [95%CI 0.03–0.26], $p = 0.0157$). This difference was not significant when the FLEX and NC groups were compared (NC-FLEX = 0.11; [95% CI: 0.001–0.23]; $p = 0.0528$), nor when PCVM and FLEX groups were compared (FLEX-PCVM = 0.03; [95% CI: 0.09–0.14]; $p = 0.6507$).

Table 3 Distribution of the lung lesion scores by treatment (n [%]), according to the Madec scoring system and the extrapolation to the Goodwin scoring system

		PCVM group ($N = 173$)	FLEX group ($N = 163$)	NC group ($N = 182$)
Madec scoring system (max. 28)	Missing[a]	20 [11.6]	18 [11.0]	28 [15.4]
	Score 0	142 [82.1]	133 [81.6]	131 [72.0]
	Score 1–3	10 [5.8]	9 [5.5]	17 [9.3]
	Score 4–6	1 [0.6]	2 [1.2]	4 [2.2]
	Score 7–9	0 [0.0]	0 [0.0]	1 [0.5]
	Score 8–12	0 [0.0]	1 [0.6]	1 [0.5]
	Maximum score	5	10	11
	Proportion of lungs with EP-like lesions	6.3%	7.4%	12.6%
Goodwin scoring system (max. 55)	Score 0	142 [82.1]	133 [81.6]	131 [72.0]
	0 < Score ≤ 5	8 [4.6]	9 [5.5]	15 [8.2]
	5 < Score ≤ 10	2 [1.2]	2 [1.2]	5 [2.7]
	Score > 10	1 [0.6]	1 [0.6]	3 [1.6]
	Maximum score	12.5	21.25	25

[a]Missing animals were those that had been slaughtered before the lung scoring team arrived

M. hyopneumoniae serology, performed with the Swine HerdChek® M. hyo IDEXX kit, confirmed that *M. hyopneumoniae* exposure occurred during the finishing period, with a limited challenge (3% of positive pigs in the NC group on week 22). The fact that the reduction in the severity of EP-like lesions was only significant in the group vaccinated with Porcilis® PCV M Hyo might have an economic significance, considering that a significant (*p* < 0.001) negative correlation has been demonstrated between pneumonia score and growth, with an ADWG loss of about 0.7% for each point of pneumonia increase [22].

For the analysis of the Average Daily Weight Gain (ADWG), a sample size of 300 in each treatment group had 80% power to detect a difference in means of 25 g/d between vaccinated and control groups. This size was not achieved at inclusion, but the measured ADWG over the finishing period exceeded this value (see Table 4). Hence, a mixed ANOVA model[7] was used for statistical analysis. All animals were weighed individually with a calibrated scale. The weighing prior to slaughter was done on the same day for all animals of the same farrowing batch, one or a few days before the first pigs of that same batch were shipped to slaughter.

There was no statistically significant difference in the ADWG over the nursery period between groups (data not shown), confirming that neither vaccine has a detectable negative impact on growth performance shortly after injection. Over the finishing period (10–22 weeks of age), there was a highly significant difference between both vaccinated groups and the NC group (*p* = 0.0004), but not between the PCVM and FLEX groups (see Table 4). Overall (weeks 3–22), the difference between both vaccinated groups and the NC group was also highly significant (*p* = 0.0014). Although not statistically significant, both during finishing and overall, ADWG was numerically higher in the PCVM group than in the FLEX group. ADWG, a primary efficacy parameter for the prevention against PCV2 and *M. hyopneumoniae* infections, was significantly higher in

the finishing period for both vaccinated groups, compared to the control group, which confirms the interest of early vaccination of piglets with a bivalent vaccine on a farm where both pathogens are circulating.

The estimation of the improvement of the farmer's income was based on the results in the PCVM group (ADWG and mortality) and the average Dutch economical production figures, compiled by the Wageningen Economic Research institute: the 38 g/d improvement of the ADWG corresponds to €1.37 more income per finisher; the 2-point lower mortality rate produces a €1.47 gain. In total, the trial at least allowed to estimate an income improvement of € 2.84 per finisher.[8] This is probably a conservative estimate, since individual feed intake could not be measured and potential gains in food conversion rate (FCR) are not included in the present economical calculation.

Conclusion

On a conventional Dutch farrow-to-finish farm with good management and a good health status, where PCV2 and *M. hyopneumoniae* were diagnosed as the prominent infectious risk factors for respiratory disease, a randomised field trial was performed. Three treatments were compared: piglets vaccinated at 3 weeks of age with Porcilis® PCV M Hyo bivalent ready-to-use vaccine, or with the FLEX combination vaccine (doses of the CircoFLEX® and MycoFLEX® vaccines mixed into a single injection), or with a placebo injection. Both vaccines significantly reduced the negative effect of both pathogens on growth performance, as measured by the ADWG over the finishing period, and overall. A significant reduction in the severity of the pneumonia-like lesions was only observed in the pigs vaccinated with Porcilis® PCV M Hyo. When viremia was expressed as AUC per group, the PCVM group had a significantly lower AUC value than both other groups. The FLEX group had a significantly lower AUC value than the NC group. This study further supports safety and efficacy data of Porcilis® PCV M Hyo bivalent ready-to-use vaccine.

Table 4 Average Daily Weight gain improvement/reduction between treatment groups over the finishing period and overall (* *p* = 0.0004 ** *p* = 0.0014)

Compared groups	ADWG over the finishing period (g/d)	Reduction of ADWG over the finishing period	Wean-to-finish ADWG (g/d)	Reduction of ADWG from wean-to-finish
PCVM vs. NC	PCVM: 842	−38 g/day* and 95% CI [−57, −19]	PCVM: 660	−24 g/day** and 95% CI [−37, −11]
	NC: 803		NC: 634	
FLEX vs. NC	FLEX: 827	−26 g/day* and 95% CI [−44, −7]	FLEX: 650	−17 g/day** and 95% CI [−30, −3]
	NC: 803		NC: 634	
PCVM vs. FLEX	PCVM: 842	−12 g/day and 95% CI [−31, 7]	PCVM: 660	−8 g/day and 95% CI [−21, 6]
	FLEX: 827		FLEX: 650	

Endnotes

[1]Van Dongen F. in Proceedings of the 24th International Pig Veterinary Society, Dublin Ireland, 7–10 June 2016, p. 287.

[2]Vangroenweghe F. in Proceedings of the 24th International Pig Veterinary Society, Dublin Ireland, 7–10 June 2016, p. 151.

[3]This EPAR is freely available online on the website of EMA: http://www.ema.europa.eu/ema/index.jsp?curl=pages/medicines/veterinary/medicines/003796/vet_med_000307.jsp&mid=WC0b01ac058008d7a8.

[4]The summary of the European public assessment report of this vaccine is available online at http://www.ema.europa.eu/docs/en_GB/document_library/EPAR_-_Summary_for_the_public/veterinary/003796/WC500177275. pdf

[5]The summary of the European public assessment report of this vaccine is available online at http://www.ema.europa.eu/docs/en_GB/document_library/EPAR_-_Product_Information/veterinary/000126/WC500062388.pdf

[6]Both analyses included the sow as random effect and treatment as fixed effect.

[7]The model considered the dam as a random effect and treatment, gender and their interaction as fixed effects. The initial weight was included in the model as a covariate.

[8]Vaccination cost was not included in this calculation.

Abbreviations

ADWG: Average daily weight gain; FCR: Food conversion rate; LLS: Lung lesion score; PCR: Polymerase chain reaction; PCV2: Porcine circovirus type 2; PRRS: Porcine reproductive and respiratory syndrome; PRRSV: Porcine reproductive and respiratory syndrome virus; RTU: Ready-to-use; SIV: Swine influenza virus

Acknowledgements

The authors are grateful to the farm owner and his stockmen, for agreeing to engage in the trial and for working in good cooperation with the investigation team, to J.Hijink (Hijdeporc B.V.) for performing the lung checks, and to D. Dufe for support in the statistical analysis. The authors also wish to address special thanks to Vion Company for excellence of cooperation spirit and for enabling us to perform the slaughterhouse checks, and to Antonio Arts (Vion Company) also regarding the slaughterhouse checks.

Funding

Intervet Nederland BV funded the study.

Authors' contributions

KL was Clinical Investigator and wrote the results section; GV and JR designed the study; JR reviewed the manuscript. All authors read and approved the final manuscript.

Competing interests

With the exception of the primary author, all other authors of this short report are employees from the company sponsor.

Author details

[1]De Graafschapdierenartsen bv, Schimmeldijk 1 Vorden, 7251 MX Vorden, The Netherlands. [2]MSD Animal Health, Wim de Korverstraat 35, 5831 AN Boxmeer, The Netherlands. [3]Merck Animal Health, 2 Giralda Farms, Madison, NJ 07940, USA.

References

1. Segalés J. Porcine circovirus type 2 (PCV2) infections: clinical signs, pathology and laboratory diagnosis. Virus Res. 2012;164(1–2):10–9.
2. Clark LK, Armstrong CH, Scheidt AB, Van Alstine WG. The effect of Mycoplasma hyopneumoniae infection on growth in pigs with or without environmental constraints. J Swine Health Prod. 1993;1(6):10–4.
3. Meng XJ. Porcine circovirus type 2 (PCV2): pathogenesis and interaction with the immune system. Annu Rev Anim Biosci. 2013;1:43–64.
4. Simionatto S, Marchioro SB, Maes D, Dellagostin OA. Mycoplasma hyopneumoniae: from disease to vaccine development. Vet Microbiol. 2013; 165(3–4):234–42.
5. Ren L, Chen X, Ouyang H. Interactions of porcine circovirus 2 with its hosts. Virus Genes. 2016;52(4):437–44.
6. Mebus CA, Underdahl NR. Scanning electron microscopy of trachea and bronchi from gnotobiotic pigs inoculated with Mycoplasma hyopneumoniae. Am J Vet Res. 1977;38(8):1249–54.
7. Shen Y, Hu W, Wei Y, Feng Z, Yang Q. Effects of Mycoplasma hyopneumoniae on porcine nasal cavity dendritic cells. Vet Microbiol. 2017; 198:1–8.
8. L'Ecuyer C, Boulanger P. Enzootic pneumonia in pigs: identification of a causative mycoplasma in infected pigs and in cultures by immunofluorescent staining. Can J Comp Med. 1970;34(1):38–46. https://www.ncbi.nlm.nih.gov/pmc/articles/PMC1319418/pdf/compmed00061-0042.pdf
9. Thacker EL. Immunology of the porcine respiratory disease complex. Vet Clin North Am Food Anim Pract. 2001;17(3):551–65.
10. Segalés J. Best practice and future challenges for vaccination against porcine circovirus type 2. Expert Rev Vaccines. 2015;14(3):473–87.
11. Maes D, Sibila M, Kuhnert P, Segalés J, Haesebrouck F, Pieters M. Update on Mycoplasma hyopneumoniae infections in pigs: Knowledge gaps for improved disease control. Transbound Emerg Dis. 2017. doi:10.1111/tbed.12677.
12. Fablet C, Marois-Créhan C, Simon G, Grasland B, Jestin A, Kobisch M, Madec F, Rose N. Infectious agents associated with respiratory diseases in 125 farrow-to-finish pig herds: a cross-sectional study. Vet Microbiol. 2012;157(1–2):152–63.
13. Meyns T, Van Steelant J, Rolly E, Dewulf J, Haesebrouck F, Maes D. A cross-sectional study of risk factors associated with pulmonary lesions in pigs at slaughter. Vet J. 2011;187(3):388–92.
14. Wellenberg GJ, Bouwkamp FT, Wolf PJ, Swart WA, Mombarg MJ, de Gee AL. A study on the severity and relevance of porcine circovirus type 2 infections in Dutch fattening pigs with respiratory diseases. Vet Microbiol. 2010;142(3–4):217–24.
15. Fachinger V, Bischoff R, Jedidia SB, Saalmüller A, Elbers K. The effect of vaccination against porcine circovirus type 2 in pigs suffering from porcine respiratory disease complex. Vaccine. 2008;26(11):1488–99.
16. Garcia-Morante B, Segalés J, Fraile L, Pérez de Rozas A, Maiti H, Coll T, Sibila M. Assessment of Mycoplasma hyopneumoniae-induced pneumonia using different lung lesion scoring systems: a comparative review. J Comp Pathol. 2016;154(2–3):125–34.
17. Opriessnig T, Giménez-Lirola LG, Halbur PG. Polymicrobial respiratory disease in pigs. Anim Health Res Rev. 2011;12(2):133–48.

18. Chae C. Porcine respiratory disease complex: interaction of vaccination and porcine circovirus type 2, porcine reproductive and respiratory syndrome virus, and Mycoplasma hyopneumoniae. Vet J. 2016;212:1–6.
19. Madec F, Kobisch M. Lung lesion scoring of finisher pigs at the slaughterhouse [in French]. Journées de la Recherche Porcine. 1982;14:405–12.
20. Witvliet M, Holtslag H, Nell T, Segers R, Fachinger V. Efficacy and safety of a combined porcine Circovirus and Mycoplasma hyopneumoniae vaccine in finishing pigs. Trials in Vaccinology. 2015;4:43–9.
21. Goodwin RF, Hodgson RG, Whittlestone P, Woodhams RL. Some experiments relating to artificial immunity in enzootic pneumonia of pigs. J Hyg (Lond). 1969;67(3):465–76. http://www.ncbi.nlm.nih.gov/pmc/articles/PMC2130744/pdf/jhyg00097-0090.pdf
22. Pagot E, Pommier P, Keïta A. Relationship between growth during the fattening period and lung lesions at slaughter in swine. Revue Méd Vét. 2007;158(5):253–9. http://www.revmedvet.com/2007/RMV158_253_259.pdf

13

Genetic resistance - an alternative for controlling PRRS?

Gerald Reiner

Abstract

PRRS is one of the most challenging diseases for world-wide pig production. Attempts for a sustainable control of this scourge by vaccination have not yet fully satisfied. With an increasing knowledge and methodology in disease resistance, a new world-wide endeavour has been started to support the combat of animal diseases, based on the existence of valuable gene variants with regard to any host-pathogen interaction. Several groups have produced a wealth of evidence for natural variability in resistance/susceptibility to PRRS in our commercial breeding lines. However, up to now, exploiting existing variation has failed because of the difficulty to detect the carriers of favourable and unfavourable alleles, especially with regard to such complex polygenic traits like resistance to PRRS. New hope comes from new genomic tools like next generation sequencing which have become extremely fast and low priced. Thus, research is booming world-wide and the jigsaw puzzle is filling up – slowly but steadily. On the other hand, knowledge from virological and biomedical basic research has opened the way for an "intervening way", i.e. the modification of identified key genes that occupy key positions in PRRS pathogenesis, like *CD163*. *CD163* was identified as the striking receptor in PRRSV entry and its knockout from the genome by gene editing has led to the production of pigs that were completely resistant to PRRSV – a milestone in modern pig breeding. However, at this early step, concerns remain about the acceptance of societies for gene edited products and regulation still awaits upgrading to the new technology. Further questions arise with regard to upcoming patents from an ethical and legal point of view. Eventually, the importance of *CD163* for homeostasis, defence and immunity demands for more insight before its complete or partial silencing can be answered. Whatever path will be followed, even a partial abolishment of PRRSV replication will lead to a significant improvement of the disastrous herd situation, with a significant impact on welfare, performance, antimicrobial consumption and consumer protection. Genetics will be part of a future solution.

Keywords: PRRS, Disease resistance, Gene editing, *CD163*

Background

The production of PRRS resistant pigs by gene editing has produced a milestone in pig breeding and a big hope for a sustainable combat of an important disease. However, much remains to be done to reach the demands of practical breeding. While gene editing methods try to modify genes that play important roles in the pathogenesis of a disease, functional genome analysis and association studies intend to detect and exploit naturally existing genetic variation in such genes. Both approaches are in process at a world-wide endeavor to improve resistance of pigs to infectious diseases. The aim of this review is to provide insight into status and potential of these applications with regrd to PRRS, with a glimpse on future and existing concerns. Conclusions are based on the existing literature.

Genetic resistance as a first choice of prophylaxis

Breeding for disease-resistant pigs might be the *ultima ratio* in combatting infectious diseases. Regardless of whether pigs would be resistant *sensu stricto*, (i.e. the absolute prevention of an infection, or just tolerating the infection) minimal amplification and shedding of the pathogen and minimal effects on health and performance could be achieved. Thus, the infectious pressure in and between herds could be efficiently reduced, followed by diminished disease incidence, improved performance and

Correspondence: gerald.reiner@vetmed.uni-giessen.de
Department of Veterinary Clinical Sciences, Swine Clinic,
Justus-Liebig-University, Frankfurter Strasse 112, 35392 Giessen, Germany

product quality, reduced antibiotic treatment, improved consumer protection and increased animal welfare [90].

Genetic resistance in practical breeding

Disease-resistant breeds, populations or animals are of considerable importance to livestock. Prime examples are resistance to coccidiosis and Marek's disease in fowl (e.g. [20]), to trypanosomiasis [77] and ticks [81] in cattle at tropical sites, to mastitis in dairy cattle (e.g. [41]), and to gastro-intestinal nematodes in sheep [109]. In pigs, however, examples of genetic resistance in commercial breeding programmes are sparse. Two examples are resistance to fimbriated F18 [121] and F4 [49] *Escherichia coli*. They represent rare cases of single-gene controlled genetic resistance. F18 fimbriated E.coli cause post-weaning diarrhoea and oedema disease [73] and resistance is realised by a receptor variant that does not bind any type of E.coli F18 fimbriae. Similarly, the right F4 receptor variant gives resistance to neonatal diarrhoea caused by most of F4-fimbriated E.coli. Other examples include the breeding for improved immune responsiveness, i.e. a higher general reactivity in humoral and cellular immunity in pigs (e.g. [129]). In spite of the currently limited commercial applications in swine, a wide range of genetic variation has been observed in genetic resistance to different bacterial, viral and parasitic diseases. A comprehensive search for disease resistance might identify differences in susceptibility/resistance in any host-species with regard to any relevant pathogen [90]. However, most of this genetic variation cannot be used in practical breeding, because of the difficulty in recognising favourable and unfavourable gene variants within the breeders. Their identification is impeded by highly variable and influential farm-specific environmental effects (e.g., pathogen load, immunity, housing, feeding and management conditions), the polygenic inheritance mode of most resistance traits, the limited availability of animal models and limited detailed knowledge of pathogenesis for most porcine diseases.

Improving genetic disease resistance

While classical breeding is, thus generally inappropriate for efficient improvement of genetic resistance, evolved knowledge of the porcine genome combined with new tools and technologies – developed in the context of genome projects – have created new opportunities to dissect the genetic control of complex traits, including host responses to infection [4]. Alternatively to classical breeding, responsible gene variants can be identified via experiments in selected populations that vary significantly in resistance/susceptibility, under standardised environmental conditions, including time point of challenge and quantity of the pathogen. Once the responsible gene variants are identified, causal variants in experimental populations need to be validated in commercial farms to confirm segregation and association, prior to application in selection. Then, breeders can be selected via marker-assisted and genomic selection [74]. Provided there is societal consent, desirable gene variants can even be introduced into breeding populations via genetic engineering (e.g., [84]). In addition, understanding the molecular basis of genetic resistance will help improving the knowledge of the underlying mechanisms of disease and disease resistance, thus promoting new and enhanced developments in diagnostics, therapy and prophylaxis.

Examples on the way

We have seen there are limited examples of applicable gene variants already in the field to improve genetic resistance in swine [49, 121]. However, the search for significant and applicable gene variants has developed into an ever-expanding and successful branch of clinical research, including viral (Pseudorabiesvirus [88]; Influenza A (e.g. [143]); bacterial (*Haemophilus parasuis* [131]; *Actinobacillus pleuropneumoniae* [93, 94]; *Mycoplasma hyopneumoniae* (e.g., [108]); *Streptococcus suis* [136]) and parasitic diseases (*Sarcocystis* [89]; *Ascaris suum* [100, 101]). More than 2,500 quantitative trait loci (QTL) have been published for health parameters in the pig, among them 400 for resistance/susceptibility against a broad range of pathogens (http://www.animalgenome.org/QTLdb/; current status: October 2016). QTL are gene loci which participate in the control of quantitative distributed traits such as milk yield, growth performance and disease resistance. The most remarkable results have been seen in resistance to PRRSV.

Porcine Reproductive and Respiratory Syndrome (PRRS)

PRRS is one of the most devastating diseases in swine, worldwide (for overview see [147]). The disease causes respiratory and reproduction failures. Losses for the US pig industry were estimated at over $ 650 million annually, excluding costs for diagnosis, vaccination, treatment and biosecurity [44]. PRRSV is a single stranded RNA virus from the *Arteriviridae* family and it can be found in two genotypes (US [type 2] and EU [type 1]). Each genotype comprises of thousands of genetic and antigenic heterogenic strains [147]. PRRSV replicates in cells of the monocyte/macrophage lineage, especially in activated macrophages. Its high variability and its ability for immune evasion make it extremely difficult to design sustainable vaccines, especially under heterologous situations (Wilkinson et al. [130]). Thus, other solutions are searched for to combat the disease, among them the use of genetic resistant pigs.

Natural genetic disease resistance against PRRS in swine breeds and populations

Halbur et al. [38] provided initial indications of genetic differences in susceptibility/resistance of pigs against PRRS. Duroc pigs showed lower performance combined with an increased severity of lung lesions and antibody titres after infection with PRRSV than Meishan pigs. Clinical abortion rates were found to be associated with IFNγ and influenced by sows' genetics [67]. A genetic background for differences in performance, severity of lesions, viral titres, infected macrophages and immunological parameters has also been described by Petry et al. [85], Vincent et al. [119, 120], Doeschl-Wilson et al. [26] and Reiner et al. [91], although differences were often small and partially inconsistent over time. Lean lines (Duroc and Hampshire) have been found to be more susceptible than lines selected for higher reproductivity. Ait-Ali et al. [1] reported on favourable macrophages in Landrace pigs and assumed the density and distribution of CD169 and IL-8 levels to be critical factors. High levels of IL-8 and low levels of IFNγ were also associated with PRRSV resistance by Petry et al. [86].

PRRS resistance: tracking down the molecular basis by genome-wide genetic association and differential expression studies

These results provided enough evidence for a genetic background of PRRS resistance and remarkable differences in susceptibility between breeds or at least populations. For the next step, pigs differing at most in susceptibility/resistance were used in experiments to take a detailed look at their genetic peculiarities. Three major setups were applied initially: QTL analysis [39] and genome-wide association study (GWAS) were used to identify chromosomal areas and eventually single nucleotide polymorphisms (SNPs) associated with PRRS phenotypes (e.g., degree of viremia, lung lesions and performance after PRRSV infection [13–15], antibody response [105]) and differential expression experiments to detect genes via differences in their expression levels in susceptible and resistant pigs [103, 104]. The most significant results have been achieved by Joan Lunney (USDA), Bob Rowland (Kansas State University) and colleagues, particularly in the context of the PRRS Host Genetics Consortium (PHGC, for a review, see [69]).

Based on up to 60,000 SNP markers together with new statistical tools, more than 30 QTL for resistance against PRRS have been mapped to 11 chromosomes http://www.animalgenome.org/QTLdb/ [13, 15]. As part of the PRRS Host Genetics Consortium, a genome-wide association study based on 190 pigs from a commercial breeding line and the Illumina PorcineSNP60 BeadChip detected associations with viral load and body weight after PRRSV infection. A major QTL region was mapped to chromosome 4 (SSC4), explaining 16 % of genetic variance for virus load with a frequency for the favourable allele of 0.16 and a heritability of 0.30 [13].

One of the most limiting factors in association studies has been the density of gene markers. Next generation sequencing is a recent technological breakthrough that is speeding up the genetics and genomics of a broad range of traits, conferring new opportunities for high-throughput low cost genotyping. Costs for sequencing have dropped by 1:100,000 during the last 15 years. Marker density can be increased by 10^4 to 10^5 as compared to conventional SNP-chips which has led to the concept of genotyping by sequencing (for overview see [51]). Such technics may help to raise our understanding of host-PRRSV interaction to a higher end much more complex level, including the complete genomic information of both the host and the virus. Next generation sequencing will have a high impact on the understanding of the virus' adaption to replication in the host [18, 68].

GBP5 is an important candidate gene for PRRS resistance

The highest linkage disequilibrium was found for SNP WUR10000125. The interferon-induced guanylate-binding protein 5 gene (GBP5) was identified as the most likely candidate in a total of eight consecutive and independent trials [13–15]. This gene was differentially expressed and validated in different pig populations [53] and an intronic SNP (rs340943904) (close to WUR10000125, but not on the 60 k SNP chip) was found to be responsible for introducing a splicing site that truncated the C-terminal 88 amino acids in the recessive A-allele. GBP5 is involved in immune response to bacterial and viral infection in different species, namely in the inflammatory response and the assembly of the inflammasome in mammals [107], which strongly depends on the C-terminal 67 amino acids which are highly conserved between species [12]. Although the exact role of GBP5 in PRRSV defence remains to be identified, this SNP is the putative quantitative trait nucleotide (QTN) (i.e., the SNP most likely to be responsible for the QTL on SSC4). In addition, Boddicker et al. [14] only found small effects for resistance to PRRS on SSC1, 5, 7 and X. Further research is needed to show the generality of these findings in other global pig breeds.

A second approach to detect underlying molecular differences in PRRS susceptibility/resistance was performed via microarray-based gene expression analysis, in vivo [2, 6, 9, 11, 36, 42, 46, 75, 103, 104, 137–141, 146] or in vitro [98, 99]. Several immune response pathways were upregulated after infection and several hundreds of differentially expressed genes were detected, but this did not lead to a simple identification of directly responsible genes. One major concern with differential expression (DE) studies is that many differentially expressed genes (A) do not necessarily need to carry the responsible mutation. Instead, their differential expression is achieved via the products of other genes (B) that regulate gene expression by binding to the promoter, the 5′ and 3′ untranslated region or to other regulatory elements of the A genes. These B genes, however, do not necessarily need to be differentially expressed, provided the relevant mutation leads to an amino acid exchange, resulting in altered efficiency of the gene products of genes B at the promoters of genes A. Thus, they may not be detected in DE studies. Thus, the strength of DE studies lies mainly in the detection of the gene networks and pathways involved and in integrating the analysis of genetic and DE data.

The role of genetic variation in type I interferon genes

Type I interferons are a heterogeneous group of cytokines, important in antiviral response. Genetic variation has been linked to susceptibility to viral diseases, and PRRSV has been found to suppress type I IFN production as a major strategy for evading the immune system [60, 80, 82]. Sang et al. [97] discovered more than 100 polymorphisms in 39 functional genes from the type I interferon family. More than 20 polymorphic mutants have been linked with differing anti-PRRSV activities in vitro [97].

Genetic variation in autochtonous breeds may contribute genetic resistance against PRRS

Rare breeds, often autochthonous to some regions or countries and poorly adapted to modern pig production, are a valuable source of rare gene variants with sometimes unexpected effects. Rare or even lost SNPs might be (re-)introduced via gene editing methods or by genetic introgression. However, this requires knowledge of these effects and, therefore, the breeds carrying the rare SNPs. One potential example was provided by Li et al. [62] who identified an *Mx1* (myxovirus resistance protein 1) promoter variation, potentially associated with PRRS resistance. *Mx1* exhibits potent anti-RNA viral activity [7, 78] and is involved in early host defence against PRRSV [19, 145]. A second candidate gene, potentially involved in PRRSV resistance, with the valuable allele preferentially restricted to Chinese autochthone breeds, is the ubiquitin-specific protease 18 (*USP18*; [63]).

The role of microRNA genes

MicroRNAs are small non-coding RNA, involved in post-transcriptional gene regulation [92]. They modify mRNA stability by interaction with its 3′ untranslated region and have been shown to be involved in viral pathogenesis in pigs, e.g. swine influenza virus and pseudorabies virus (He et al. [40]; Anselmo et al. [5]; Loveday et al. [66]). Up to now, no microRNA variability has been described in association with PRRS resistance/susceptibility.

However, the porcine microRNAome has been studied in PRRSV-infection and the expression of several microRNAs is altered by PRRSV infection [42, 47, 64]. These results could lead to microRNA-based anti-PRRSV therapies in the future.

Support from basic virus research: the PRRSV receptors

Most genes and molecules involved in PRRS pathogenesis escape detection via genetic and genomic methods, if they are not variable in sequence or expression, or if this variability is not present in the studied populations. Thus, basic virus research is of high importance in the attempt to resolve the pathogenesis of PRRS and to detect candidate genes for PRRS-resistance.

At least six cellular molecules have been described so far as putative receptors for PRRSV, including *CD163*, the cysteine-rich scavenger receptor (SRCR; [17]), sialoadhesin (*CD169*; siglec-1; [29]), *CD151* [106], heparin sulfate [50], vimentin [52] and *CD209* [45], reviewed by Zhang and Yoo [144].

CD163

CD163 is restrictively expressed in cells from the monocyte/macrophage lineage, and significant expression is exclusively found in activated (major) tissue macrophages, together with complement and Fc receptors, other scavenger receptors, and receptors for mediators, adhesion molecules and growth factors [3, 112]. Macrophages not or only newly involved in inflammation and defence do not express *CD163* to any substantial degree [8, 118]. Activation of TLRs (e.g., TLR4) by LPS or other pathogen-associated molecular patterns (PAMPs) increases IL10 [125], one of the strongest upregulators of *CD163* in humans [133]. A second important activator of *CD163* is stress (glucocorticoids) [43, 112].

One major function of *CD163* is in the receptor-mediated endocytosis that delivers extracellular substrates to the endo- and lysosomes of scavenger cells for intracellular metabolism and activation of ligand-specific signal pathways that direct the right answer to the respective substrate [113]. While ligands are delivered to early endosomes, *CD163* recycles to the plasma membrane for new rounds of endocytosis [102]. These events are best recognized regarding the elimination of toxic cell-free haemoglobin from the serum as an important physiological metabolic pathway [56, 102]. Another role of the scavenger receptor seems to be the receptor-mediated internalisation of pathogens, and coincidentally its role as an innate immune sensor for Gram-positive and Gram-negative bacteria, linking bacterial infection with inflammation (e.g., via pro-inflammatory cytokines like TNFα [116]). However, some pathogens have developed mechanisms to evade these physiological processes and use the receptor to enter their host cells, namely African swine fever virus (ASFV; [96]) and PRRSV [17, 83, 114].

CD163 and PRRSV

CD163 has been well documented as attachment and internalization receptor in ASFV [96], the PRRSV-related Simian Haemorrhagic Fever Virus (SHFV; [16]) and PRRSV [17]. PRRSV was first identified to enter the cell via a common receptor-dependent endocytosis [55], relying on the clathrin-mediated pathway and a low pH and shifting the virus from the cell surface to early endosomes [79]. The receptor was found to be responsible for the highly specific tropism of the virus [54]. Since then, several attachment factors have been studied extensively as potential PRRSV receptors and CD163 and CD169 were identified the most likely candidates involved. However, only CD163 has been shown capable of conferring PRRSV permissiveness to cell lines unsusceptible to PRRSV, even in the absence of CD169 (e.g., [17, 83, 113, 114, 116, 123, 124]). It was shown that PRRSV permissivity was conferred by CD163 independent of the PRRSV genotype involved (1 [EU] or 2 [US]) [17, 61]. Down-regulation of CD163 (but not CD169) in susceptible cells by ADAM17 was able to completely block PRRSV infection [37]. All these data show that CD163 alone can transfer PRRSV permissiveness to non-responsive cells and establish a productive replication cycle [144]. The role of CD163 was finally proven in the gene editing experiments of Prather et al. [87] and Whitworth et al. [128], who transferred PRRSV resistance to pigs by deleting CD163 sequences from the pigs' genome. However, they had no success when deleting CD169.

The central role of CD163 in PRRSV replication has never been in debate. There was just some discussion about the step where the binding between CD163 and PRRSV would take place. Van Gorp et al. [113–116] provided evidence for first interactions between PRRSV and CD163 during virus uncoding in early endosomes. However, the lack of measureable amounts of CD163 in contact with PRRSV on the cell surface might be due to a fast cycling process of CD163 between cell surface and endosomes as described by Schaer et al. [102] and Zhang and Yoo [144]. Minor differences between experiments in terms of efficiency of PRRSV replication seem to be more a matter of receptor interaction and membrane lipid environment than of differences between PRRSV genotype, although variability of the pathogen itself also affects the quantitative outcome of PRRSV replication.

The fact that not all cells that express CD163 can be infected by PRRSV which is important for realisation of PRRSV-specific cell tropism [144] and that PRRSV shows a restricted tropism for subsets of porcine macrophages in vivo might be a question of CD163 quantity or of interaction with other, maybe until now not identified co-receptors [34]. The expression of CD163 on macrophages in different microenvironments in vivo, may determine the replication efficiency and subsequent virulence of PRRSV [83].

CD163 domains

CD163 consists of nine cysteine-rich tandem repeats, forming the extracellular scavenger receptor, a transmembrane domain and the intracellular cytoplasmic tail. Different from the situation with haemoglobin (domains 2 and 3; [30]), the essential parts of CD163 in PRRSV entry seems to be related to domain 5, the two proline-serine-threonine (PST)-rich regions and a few others, but not with the complete receptor [113]. The first 4 N-terminal domains and the C-terminal 223 residues (cytoplasmic tail) [59] are not relevant for PRRSV-replication. The transmembrane domain is essential, but not specific [127]. The interacting PRRSV glycoproteins responsible for receptor binding and infection are GP2a, GP3, GP4 and E, [110]. GP4 and GP2a are especially important [21]. Replacing ORFs 2a to 4 with EAV ORFs keeps the virus viable and infectious, but protects macrophages from infection [110].

Glycosylation of GP2a and GP4 by glycans can have different effects on PRRSV replication, depending on the PRRSV genotype [22, 126, 134]. However, transitions are fluent, because of the role of lipids and cholesterol from the lipid rafts of the outer plasma membrane that interact with embedded proteins and receptors [28, 142]. As a putative ion channel protein, the E protein is involved in decreasing pH values as a further part of a successful uncoating process [58].

Supporting receptors

Sialoadhesin (CD169) is a transmembrane glycoprotein, a lectin, restricted to activated tissue macrophages [76, 132] and involved in cell-cell interaction. Expression can be induced in macrophages by IFNα and IFNγ during the inflammatory process [95]. The receptor facilitates pathogen interactions and uptake of sialylated pathogens (e.g., HIV [95] and PRRSV [25, 29, 117]. Especially the amino acids S107 and R116 bind sialic acid of PRRSV GP5 [25, 48, 111]. Sialoadhesin seems to facilitate attachment of PRRSV, eventually together with heparin sulfate, and internalisation, but not replication of the virus [24, 114, 116]. A gene editing experiment that deleted CD169 found full PRRSV-permissive macrophages and unaltered viremia and antibody production in the pigs [87]. The authors conclude that sialoadhesin is not required for PRRSV infection and that the absence of the CD169 gene neither prevents PRRS nor alters PRRS pathogenesis.

Heparin sulfate is widely distributed on the surface of most mammalian cells. Heparin sulfate, heparin-like proteins and proteoglycans bind to GP5/M heterodimers and the M complex of PRRSV in a virus-dependent manner [23, 50]. Together with sialoadhesin, heparin sulfate seems to propagate the interaction between PRRSV and its specific receptor(s), but heparin sulfate is not necessarily required for PRRSV entry [23].

CD151 is involved in numerous cell functions and cell signalling [32]. Silencing the gene made susceptible cells resistant, while overexpression made resistant cells susceptible to PRRSV, making *CD151* a key receptor for PRRSV infection [106]. Blocking *CD151* by microRNA (miR506) prevents the cells from being infected [135]. However, *CD151* is restricted to the erythroid cell lineage and is not expressed on macrophages.

Vimentin and *CD209* are further putative receptors that might be involved in varying efficiency of PRRSV binding and replication [45, 52].

A gene editing breakthrough in PRRS resistance?
All these results regarding PRRSV receptors finally led to gene editing experiments and the knockout of PRRSV-receptor function in *CD169* [87] and *CD163* [128] in gene-edited pigs. Loss of *CD169* did not affect PRRSV replication, but gene-edited pigs without *CD163*-receptor function were protected from PRRSV. The pigs showed no fever, respiratory or other clinical signs, and no lung pathology, viremia or antibody response after inoculation with a NVSL 97–7895 PRRSV isolate in a controlled study. In addition, no problems occurred during pregnancy and growth of the piglets until challenged with the PRRSV isolate at the age of 3 weeks.

What is gene editing?
The goal of improving livestock genomes by direct manipulation is old. Its development was accompanied by serious problems in terms of site-specificity (precision), efficiency of the methods used and a lack of acceptance in wider society. Thus, unlike transgenic crops, no transgenic livestock has ever gained commercial approval [57]. All these problems may have been overcome with the introduction of gene editing via CRISPR/CAS9 [27]. The system combines an endonuclease with a specific short guiding (sg) RNA sequence. Like a primer in PCR, this sequence provides accurate specificity, while the linked enzyme can cleave and modify the DNA at exactly the position targeted by the sgRNA sequence. The key-step of this method is the double strand break in DNA and the interaction with cellular DNA repair mechanisms that leads to a high degree of failures (50 %) when joining the ends or even higher, when homology directed repair is induced by the introduction of the desired new sequence [27]. The system can also be used in a multiplex manner to edit different genes in one step. However, comparable to the amplification of

incorrect sequences by primer mismatching in PCR, care must be taken not to introduce unintended mutations anywhere in the genome at off-target sites. New methods have been developed to minimise the off-target size problem [71]. Originally, the CRSISPR Cas9 system was part of natural, sequence-specific immunity in bacteria, responsible for the introduction of DNA double-strand breaks into invading plasmids and phages [35]. Taken together, concerns about the precision and efficiency of transgenics have been overcome by this new method in previously inconceivable way. The first genome editing experiment in pigs succeeded to resilience the African Swine Fever receptor by its warthog homologue [65].

Concerns about gene edition as a tool to generate genetic resistance to combat PRRS
Gene editing and regulation by authorities
Gene editing can introduce mutations to the genome without adding any footprints associated with the technology. Thus, genome modifications cannot be distinguished from natural mutations [57]. Further, vectors to introduce foreign DNA into transgenic organisms, which might prove hazardous to consumers, are no longer needed. Both factors have led to the enthusiastic acceptance of gene editing by most researchers, the scientific community and the industry. Unlike transgenic organisms, gene-edited plants and animals may not need regulatory oversight [70, 122], provided the human germ line is not involved. Animals and products might not even be classified as genetically modified organisms (GMO). However, as the methodology explodes and a vast number of gene-edited livestock will be produced in the coming years, societal interpretation is currently difficult to predict. However, restrictions are likely.

Patenting gene-edited PRRS resistance
A second concern is related to upcoming patents. Generally, societies have to decide whether naturally occurring receptors or gene variants with a potential to improve health and welfare should be reserved exclusively for certain companies. The future always brings changes and the ability of populations and species to change is based on their genetic variability. As any individual can carry a maximum of two alleles at any position in the genome, resource populations often lose rare alleles with decreasing population size. These alleles, once lost, cannot be reintroduced by gene editing, as their favourable effects have never been documented. A single breed is not enough to fulfil the different demands of diversified markets worldwide. A chance to become resistant to PRRS needs to be retained for other breeds, lines and populations too.

Side-effects of CD163-edited knockout pigs
The facts outlined above for *CD163* show that this protein has not evolved solely as a PRRSV receptor, but

with a broad spectrum of tasks, including the elimination of pathogens other than PRRSV and the regulation of the immune system. *CD163* awaits the discovery and evaluation of further involvements and mechanisms. Any knockout of *CD163* as a whole or in part needs meticulous investigation of impacted pigs under field conditions, including the effects of other pathogens and adverse conditions. Work is currently in progress and results are expected in future.

Stability of the genetic resistance in the CD163 knockout pig

Will *CD163* knockout protect against other and upcoming PRRSV strains? One common concern surrounding disease resistance is whether pathogens will be able to adapt to host resistance like they acquire resistance to antibiotics. Acquiring resistance is possible in theory, but the method is unlikely to be similar, because there are no plasmids harbouring information for an arbitrary switch to new tropism. Some examples of single mutations provoked tissue or even species shift under "natural" conditions, although species shifts are very rare events in the evolution of most viruses [33]. A prime example is the Influenza A virus (e.g. [72]). Other examples arise from the *Coronaviridae* (e.g., SARS [31]) and TGE/PRCV [10] viruses.

The specific risk for the development of mutations that could alter cell or even species tropism might be high in PRRSV-infected pig herds. As a RNA virus, PRRSV has high mutation rates and the herd situation generally provides conditions that lead to the crowding of different pathogens or strains. Forsberg et al. [33] conclude that a supposed interspecies transmission for PRRSV took place before 1981. However under the conditions of current pig-PRRSV-interaction - including a high degree of adaptation of the virus to its host, an unmanageable multitude of strains and genotypes and highest burdens within pigs and herds - mutations in the PRRSV genome that might overcome *CD163* could arise within a much shorter period.

The tremendous all-or-nothing-principle of *CD163* on PRRSV replication could provide an unique and widespread solution to the PRRS problem. However, because only one receptor is involved, it runs a strong risk of being overcome by one or few SNPs. Work by Frydas et al. [34] indicates that tropism of PRRSV may change, at least for type 1. The fact that some isolates infected significantly more cells in nasal mucosa than others, suggests the potential existence of additional receptors. Up to now, the *CD163*-knockout experiment was only conducted with type 2 isolates.

On the other hand, differences in oligo- or polygenic pathways that are involved in the immune answer to PRRSV infection are much more complex. This complexity hinders their elucidation and the all-or-nothing-

principle of resistance. However, if such natural resistance could be implemented, the odds that PRRSV would overcome these genetic changes would decrease. It is impossible to predict exactly what will happen. Some good examples arise from indigenous (autochthone) breeds, evolved under endemic disease challenge. Such breeds have developed sustainable resistance that makes them superior to others. This aspect further underlines the necessity to preserve genetic and breed diversity in swine.

Conclusion

The detection and knockout of CD163 as the receptor responsible for PRRSV replication in pigs is a milestone in modern pig production. Complete or even partial elimination of PRRSV replication would lead to a significant improvement in the disastrous situation in infected herds, with significant impact on welfare, production efficiency, performance and consumer protection. However, the complete function of the receptor and its reasonable modification still requires elucidation, and the evaluation of other gene variants involved in immunological pathways is just beginning. Thus, the future will see combined efforts to develop and transfer new knowledge to the herd level. The degree of success in using genetic resistance as an alternative in controlling PRRS will be measured in terms of microbiological and health parameters, but also in terms of availability for pig populations all over the world.

Acknowledgements
Not applicable.

Funding
No funding.

Author's contribution
100 % by the author.

Competing interests
The author declares that he has no competing interests.

References
1. Ait-Ali T, Wilson AD, Westcott DG, Clapperton M, Waterfall M, Mellencamp MA, Drew TW, Bishop SC, Archibald AL. Innate immune response to replication of porcine reproductive and respiratory syndrome virus in isolated swine alveolar macrophages. Viral Immunol. 2007;20:105–18.
2. Ait-Ali T, Wilson AD, Carre W, Westcott DG, Frossard JP, Mellencamp MA, Mouzaki D, Matika O, Waddington D, Drew TW, Bishop SC, Archibald AL. Host inhibits replication of European porcine reproductive and respiratory

syndrome virus in macrophages by altering differential regulation of type-I interferon transcriptional response. Immunogenetics. 2011;63:437–48.

3. Akila P, Prashant V, Suma MN, Prashant SN, Chaitra TR. *CD163* and its expanding functional repertoire. Clin Chim Acta. 2012;413:669–74.

4. Andersson L, Georges M. Domestic-animal genomics: deciphering the genetics of complex traits. Nat Rev Genet. 2004;5:202–12.

5. Anselmo A, Flori L, Jaffrezic F, Rutigliano T, Cecere M, Cortes-Perez N, Lefèvre F, Rogel-Gaillard C, Giuffra E, Ouzounis C. Co-Expression of Host and Viral MicroRNAs in Porcine Dendritic Cells Infected by the Pseudorabies Virus. PLoS One. 2011;6(3):e17374.

6. Arceo ME, Ernst CW, Lunney JK, Choi I, Raney NE, Huang T, Tuggle CK, Rowland RRR, Steibel JP. Characterizing differential individual response to porcine reproductive and respiratory syndrome virus infection through statistical and functional analysis of gene expression. Front Genet. 2012;3:321.

7. Asano A, Ko JH, Morozumi T, Hamashima N, Watanabe T. Polymorphisms and the antiviral property of porcine MX1 protein. J Vet Medic Sci. 2002;64:1085–9.

8. Backe E, Schwarting R, Gerdes J, Ernst M, Stein H. Ber-MAC3: new monoclonal antibody that defines human monocyte macrophage differentiation antigen. J Clin Pathol. 1991;44:936–45.

9. Badaoui B, Rutigliano T, Anselmo A, Vanhee M, Nauwynck H, Giuffra E, Botti S. RNA-sequence analysis of primary alveolar macrophages after in vitro infection with porcine reproductive and respiratory syndrome virus strains of differing virulence. PLoS One. 2014;9:e91918.

10. Ballesteros ML, Sanchez CM, Enjuanes L. Two amino acid changes at the N-terminus of Transmissible Gatsroenteritis Coronavirus spike protein results in the loss of enteric tropism. Virology. 1997;227:378–88.

11. Bates JS, Petry DB, Eudy J, Bough L, Johnson RK. Differential expression in lung and bronchial lymph node of pigs with high and low responses to infection with porcine reproductive and respiratory syndrome virus. J Anim Sci. 2008;86:3279–89.

12. Biasini M, Bienert S, Waterhouse A, Arnold K, Studer G, Schmidt T, Kiefer F, Cassarino TG, Bertoni M, Bordoli L, Schwede T. SWISS-MODEL: modelling protein tertiary and quaternary structure using evolutionary information. Nucl Acids Res. 2014;42:W252–8.

13. Boddicker N, Waide EH, Rowland RR, Lunney JK, Garrick DJ, Reecy JM, Dekkers JCM. Evidence for a major QTL associated with host response to porcine reproductive and respiratory syndrome virus challenge. J Anim Sci. 2012;90:1733–46.

14. Boddicker NJ, Bjorkquist A, Rowland RR, Lunney JK, Reecy JM, Dekkers JC. Genome-wide association and genomic prediction for host response to porcine reproductive and respiratory syndrome virus infection. Genet Sel Evol. 2014;46:18.

15. Boddicker NJ, Garrick DJ, Rowland RR, Lunney JK, Reecy JM, Dekkers JC. Validation and further characterization of a major quantitative trait locus associated with host response to experimental infection with porcine reproductive and respiratory syndrome virus. Anim Genet. 2013;45:48–58.

16. Cai Y, Postnikova EN, Bernbaum JG, Yu SQ, Mazur S, Deiuliis NM, Radoshitzky SR, Lackemeyer MG, McCluskey A, Robinson PJ, Haucke V, Wahl-Jensen V, Bailey AL, Lauck M, Friedrich TC, O'Connor DH, Goldberg TL, Jahrling PB, Kuhn JH. Simian hemorrhagic fever virus cell entry is dependent on *CD163* and uses a clathrin-mediated endocytosis-like pathway. J Virol. 2015;89:844–56.

17. Calvert JG, Slade DE, Shields SL, Jolie R, Mannan RM, Ankenbauer RG, Welch S-KW. *CD163* expression confers susceptibility to porcine reproductive and respiratory syndrome viruses. J Virol. 2007;81:7371–9.

18. Chen N, Dekkers JCM, Ewen CL, Rowland RRR. Porcine reproductive and respiratory syndrome virus replication and quasispecies evolution in pigs that lack adaptive immunity. Virus Res. 2015;195:246–9.

19. Chung HK, Lee JH, Kim SH, Chae C. Expression of interferon-alpha and MX1 protein in pigs acutely infected with porcine reproductive and respiratory syndrome virus (PRRSV). J Comp Pathol. 2004;130:299–305.

20. Cole RK. Studies on genetic resistance to Marek's disease. Avian Dis. 1968;12:9–28.

21. Das PB, Dinh PX, Ansari IH, de Lima M, Osorio FA, Pattnaik AK. The minor envelope glycoproteins GP2a and GP4 of porcine reproductive and respiratory syndrome virus interact with the receptor *CD163*. J Virol. 2010;84:1731–40.

22. Das PB, Vu HL, Dinh PX, Cooney JL, Kwon B, Osorio FA, Pattnaik AK. Glycosylation of minor envelope glycoproteins of porcine reproductive and respiratory syndrome virus in infectious virus recovery, receptor interaction, and immune response. Virology. 2011;410:385–94.

23. Delputte PL, Vanderheijden N, Nauwynck HJ, Pensaert MB. Involvement of the matrix protein in attachment of porcine reproductive and respiratory syndrome virus to a heparinlike receptor on porcine alveolar macrophages. J Virol. 2002;76:4312–20.

24. Delputte PL, Costers S, Nauwynck HJ. Analysis of porcine reproductive and respiratory syndrome virus attachment and internalization: distinctive roles for heparan sulphate and sialoadhesin. J Gen Virol. 2005;86:1441–5.

25. Delputte PL, Van Breedam W, Barbe F, Van Reeth K, Nauwynck HJ. IFN- α treatment en- hances porcine arterivirus infection of monocytes via upregulation of the porcine arterivirus receptor sialoadhesin. J Interf Cytokine Res. 2007;27:757–66.

26. Doeschl-Wilson AB, Kyriazakis I, Vincent A, Rothschild MF, Thacker E, Galina-Pantoja L. Clinical and pathological responses of pigs from two genetically diverse commercial lines to porcine reproductive and respiratory syndrome virus infection. J Anim Sci. 2009;87:1638–47.

27. Doudna JA, Charpentier E. The new frontier of genome engineering with CRISPR-Cas9. Science. 2014;346:1258096-1–9.

28. Du Y, Pattnaik AK, Song C, Yoo D, Li G. Glycosyl-phosphatidylinositol (GPI)-anchored membrane association of the porcine reproductive and respiratory syndrome virus GP4 glycoprotein and its co-localization with *CD163* in lipid rafts. Virology. 2012;424:18–32.

29. Duan X, Nauwynck HJ, Pensaert MB. Effects of origin and state of differentiation and activation of monocytes/macrophages on their susceptibility to porcine reproductive and respiratory syndrome virus (PRRSV). Arch Virol. 1997;142:2483–97.

30. Fabriek BO, van Bruggen R, Deng DM, Ligtenberg AJ, Nazmi K, Schornagel K, Vloet RP, Dijkstra CD, van den Berg TK. The macrophage scavenger receptor *CD163* functions as an innate immune sensor for bacteria. Blood. 2009;113:887–92.

31. Feng H-P. Crossing the species barrier. Nature Struct Mol Biol. 2005;12:831.

32. Fitter S, Sincock PM, Jolliffe CN, Ashman LK. Transmembrane 4 superfamily protein *CD151* (PETA-3) associates with beta 1 and alpha IIb beta 3 in tegrins in haemopoietic cell lines and modulates cell–cell adhesion. Biochem J. 1999;338:61–70.

33. Forsberg R, Oleksiewicz MB, Petersen AMK, Hein J, Botner A, Storgaard T. A molecular clock dates the common ancestor of european-type porcine reproductive and respiratory syndrome virus at more than 10 years before the Emergence of Disease. Virology. 2001;289:174–9.

34. Frydas IS, Verbeeck M, Cao J, Nauwynck HJ. Replication characteristics of porcine reproductive and respiratory syndrome virus (PRRSV) European subtype 1 (Lelystad) and subtype 3 (Lena) strains in nasal mucosa and cells of the monocytic lineage: indications for the use of new receptors of PRRSV (Lena). Vet Res. 2013;44:73.

35. Garneau JE, Dupuis M-E, Villion M, Romero DA, Barrangou R, Boyaval P, Fremaux C, Horvath P, Magadán AH, Moineau S. The CRISPR/Cas bacterial immune system cleaves bacteriophage and plasmid DNA. Nature. 2010;468:67–71.

36. Genini S, Delputte PL, Malinverni R, Cecere M, Stella A, Nauwynck HJ, Giuffra E. Genome-wide transcriptional response of primary alveolar macrophages following infection with porcine reproductive and respiratory syndrome virus. J Gen Virol. 2008;89:2550–64.

37. Guo L, Niu J, Yu H, Gu W, Li R, Luo X, Huang M, Tian Z, Feng L, Wang Y. Modulation of *CD163* expression by metalloprotease ADAM17 regulates porcine reproductive and respiratory syndrome virus entry. J Virol. 2014;88:10448–58.

38. Halbur P, Rothschild MF, Thacker B. Differences in susceptibility of Duroc, Hampshire and Meishan pigs to infection with a highvirulence strain (VR2385) of porcine reproductive and respiratory syndrome virus (PRRS). J Anim Breed Genet. 1998;115:181–9.

39. Haley CS, Andersson L. Linkage mapping of quantitative trait loci in plants and animals. In: Dear PH, editor. Genome mapping. Oxford: IRL Press; 1997. p. 49–71.

40. He T, Feng G, Chen H, Wang L, Wang Y. Identification of host encoded microRNAs interacting with novel swine-origin influenza A (H1N1) virus and swine influenza virus. Bioinformation. 2009;4(3):112–118.

41. Heringstad B, Klemetsdal G, Ruane J. Selection for mastitis resistance in dairy cattle: a review with focus on the situation in the nordic countries. Livest Prod Sci. 2000;64:95–106.

42. Hicks JA, Yoo D, Liu HC. Characterization of the microRNAome in porcine reproductive and respiratory syndrome virus infected macrophages. Plos One. 2013;8:e82054.

43. Högger P, Dreier J, Droste A, Buck F, Sorg C. Identification of the Integral Membrane Protein RM3/1 on Human Monocytes as a Glucocorticoid-Inducible Member of the Scavenger Receptor Cysteine-Rich Family (*CD163*). J Immunol. 1998;161:1883–90.

44. Holtkamp DJ, Kliebenstein J, Neumann EJ, Zimmerman JJ, Rotto HF, Yoder TK, Wang C, Yeske PE, Mowrer CL, Haley CA. Assessment of the economic

impact of porcine reproductive and respiratory syndrome virus on United States pork producers. J Swine Health Prod. 2013;21:72–84.

45. Huang YW, Dryman BA, Li W, Meng XJ. Porcine DC-SIGN: molecular cloning, gene structure, tissue distribution and binding characteristics. Dev Comp Immunol. 2009;33:464–80.

46. Islam MA, Große-Brinkhaus C, Pröll MJ, Uddin MJ, Rony SA, Tesfaye D, Tholen E, Hölker M, Schellander K, Neuhoff C. Deciphering transcriptome profiles of peripheral blood mononuclear cells in response to PRRSV vaccination in pigs. BMS Genomics. 2016;17:641.

47. Jia X, Bi Y, Li J, Xie Q, Yang H, Liu W. Cellular microRNA miR-26a suppresses replication of porcine reproductive and respiratory syndrome virus by activating innate antiviral immunity. Sci Rep. 2015;5:10651.

48. Jiang Y, Khan FA, Pandupuspitasari NS, Kadariya I, Cheng Z, Ren Y, Chen X, Zhou A, Yang L, Kong D, Zhang S. Analysis of the binding sites of porcine sialoadhesin receptor with PRRSV. Int J Mol Sci. 2013;14:23955–79.

49. Jorgensen CB, Cirera S, Archibald A, Andersson L, Fredholm M, Edfors-Lilja I. Porcine polymorphisms and methods for detecting them. International application publish under the patent cooperation treaty (PCT). 2003. PCT/DK2003/000807 or WO2004/048606 A2.

50. Jusa ER, Inaba Y, Kouno M, Hirose O. Effect of heparin on in fection of cells by porcine reproductive and respiratory syndrome virus. Am J Vet Res. 1997;58:488–91.

51. Kim C, Guo H, Kong W, Chandnani R, Shuang LS, Paterson AH. Application of genotyping by sequencing technology to a variety of crop breeding programs. Plant Sci. 2016;242:14–22.

52. Kim J-K, Fahad AM, Shanmukhappa K, Kapil S. Defining the Cellular Target(s) of Porcine Reproductive and Respiratory Syndrome Virus Blocking Monoclonal Antibody 7G10. J Virol. 2006;133:477–83.

53. Koltes JE, Fritz-Waters E, Eisley CJ, Choi I, Bao H, Kommadath A, Serão NVL, Boddicker NJ, Abrams SM, Schroyen M, Loyd H, Tuggle CK, Plastow GS, Guan L, Stothard P, Lunney JK, Liu P, Carpenter S, Rowland RRR, Dekkers JCM, Reecy JM. Identification of a putative quantitative trait nucleotide in guanylate binding protein 5 for host response to PRRS virus infection. BMC Genomics. 2015;16:412.

54. Kreutz LC. Cellular membrane factors are the major determinants of porcine reproductive and respiratory syndrome virus tropism. Virus Res. 1998;53:121–8.

55. Kreutz LC, Ackermann MR. Porcine reproductive and respiratory syndrome virus enters cells through a low pH-dependent endocytic pathway. Virus Res. 1996;42:137–47.

56. Kristiansen M, Graversen JH, Jacobsen C, Sonne O, Hoffman HJ, Law SK, Moestrup SK. Identification of the haemoglobin scavenger receptor. Nature. 2001;409:198–201.

57. Laible G, Wei J, Wagner S. Improving livestock for agriculture – technological progress from random transgenesis to precision genome editing heralds a new era. Biotechn J. 2015;10:109–20.

58. Lee C, Yoo D. The small envelope protein of porcine reproductive and respiratory syndrome virus possesses ion channel protein-like properties. Virology. 2006;355:30–43.

59. Lee YJ, Lee C. Deletion of the cytoplasmic domain of CD163 enhances porcine reproductive and respiratory syndrome virus replication. Arch Virol. 2010;155:1319–23.

60. Lee SM, Schommer SK, Kleiboeker SB. Porcine reproductive and respiratory syndrome virus field isolates differ in in vitro interferon phenotypes. Vet Immunol Immunopathol. 2004;102:217–31.

61. Lee YJ, Park CK, Nam E, Kim SH, Lee OS, Leedu S, Lee C. Generation of a porcine alveolar macrophage cell line for the growth of porcine reproductive and respiratory syndrome virus. J Virol Methods. 2010;163:410–5.

62. Li L, Gao F, Jiang Y, Yu L, Zhou Y, Zheng H, Tong W, Yang S, Xia T, Qu Z, Tong G. Cellular miR-130b inhibits replication of porcine reproductive and respiratory syndrome virus in vitro and in vivo. Sci Rep. 2015;5:17010.

63. Li Y, Sun Y, Xiang F, Kang L, Wang P, Wang L, Liu H, Li Y, Jiang Y. Identification of a single nucleotide polymorphism regulating the transcription of ubiquitin specific protease 18 gene related to the resistance t porcine reproductive and respiratory syndrome virus infection. Vet Immunol Immunopathol. 2014;162:65–71.

64. Li Y, Liang S, Liu H, Sun Y, Kang L, Jiang Y. Identification of a short interspersed repetitive element insertion polymorphism in the porcine Mx1 promoter associated with resistance to porcine reproductive and respiratory syndrome virus infection. Anim Genet. 2015;46:437–40.

65. Lillico SG, Proudfoot C, King TJ, Tan W, Zhang L, Mardjuki R, Paschon DE, Rebar EJ, Urnov FD, Mileham AJ, McLaren DG, Whitelaw BA. Mammalian interspecies substitution of immune modulatory alleles by genome editing. Sci Rep. 2016;6:21645.

66. Loveday E-K, Svinti V, Diederich S, Pasick J, Jean F. Temporal- and Strain-Specific Host MicroRNA Molecular Signatures Associated with Swine-Origin H1N1 and Avian-Origin H7N7 Influenza A Virus Infection. J Virol. 2012;86(11): 6109–6122.

67. Lowe JE, Husmann R, Firkins LD, Zuckermann FA, Goldberg TL. Correlation of cell-mediated immunity against porcine reproductive and respiratory syndrome virus with protection against reproductive failure in sows during outbreaks of porcine reproductive and respiratory syndrome in commercial herds. J Am Vet Med Assoc. 2005;226:1707–11.

68. Lu ZH, Brown A, Wilson AD, Calvert JG, Balasch M, Fuentes-Utrilla P, Loecherbach J, Turner F, Talbot R, Archibald AL, Ait-Ali T. Genomic variation in macrophage-cultured European porcine reproductive and respiratory syndrome virus Olot/91 revealed using ultra-deep next generation sequencing. Virol J. 2014;11:42.

69. Lunney JK, Fang Y, Ladinig A, Chen N, Li Y, Rowland B, Renukaradhya GJ. Porcine Reproductive and Respiratory Syndrome Virus (PRRSV): Pathogenesis and interaction with the immune system. Annu Rev Anim Biosci. 2016;4:15.1–15.26.

70. Lusser M, Davies HV. Comparative regulatory approaches for groups of new plant breeding techniques. New Biotechn. 2013;30:437–46.

71. Mali P, Aach J, Benjamin Stranges P, Esvelt KM, Moosburner M, Kosuri S, Yang L, Church GM. CAS9 transcriptional activators for target specificity screening and paired nickases for cooperative genome engineering. Nature Biotechn. 2013;31:833–8.

72. Mänz B, Schwemmle M, Brunotte L. Adaptation of avian Influenza A Virus polymerase in mammals to overcome the host species barrier. J Virol. 2013;87:7200–9.

73. Meijerink E, Fries R, Vögeli P, Masabanda J, Wigger G, Stricker C, Neuenschwander S, Bertschinger HU, Stranzinger G. Two a(1,2) fucosyltransferase genes on porcine chromosome 6q11 are closely linked to the blood group inhibitor (S) and Escherichia coli F18 receptor (ECF18R) loci. Mamm Genome. 1997;8:736–41.

74. Meuwissen TH, Van Arendonk JA. Potential improvements in rate of genetic gain from marker-assisted selection in dairy cattle breeding schemes. J Dairy Sci. 1992;75:1651–9.

75. Miller LC, Fleming D, Arbogast A, Bayles DO, Guo B, Lager KM, Henningson JN, Schlink SN, Yang H-C, Faaberg KS, Kehrli ME. Analysis of the swine tracheobronchial lymph node transcriptomic response to infection with a Chinese highly pathogenic strain of porcine reproductive and respiratory syndrome virus. BMC Vet Res. 2012;8:208.

76. Munday J, Floyd H, Crocker PR. Sialic acid binding receptors (siglecs) expressed by macrophages. J Leu ko c Biol. 1999;66:705–11.

77. Murray M, Stear MJ, Trail JCM, Diteran GD, Agyemang K, Dwinger RH. Trypanosomiasis in cattle. Prospects for control. In: Axford RFE, Bishop SC, Nicholas FW, Owen JB, editors. Breeding for disease Resistance in farm animals. Wallingford: CABI; 2000. p. 203–23.

78. Nakajima E, Morozumi T, Tsukamoto K, Watanabe T, Plastow G, Mitsuhashi T. A naturally occurring variant of porcine Mx1 associated with increased susceptibility to influenza virus in vitro. Biochem Genet. 2007;45:11–24.

79. Nauwynck HJ, Duan X, Favoreel HW, Van Oostveldt P, Pensaert MB. Entry of porcine re- productive and respiratory syndrome virus into porcine alveolar macrophages via receptor-mediated endocytosis. J Gen Virol. 1999;80:297–305.

80. Neumann EJ, Kliebenstein JB, Johnson CD, Mabry JW, Bush EJ, Seitzinger AH, Green AL, Zimmerman JJ. Assessment of the economic im pact of porcine reproductive and respiratory syndrome on swine production in the United States. J Am Vet Med Assoc. 2005;227:385–92.

81. Nicholas FW. Veterinary genetics. Oxford: Oxford University Press; 1987.

82. Patel D, Nan Y, Shen M, Ritthipichai K, Zhu X, Zhang Y-J. Porcine reproductive and respiratory syndrome virus inhibits type I interferon signalling by blocking STAT1/STAT2 nuclear translocation. J Virol. 2010;84:11045–55.

83. Patton JB, Rowland RR, Yoo D, Chang KO. Modulation of CD163 receptor expression and replication of porcine reproductive and respiratory syndrome virus in porcine macrophages. Virus Res. 2009;140:161–71.

84. Petersen B, Niemann H. Molecular scissors and their application in genetically modified farm animals. Transgen Res. 2015;24:381–96.

85. Petry DB, Holl JW, Weber JS, Doster AR, Osorio FA, Johnson RK. Biological responses to porcine respiratory and reproductive syndrome virus in pigs of two genetic populations. J Anim Sci. 2005;83:1494–502.

86. Petry DB, Lunney J, Boyd P, Kuhar D, Blankenship E, Johnson RK. Differential immunity in pigs with high and low responses to porcine reproductive and respiratory syndrome virus infection12. J Anim Sci. 2007;85:2075–92.

87. Prather RS, Rowland RR, Ewen C, Trible B, Kerrigan M, Bawab B, Tesona JM, Maoa J, Leea K, Samuela MS, Whitwortha KM, Murphya CN, Egena T, Green JA. An intact sialoadhesin (Sn/SIGLEC1/CD169) is not required for attachment/internalization of the porcine reproductive and respiratory syndrome virus. J Virol. 2013;87:9538–46.

88. Reiner G, Melchinger E, Kramarova M, Pfaff E, Büttner M, Saalmüller A, Geldermann H. Detection of quantitative trait loci for resistance/susceptibility to pseudorabies virus in swine. J Gen Virol. 2002;83:167–72.

89. Reiner G, Willems H, Berge T, Fischer R, Köhler F, Hepp S, Hertrampf B, Kliemt D, Daugschies A, Zahner H, Geldermann H, Mackenstedt U. Mapping of quantitative trait loci for resistance/susceptibility to Sarcocystis miescheriana in swine. Genomics. 2007;89:638–46.

90. Reiner G. Investigations on genetic disease resistance in swine-A contribution to the reduction of pain, suffering and damage in farm animals. Appl Anim Behav Sci. 2009;118:217–21.

91. Reiner G, Willems H, Pesch S, Ohlinger VF. Variation in resistance to the Porcine Reproductive and Respiratory Syndrome Virus (PRRSV) in Pietrain and Miniature pigs. J Anim Breed Genet. 2010;127:100–6.

92. Reiner G. MicroRNA (miRNA): seminal biomarkers for disease diagnostics in swine? Berl Münch Tierärztl Wschr. 2011;124:10–5.

93. Reiner G, Bertsch N, Hoeltig D, Selke M, Willems H, Gerlach GF, Tuemmler B, Probst I, Herwig R, Drungowski M, Waldmann KH. Identification of QTL affecting resistance/susceptibility to acute Actinobacillus pleuropneumoniae infection in swine, Mamm. Genome. 2014;25:180–91.

94. Reiner G, Dreher F, Drungowski M, Hoeltig D, Bertsch N, Selke M, Willems H, Gerlach GF, Probst I, Tuemmler B, Waldmann KH, Herwig R. Pathway deregulation and expression QTLs in response to Actinobacillus pleuropneumoniae infection in swine. Mamm Genome. 2014;25:600–17.

95. Rempel H, Calosing C, Sun B, Pulliam L. Sialoadhesin expressed on IFN-induced monocytes binds HIV-1 and enhances in fectivity. PLoS One. 2008;3:e1967.

96. Sanchez-Torres C, Gomez-Puertas P, Gomez-del-Moral M, Alonso F, Escribano JM, Ezquerra A, Dominguez J. Expression of porcine CD163 on monocytes/macrophages correlates with permissiveness to African swine fever infection. Arch Virol. 2003;148:2307–23.

97. Sang Y, Rowland RRR, Blecha F. Porcine type I interferons: polymorphic sequences and activity against PRRSV. BMC Proc. 2011;5 Suppl 4:58.

98. Sang Y, Brichalli W, Rowland RRR, Blecha F. Genome-wide analysis of antiviral signature genes in porcine macrophages at different activation statuses. PLoS One. 2014;9:e87613.

99. Sang Y, Rowland RRR, Blecha F. Antiviral regulation in porcine monocytic cells at different activation statuses. J Virol. 2014;88:11395–410.

100. Scallerup P, Nejsum P, Jorgensen CB, Göring HHH, Karlskov-Mortensen P, Archibald AL, Fredholm M, Thamsborg SM. Detection of a quantitative trait locus associated with resistance to Ascaris suum infection in pigs. Int J Parasitol. 2012;42:383–91.

101. Scallerup P, Thamsborg SM, Jorgensen CB, Enemark HI, Yoshida A, Göring HHH, Fredholm M, Nejsum P. Functional study of a genetic marker allele associated with resistance to Ascaris suum in pigs. Parasitology. 2014;141:777–87.

102. Schaer CA, Schoedon G, Imhof A, Kurrer MO, Schaer DJ. Constitutive endocytosis of CD163 mediates haemoglobin-heme uptake and determines the noninflammatory and protective transcriptional response of macrophages to hemoglobin. Circ Res. 2006;99:943–50.

103. Schroyen M, Steibel JP, Koltes JE, Choi I, Eisley C, Fritz-Waters E, Reecy JM, Rowland RRR, Lunney JK, Ernst CW, Tuggle CK. Whole blood microarray analysis of pigs showing extreme phenotypes after a porcine reproductive and respiratory syndrome virus infection. BMC Genom. 2015;16:516.

104. Schroyen M, Eisley C, Koltes JE, Fritz-Waters E, Choi I, Plastow GS, Guan L, Stothard P, Bao H, Kommadath A, Reecy JM, Lunney JK, Rowland RRR, Dekkers JCM, Tuggle CK. Bioinformatic analyses in early host response to Porcine Reproductive and Respiratory Syndrome Virus (PRRSV) reveals pathway differences between pigs with alternate genotypes for a major host response QTL. BMC Genomics. 2016;17:196.

105. Serao NVL, Kemp RA, Mote BE, Willson P, Harding JCS, Bishop SC, Plastow G, Dekkers JCM. Genetic and genomic basis of antibody response to porcine reproductive and respiratory syndrome (PRRS) in gilts and sows. Genet Sel Evol. 2016;48:51.

106. Shanmukhappa K, Kim JK, Kapil S. Role of CD151, Atetraspanin, in porcine reproductive and respiratory syndrom e virus infection. Virol J. 2007;4:62.

107. Shenoy AR, Wellington DA, Kumar P, Kassa H, Booth CJ, Cresswell P, MacMicking JD. GBP5 Promotes NLRP3 Inflammasome Assembly and Immunity in Mammals. Science. 2012;336:481–5.

108. Shimazu T, Borjigin L, Katayama Y, Li M, Satoh T, Watanabe K, Kitazawa H, Roh S-G, Aso H, Kazuo K, Suda Y, Sakuma A, Nakajo M, Suzuki K. Genetic selection for resistance to mycoplasmal pneumonia of swine (MPS) in the Landrace line influences the expression of soluble factors in blood after MPS vaccine sensitization. Anim Sci J. 2014;85:365–73.

109. Stear MJ, Wakelin D. Genetic resistance to parasitic infection. Rev Sci Tech. 1998;17:143–53.

110. Tian D, Wei Z, Zevenhoven-Dobbe JC, Liu R, Tong G, Snijderb EJ, Yuan S. Arterivirus minor envelope proteins are a major determinant of viral tropism in cell culture. J Virol. 2012;86:3701–12.

111. Van Breedam W, Van Gorp H, Zhang JQ, Crocker PR, Delputte PL, Nauwynck HJ. The M/GP(5) glycoprotein complex of porcine reproductive and respiratory syndrome virus binds the sialoadhesin receptor in a sialic acid-dependent manner. PLoS Pathog. 2010;6:e1000730.

112. Van den Heuvel MM, Tensen CP, van As JH, Van den Berg TK, Fluitsma DM, Dijkstra CD, Dopp EA, Droste A, Van Gaalen FA, Sorg C, Högger P, Beelen RH. Regulation of CD 163 on human macrophages: cross-linking of CD163 induces signalling and activation. J Leukoc Biol. 1999;66:858–66.

113. Van Gorp H, Delputte PL, Nauwynck HJ. Scavenger receptor CD163, a Jack-of-all-trades and potential target for cell-directed therapy. Mol Immunol. 2010;47:1650–60.

114. Van Gorp H, Van Breedam W, Delputte PL, Nauwynck HJ. Sialoadhesin and CD163 join forces during entry of the porcine reproductive and respiratory syndrome virus. J Gen Virol. 2008;89:2943–53.

115. Van Gorp H, Van Breedam W, Delputte PL, Nauwynck HJ. The porcine reproductive and respiratory syndrome virus requires trafficking through CD163-positive early endosomes, but not late endosomes, for productive in fection. Arch Virol. 2009;154:1939–43.

116. Van Gorp H, Van Breedam W, Van Doorsselaere J, Delputte PL, Nauwynck HJ. Identification of the CD163 protein domains involved in infection of the porcine reproductive and respiratory syndrome virus. J Virol. 2010;84:3101–5.

117. Vanderheijden N, Delputte PL, Favoreel HW, Vandekerckhove J, Van Damme J, van Woensel PA, Nauwynck HJ. Involvement of sialoadhesin in entry of porcine reproductive and respiratory syndrome virus into porcine alveolar macrophages. J Virol. 2003;77:8207–15.

118. Verschure PJ, Vannoorden CJF, Dijkstra CD. Macrophages and dendritic cells during the early stages of antigen-induced arthritis in rats – immunohistochemical analysis of cryostat sections of whole knee-joint. Scand J Immunopathol. 1989;29:371–81.

119. Vincent AL, Thacker BJ, Halbur PG, Rothschild MF, Thacker EL. In vitro susceptibility of macrophages to porcine reproductive and respiratory syndrome virus varies between genetically diverse lines of pigs. Viral Immunol. 2005;18:506–12.

120. Vincent AL, Thacker BJ, Halbur PG, Rothschild MF, Thacker EL. An investigation of susceptibility to porcine reproductive and respiratory syndrome virus between two genetically diverse commercial lines of pigs. J Anim Sci. 2006;84:49–57.

121. Vögeli P, Meijerink E, Fries R, Neuenschwander S, Vorlander N, Stranzinger G, Bertschinger HU. A molecular test for the detection of E. coli F18 receptors: a breakthrough in the struggle against edema disease and post-weaning diarrhea. Schweizer Arch Tierheilk. 1997;139:479–84.

122. Waltz E. Tiptoeing around transgenetics. Nat Biotechnol. 2012;30:215–17.

123. Wang L, Zhang H, Suo X, Zheng S, Feng W-H. Increase of CD163 but not sialoadhesin on cultured peripheral blood monocytes is coordinated with enhanced susceptibility to porcine reproductive and respiratory syndrome virus infection. Vet Immunol Immunopathol. 2011;141:209–20.

124. Wang X, Wei R, Li Q, Liu H, Huang B, Gao J, Mu Y, Wang C, Hsu WH, Hiscox JA, Zhou E-M. PK-15 cells transfected with porcine CD163 by PiggyBac transposon system are susceptible to porcine reproductive and respiratory syndrome virus. J Virol Methods. 2013;193:383–90.

125. Weaver LK, Pioli PA, Wardwell K, Vogel SN, Guyre PM. Up-regulation of human monocyte CD163 upon activation of cell-surface Toll-like receptors. J Leukoc Biol. 2007;81:663–71.

126. Wei Z, Tian D, Sun L, Lin T, Gao F, Liu R, Tong G, Yuan S. Influence of N-linked glycosylation of minor proteins of porcine reproductive and respiratory

syndrome virus on infectious virus recovery and receptor interaction. Virology. 2012;429:1–11.

127. Welch SK, Calvert JG. A brief review of *CD163* and its role in PRRSV infection. Virus Res. 2010;154:98–103.

128. Whitworth KM, Rowland RRR, Exen, CL, Trible BR, Kerrigan MA, Cino-Ozuna AG, Samuel MS, Lightner JE, McLaren DG, Mileham AJ, Wells KD, Prather RS. Gene-edited pigs are protected from porcine reproductive and respiratory syndrome virus. Nature Biotechn. 2015;Dx.doi.org/10.1038/nbt3434

129. Wilkie BN, Mallard B. Genetic aspects of health and disease in pigs. In: Axford RFE, Bishop SC, Nicholas FW, Owen JB, editors. Breeding for disease resistance in farm animals. Wallingford: CABI; 2000. p. 379–96.

130. Wilkinson JM, Bao H, Ladinig A, Hong L, Stothard P, Lunney JK, Plastow GS, Harding JCS. Genome-wide analysis of the transcriptional response to porcine reproductive and respiratory syndrome virus infection at the maternal/fetal interface and in the fetus. BMC Genomics. 2016;17:383.

131. Wilkinson JM, Sargent CA, Galina-Pantoja L, Tucker AW. Gene expression profiling in the lungs of pigs with different susceptibilities to Glässer's disease. BMC Genomics. 2010;11:455.

132. Williams AF, Barclay AN. The immunoglobulin superfamily – domains for cell surface recognition. Annu Rev Immunol. 1988;6:381–405.

133. Williams L, Jarai G, Smith A, Finan P. IL-10 expression profiling in human monocytes. J Leukoc Biol. 2002;72:800–9.

134. Wissink EH, Kroese MV, Maneschijn-Bonsing JG, Meulenberg JJ, van Rijn PA, Rijsewijk FA, Rottier PJ. Significance of the oligosaccharides of the porcine reproductive and respiratory syndrome virus glycoproteins GP2a and GP5 for infectious virus production. J Gen Virol. 2004;85:3715–23.

135. Wu J, Peng X, Zhou A, Qiao M, Wu H, Xiao H, Liu G, Zheng X, Zhang S, Mei S. MiR-506 inhibits PRRSV replication in MARC-145 cells via *CD151*. Mol Cell Biochem. 2014;394:275–81.

136. Wu H, Gaur U, Mekchay S, Peng X, Li L, Sun H, Song Z, Dong B, Li M, Wimmers K, Ponsuksili S, Li K, Mei S, Liu G. Genome-wide identification of allele-specific expression in response to *Streptococcus suis* 2 infection in two differentially susceptible pig breeds. J Appl Genet. 2015;56:481–91.

137. Wysocki M, Chen H, Steibel JP, Kuhar D, Petry D, Bates J, Johnson R, Ernst CW, Lunney JK. Identifying putative candidate genes and pathways involved in immune responses to porcine reproductive and respiratory syndrome virus (PRRSV) infection. Anim Genet. 2012;43:328–32.

138. Xiao S, Jia J, Mo D, Wang Q, Qin L, He Z, Zhao X, Huang Y, Li A, Yu J, Niu Y, Liu X, Chen Y. Understanding PRRSV infection in porcine lung based on genome-wide transcriptome response identified by deep sequencing. PLoS One. 2010;5:e11377.

139. Xiao S, Mo D, Wang Q, Jia J, Qin L, Yu X, Niu Y, Zhao X, Liu X, Chen Y. Aberrant host immune response induced by highly virulent PRRSV identified by digital gene expression tag profiling. BMC Genomics. 2010;11:544.

140. Xing J, Xing F, Zhang C, Zhang Y, Wang N, Li Y, Yang L, Jiang C, Zhang C, Wen C, Jiang Y. Genome-wide gene expression profiles in lung tissues of pig breeds differing in resistance to porcine reproductive and respiratory syndrome virus. PLoS One. 2014;9:e86101.

141. Yang Q, Zhang Q, Tang J, Feng W-H. Lipid rafts both in cellular membrane and viral envelope are critical for PRRSV efficient infection. Virology. 2015; 484:170–80.

142. Yang T, Wilkinson J, Wang Z, Ladinig A, Harding J, Plastow G. A genome-wide association study of fetal response to type 2 porcine reproductive and respiratory syndrome virus challenge. Sci Rep. 2015;6:20305.

143. Yin XM, Liu Y, Dong WH, Zhao QH, Wu SL, Bao WB. Association of Mx1 gene polymorphism with some economic traits in Meishan pigs. Turk J Vet Anim Sci. 2015;39:389–94.

144. Zhang Q, Yoo D. PRRS virus receptors and their role for pathogenesis. Vet Microbiol. 2015;177:229–41.

145. Zhang X, Shin J, Molitor TW, Schook LB, Rutherford MS. Molecular responses of macrophages to porcine reproductive and respiratory syndrome virus infection. Virology. 1999;262:152–62.

146. Zhou P, Zhai S, Zhou X, Lin P, Jiang T, Hu X, Jiang Y, Wu B, Zhang Q, Xu X, Li J-P, Liu B. Molecular characterization of transcriptome-wide interactions between highly pathogenic porcine reproductive and respiratory syndrome virus and porcine alveolar macrophages in vivo. Int J Biol Sci. 2011;7:947–59.

147. Zimmerman JJ, Benfield DA, Dee SA, Murtaugh MP, Stadejek T, Stevenson GW, Torremorell M. Porcine reproductive and respiratory syndrome virus (porcine arterivirus). In: Zimmerman JJ, Karriker LA, Ramirez AR, Schwartz KJ, Stevenson GW, editors. Diseases of swine, 10th ed. Ames: Wiley-Blackwell; 2012. p. 461–86.

14

Modelling the within-herd transmission of *Mycoplasma hyopneumoniae* in closed pig herds

Heiko Nathues[1,2]*, Guillaume Fournie[1], Barbara Wieland[3], Dirk U. Pfeiffer[1] and Katharina D. C. Stärk[1]

Abstract

Background: A discrete time, stochastic, compartmental model simulating the spread of *Mycoplasma hyopneumoniae* within a batch of industrially raised pigs was developed to understand infection dynamics and to assess the impact of a range of husbandry practices. A 'disease severity' index was calculated based on the ratio between the cumulative numbers of acutely and chronically diseased and infectious pigs per day in each age category, divided by the length of time that pigs spent in this age category. This is equal to the number of pigs per day, either acutely or chronically infectious and diseased, divided by the number of all pigs per all days in the model. The impact of risk and protective factors at batch level was examined by adjusting 'acclimatisation of gilts', 'length of suckling period', 'vaccination of suckling pigs against *M. hyopneumoniae*', 'contact between fattening pigs of different age during restocking of compartments' and 'co-infections in fattening pigs'.

Results: The highest 'disease severity' was predicted, when gilts do not have contact with live animals during their acclimatisation, suckling period is 28 days, no vaccine is applied, fatteners have contact with pigs of other ages and are suffering from co-infections. Pigs in this scenario become diseased/infectious for 26.1 % of their lifetime. Logistic regression showed that vaccination of suckling pigs was influential for 'disease severity' in growers and finishers, but not in suckling and nursery pigs. Lack of contact between gilts and other live pigs during the acclimatisation significantly influenced the 'disease severity' in suckling pigs but had less impact in growing and finishing pigs. The length of the suckling period equally affected the severity of the disease in all age groups with the strongest association in nursery pigs. The contact between fatteners of different groups influenced the course of infection among finishers, but not among other pigs. Finally, presence of co-infections was relevant in growers and finishers, but not in younger pigs.

Conclusion: The developed model allows comparison of different prevention programmes and strategies for controlling transmission of *M. hyopneumoniae*.

Keywords: Enzootic pneumonia, Infectious disease, Epidemiology, Prevention

Background

Mycoplasma hyopneumoniae is the primary pathogen of porcine enzootic pneumonia (EP). The occurrence, the course and the severity of EP in pigs harbouring *M. hyopneumoniae* in their respiratory tract is influenced by a number of factors such as virulence of the particular

strain [1] as well as the additional co-infections with other respiratory pathogens and miscellaneous risk factors [2]. *M. hyopneumoniae* is introduced into a herd either by direct transmission following the purchase of infected pigs, or by airborne transmission [3]. Subsequently, the within-herd transmission is maintained vertically by nose-to-nose contact between sows and their offspring [4] or by horizontal route between pen mates or pigs in the same compartment [5]. If an all-in/all-out flow of pigs is not consequently implemented between production stages, transmissions of *M. hyopneumoniae* from infected older to naïve younger pigs is likely [2]. In

* Correspondence: heiko.nathues@vetsuisse.unibe.ch
[1]Veterinary Epidemiology, Economics and Public Health Group, Royal Veterinary College London, Hawkshead Lane, Hatfield, Hertfordshire AL97TA, UK
[2]Clinic for Swine, Vetsuisse Faculty, University of Berne, Bremgartenstrasse 109a, 3012 Bern, Switzerland
Full list of author information is available at the end of the article

general, pigs of every age can become infected, although in endemically infected farms mature pigs usually serve only as a reservoir for the pathogen, whereas growing pigs more often develop clinical signs of EP. For the infection of pigs with *M. hyopneumoniae* and the corresponding disease several risk factors, e.g. poor management practices, co-infections with other bacteria, viruses and/or parasites, seasonal effects, have been described [4, 6–9]. Some studies examined the role of suckling and nursery pigs and their individual risks for positivity to *M. hyopneumoniae*. Authors found that the presence of the porcine reproductive and respiratory syndrome virus (PRRSv)-EU genotype, *Pasteurella multocida*, *Haemophilus parasuis*, *Mycoplasma hyorhinis* or *Streptococcus suis* in the lung tissue of nursery pigs was significantly correlated with a higher probability of also finding *M hyopneumoniae*, whereas sow parity was not statistically related with piglet colonization in the offspring [10, 11]. Other studies focused on prevalence within different age groups [12] or follow-up of infected piglets [13], thus providing crucial knowledge for a better understanding of spread of *M. hyopneumoniae* in pig herds. Improved housing and management conditions are essential part of strategies for controlling EP [2]. Moreover, vaccination can reduce the impact of disease in endemically infected herds [14], but does not eliminate the pathogen from an infected herd [15].

In recent years, mathematical models of infectious diseases in animal populations have been widely used to gain insights about disease dynamics and the impact of control interventions. Mathematical models have, for instance, been used to enhance our knowledge about the dynamics of Methicillin-resistant *Staphylococcus aureus* [16] PRRSv [17], *Salmonella Typhimurium* [18] and transmissible gastro-enteritis in pig herds [19]. Through the identification of factors and interventions, they can be used by animal-health stakeholders – including policy-makers, veterinarians and farmers – as a decision-support tool. Models require data in order to be parameterised. In the case of *M. hyopneumoniae* a significant amount of information has been published over the last years, including the basic reproduction number (R_0) in different age groups, incubation period, etc. However, to the authors´ knowledge, no mathematical model has yet described the course of EP in a closed pig herd.

Here we use a compartmental model simulating the spread of *M. hyopneumoniae* within a batch of indoor and intensively raised pigs to assess the impact of a range of husbandry practices, industry settings and control interventions on the occurrence and spread of the pathogen. Therefore, a 'disease severity index" was calculated based on days when pigs were acutely or chronically diseased and infectious. The aims of developing this

model were gaining insights about disease dynamics and comparing different prevention programmes and strategies for controlling EP. Finally, this model shall help veterinarians and farmers as support tool in their decision making process.

Methods
Model design
In the present study, a discrete time, stochastic, compartmental model was developed, where one time-step equalled to one day. The unit of the model was the individual pig and a specific closed production batch of pigs was modelled from their birth to slaughter considering demographics of a pig population, including deaths. All piglets were born on the same day and each pig successively passed four age categories: suckling, nursery, growing and finishing. The time spent by pigs in each age category was fixed to 21 or 28 days of suckling period and 49 or 42 days of nursery period, respectively, 28 days of growing and 82 days of finishing. All pigs in a given batch were moved from one age category to the next together. For simplification, random mixing of all animals within each batch was assumed.

To model infection in the herd five successive states, i.e. compartments, were defined: susceptible (S), exposed or pre-infectious (E), acutely diseased and infectious (I_a), chronically diseased and infectious (I_c), and recovered (R) (Fig. 1). Given that there is no intra-uterine transmission [20], all suckling pigs were considered susceptible (S) after birth. In endemically infected pig herds, in which sows are frequently seropositive to *M. hyopneumoniae*, new-born suckling pigs will obtain a varying amount of maternally derived antibodies, but these do not protect against infection thus leaving the piglets fully susceptible [4]. Once infected, pigs are defined as being exposed, or pre-infectious (E) which means they are asymptomatic and do not shed the pathogen. At onset of clinical signs (coughing, etc.), pigs were considered as *'acutely diseased and infectious'* (I_a), and thereby beginning to shed the pathogen and therefore allow spread to susceptible pigs. Following this period, pigs became *'chronically diseased and infectious'* (I_c); a state in which pigs do no longer show clinical symptoms but still shed the pathogen. Finally, pigs

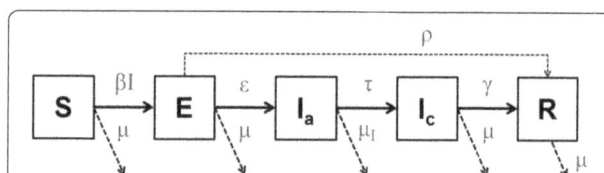

Fig. 1 Conceptual design of the compartmental model for transmission of *M. hyopneumoniae* within pig herds. (S: susceptible, E: exposed, Ia: acutely diseased and infectious, Ic: chronically diseased and infectious, R: recovered; transition parameters are explained in Table 1)

were considered to recover from the infection. These animals will have developed specific immunity [21] and no longer contributed to the transmission of *M. hyopneumoniae* within the herd. Some pre-infectious pigs were considered directly recovering from infection without experiencing symptoms or shedding the pathogen.

A pig could die at any time step during the batch cycle with its probability of survival depending on the age and the health state. The number of pigs in age category i in a given health state, surviving between time t and $t+1$, was simulated by a binomial process with the number of pigs in a given health state at time t as the number of trials, and the probability of survival ($1-_{l,i}$ for I_a and $1-_i$ for all other health states) as the probability of a success. Likewise, the transitions between infection states were simulated using binomial processes. The probability $p_{i,t}$ of a susceptible pig at time t in age category i becoming infected at time $t+1$ was dependent on $I_{a,i,t}$, $I_{c,i,t}$, $N_{i,t}$ and β_i (Eq. 1). A special situation was given for suckling pigs, which were infected by gilts and sows only. The probability of a piglet being infected by a sow increased with the duration of the suckling period. It was modelled using an exponential function (Eq. 2). The function parameters were selected in order to reproduce observed prevalence of *M. hyopneumoniae* infections in suckling pigs [22].

$$p_{i,t} = 1 - exp\left\{-\beta_i\left(I_{a,i,t} + \alpha I_{c,i,t}\right)/N_{i,t}\right\} \tag{1}$$

$I_{a,i,t}$, $I_{c,i,t}$ and $N_{i,t}$ were the number of acutely diseased and infectious pigs, chronically diseased and infectious pigs and the total number of pigs in age category i at time t, respectively. β_i was the rate of transmission for acutely diseased and infectious pigs in age category i and α was the relative infectivity of chronically compared with acutely diseased and infectious pigs, which was 0.5 by default.

$$p_{suckling,t} = 0.000251 * e^{0.1t} \tag{2}$$

t was the number of time-steps. As all piglets were born at $t = 0$, it was also interpreted as the age, in days, of the suckling pigs.

The length of time that pigs spent in each infection compartment (E, I_a and I_c) followed a normal distribution. The probability of a pig leaving an infection compartment increased with the time already spent in that compartment and was given by the cumulative distribution function (Table 1). As mentioned above, pigs leaving the E compartment could either become acutely diseased and infectious or recover from the infection. The number of pigs leaving the compartment E and directly recovering was simulated by a binomial process with the number of pigs leaving the compartment E as the number of trials and the probability ρ of not getting diseased and infectious following exposure as the probability of a success.

Table 1 Values of different, partly age-dependent transition parameters for a discrete time, stochastic compartment model estimating the within-herd transmission of *Mycoplasma hyopneumoniae* in closed pig herds

Parameter	Age group	Parameter level	Source
β	Suckling pigs	0.0005	[13]
	Nursery pigs	0.0148	
	Growing pigs	0.1497	
	Finishing pigs	0.1497	
ε	Nursery pigs	NCDF*(18, 7)	[41]
	Nursery pigs		
	Growing pigs	NCDF(13, 1.5)	[42]
	Finishing pigs		
τ	All pigs	NCDF(14, 3.5)	[42]
γ	All pigs	NCDF(28, 7)	[21]
ρ	All pigs	0.200	Expert opinion
μ	Suckling pigs	$(0.02*e^{(-0.233*x)}) + 0.002$	[23]
	Nursery pigs	$((2.0/100)/t_{Nursery\ period})$	
	Growing pigs	$((1.0/100)/t_{Growing\ period})$	
	Finishing pigs	$((1.6/100)/t_{Finishing\ period})$	
μ_l	Suckling pigs	$\mu_{[Suckling\ pigs]}$	
	Nursery pigs	$\mu*2$	
	Growing pigs	$\mu*2$	
	Finishing pigs	$\mu*2$	

*NCDF: normal cumulative distribution function with (μ, σ)

Table 1 describes transition parameters and other input parameters of the model.

Input parameters & outcome variable
Population dynamics parameters
Numbers corresponding to a one-site production system with approximately 500 producing sows and their offspring originating from a weekly batch farrowing were calculated in order to fit the model with representative numbers for an average sized herd. Based on these numbers, a standardized herd consisted of 21 farrowing groups of approximately 24 sows each (Eq. 3).

Number of sows per group (N)

$$= \frac{\text{Number of sows in the herd (n)}}{\left[\frac{\text{Length of gestation (weeks)+suckling period (weeks)+dry period (weeks)}}{\text{Farrowing rhythm (weeks)}}\right]} \tag{3}$$

Production parameters, e.g. number of life born piglets per litter or suckling pig mortality, were based on the annual report on pig production in Germany [23]. The number of piglets born live per batch was set at 293 (24 sows * 12.2 piglets born live per litter). The average proportion of pigs dying during the suckling period was

14.8 % [23], with approximately 50 % of the deaths occurring in the first four days of life [24]. Therefore, the probability of a suckling pig dying varied with the number of time steps x spent in the suckling section, and was expressed as: $\mu(x) = 0.002 + 0.02e^{-0.233x}$. Of pigs entering the nursery, growing and finishing sections, 2.0 %, 1.0 % and 2.1 % died in that section, respectively. The daily rate of death μ for each of these periods was calculated by dividing the percentage of mortality during the particular period by the number of days spent in this period. The lengths of the different production periods in the standard setting (baseline) were empirically set to 28 days for suckling (according to 91/630/EEC), 42 days for nursing, 28 days for growing and 82 days for finishing. In other scenarios, which were also analysed using the model, the suckling period was shortened to 21 days and the nursery period was then extended to 49 days.

Transition parameters

The parameters influencing the probability of moving to the next compartment were extracted from the literature, where available. For missing data, parameters were calculated from published data describing the course of *M. hyopneumoniae* infections in different age groups of pigs as described below, or were estimated based on expert opinion. For the expert opinion, 15 specialists for *M. hyopneumoniae* (5 clinicians, 5 microbiologists and 5 epidemiologists), known to the first author, were invited by email to complete an online survey. The survey closed 14 days after the invitation emails had been send. It included three semi-closed questions and one open-ended question:

- Please, imagine a case of *M. hyopneumoniae* infection with a strain of low (question 1), moderate (question 2) or high virulence (question 3):

'What do you think is the likelihood for an individual pig to recover from the infection without becoming infectious (= shedding of the pathogen)? Please provide your answer in % (0–100).'

- What do you think is the average impact of common co-infections (e.g. PRRSV, SIV & PCV2) on the transmission rate of *M. hyopneumoniae*?

'When co-infections are present, the transmission rate will increase by 0 %, 10 %, 20 %, 50 %, 100 % or 200 % (This question was to be answered in a table format for 'suckling pigs', 'nursery pigs', 'growing pigs' and 'finishing pigs')'

Parameters were adjusted to the particular age group of pigs.

The β for each age group (Table 1) was calculated from observed increases of prevalence in a longitudinal study [13]. It was assumed that *M. hyopneumoniae* prevalence (determined by PCR in bronchoalveolar lavage fluid and nasal swabs) reached 6.3 % at the end of the nursing period, 45.9 % at the end of the growing period, and 83.5 % at the end of the fattening period. Following these assumptions, the β for each group was calculated considering the overall transmission of the infection in the particular period and the length (D) of the particular infectious period (Eq. 4). The probability ρ of not becoming infectious following exposure was determined using expert opinion. Values of β were chosen to reproduce these empirical prevalences. In practice, for each successive age group, a wide range of values of β were tested. For each value of β, the spread of the pathogen within a given age group was simulated 1000 times. The average simulated prevalence of infection at the end of this production period was computed. The value of β associated with the average simulated prevalence that was the closest to the observed prevalence was then selected.

$$\beta = \frac{R_0}{D} \qquad (4)$$

In every iteration, a batch started with 293 suckling pigs. Subsequently, pigs could become exposed with α probability described in equation 1. However, β was dependent on the age group and increased, whenever pigs moved into the next age group. Pigs exposed to *M. hyopneumoniae* could become 'acutely infectious and diseased' with a probability of ε. The ε depended on the time that pigs already spent in that compartment, and was defined a normal cumulative distribution function, as described in the Table 1. Thus, the latent period was normally distributed. Instead of becoming 'acutely infectious and diseased', the pigs could also die with a probability μ or they could recover with a probability of ρ. The lengths of time that pigs remained in the infectious compartments were normally distributed. The probability τ and γ of an 'acutely infectious and diseased' pig becoming 'chronically infectious and diseased', and the probability of a 'chronically infectious and diseased' pig recovering from infection followed a normal cumulative distribution function (Table 1). Independent of the infection compartment pigs moved in the age categories from the suckling period (21/28 days) to the nursery period (42/49 days), the growing period (28 days) and finally the finishing period (82 days).

Depending on the virulence of a particular *M. hyopneumoniae* strain, exposed pigs would move directly to the compartment of recovered pigs [25]. The model was parameterised to reflect transmission of a *M. hyopneumoniae* with a substantial level of virulence. Therefore, the value for ρ was assumed low, which was also in accordance with expert opinion.

Outcome variable

For each simulation and age category, a disease severity index ($S_{Disease,i}$; Eq. 5) was calculated. It was defined as the ratio between the cumulative numbers of acutely and chronically diseased and infectious pig-days in an age category i, divided by the length of time that pigs spent in this age category i. This is equal to the number of pigs per day, either acutely or chronically infectious and diseased, divided by the number of all pigs per all days in the model (theoretical maximum is close to 100 %).

$$S_{Disease,i} = \sum_{t=0}^{T_i} (I_{a,i,t} + I_{c,i,t})/T_i \qquad (5)$$

T_i, was the length of time in days that pigs spent in an age category i.

Evaluated scenarios

The impact of different risk and protective factors on the spread of the *M. hyopneumoniae* at batch level was examined by adjusting the affected model parameters in the baseline model outlined above.

Acclimatisation of gilts (Acc)

A recent study [26] showed that one-site pig production systems are 10 times more likely to suffer from infection with *M. hyopneumoniae* followed by EP, if gilts in the particular herd do not have contact with living pigs of any age during their acclimatisation period. This risk factor was considered as a multiplier of the probability of suckling pigs becoming infected by their dam in case that no appropriate acclimatisation for gilts is implemented in the model herd. The β for suckling pigs (SP) was multiplied by 10 in order to account for this increase in the probability of the transmission of *M. hyopneumoniae* from sows and gilts to suckling pigs.

Length of suckling period (Suc)

The likelihood of transmission of *M. hyopneumoniae* from sows to their offspring increased exponentially with the length of the suckling period, which is equal to the time under exposure [22, 26, 27]. Two scenarios assuming a length of the suckling period equal to 21 and 28 days, respectively, were tested. The probability of a susceptible pig being infected by a sow on day d of its suckling period was equal to $0.000251 * e^{0.1d}$. This likelihood has been calculated considering the negativity of sucking pigs for *M. hyopneumoniae* at birth, a prevalence of 3.5 % at 28 days of age [11] and an average prevalence for the whole suckling period of less the 2 %

[10]. The corresponding data were tabled and parameters that best fit these data were selected.

Vaccination of suckling pigs against M. hyopneumoniae (Vac)

To assess impact of vaccination no special compartment for vaccinated pigs was included, since vaccination does not protect against infection [28], but with vaccinated piglets, the rate of spread of *M. hyopneumoniae* might be lower [29]. This change in the infection dynamics was considered in the model by lowering β by approximately 20 % for the age groups "suckling pigs" and "nursery pigs" in the model [30, 31], when it was assumed that suckling pigs had been vaccinated (16 scenarios out of 18).

Contact between fattening pigs of different age during restocking of compartments (Con)

The contact between pigs of different age during restocking of fattening compartments has been shown to promote the spread of the infection in this age group (OR: 13.8; [26]). In order to account for this effect, the models allowed contacts, over one day (i.e. one time-step), between outgoing finishing pigs (i.e. ending their production cycle) and growing and other finishing pigs. It created opportunities for transmission of infection from these outgoing finishing batches to batches in their growing or finishing period. This event could happen at any time during the fattening period. On the day that such contacts occurred, the probability of a pig in its growing or fattening period becoming infected was equal to:

$$p_{i,t} = 1 - exp\{-\beta_i(I_{a,i,t} + \alpha I_{c,i,t} + I_{a,O,t} + \alpha I_{c,O,t})/(N_{i,t} + N_{O,t})\}$$

Where the subscript O denoted the batch of outgoing fattening pigs. When accounting for such contacts between pigs of different age groups, successive production batches were modelled, and transmission of infection between a given batch of fattening pigs ending its production cycle, and subsequent batches of pigs which were in their fattening or growing period was simulated. A total of 100 successive batches was simulated in order to reach a stable prevalence at the end of batch production cycles, i.e. an equilibrium.

Co-infections in growing and finishing pigs (Inf)

Knowledge about the impact of co-infections on *M. hyopneumoniae* with regard to transmission of the infection, duration and severity of the disease is rare. Again, therefore expert opinion was used to assess the impact of co-infections as a multiplying factor for β in growing and finishing pigs.

Overall nine out of 15 experts answered to the questions regarding the impact of co-infections on the transmission rate of *M. hyopneumoniae*. Their estimate for suckling pigs was ranging from 0 % to 200 % increase and for nursery, growing and finishing pigs it was ranging from 10 % to 200 % increase of the transmission rate. The corresponding median values per age group were 10 %, 20 %, 50 % and 50 %, respectively. Thus, the individual values for β per age group were multiplied by 1.1, 1.2 or 1.5 in such scenarios, where the presence of co-infections was hypothesised.

Validation

The model was validated by comparing the estimated proportions of infected pigs at different stages of the batch production cycle with published figures on prevalence of *M. hyopneumoniae* in endemically infected herds at the same point in time [4, 32, 33]. Average prevalence of infection after 1000 iterations were analysed and compared to the prevalence known for that age category. Moreover, the ranges obtained after 1000 iterations, including minimum and maximum, were analysed for plausibility. Thus, length of the time-period for validation was one batch cycle, usually lasting about 180 days. A simulation with 2 % exposed suckling pigs at the end of the suckling period was used to determine the baseline of infection in the herd of the developed model. Reasons for using exactly this level of exposed piglets were observations made in different studies investigating the prevalence of *M. hyopneumoniae* in this age group [10, 11].

Sensitivity analysis

A univariate sensitivity analysis was conducted on a subset of transition parameters only to allow for realistic computing time. The selected parameters β and ρ were assumed to be of particular biological importance and, thus, they were multiplied with values between 0.2 and 2.0 in order to simulate only 20 % and up to 200 % of their impact on the model. The outcome variables for multiple comparisons were the 'severity of disease' and the proportion of 1,000 iterations not leading to any spread of infection in the herd.

The model was coded and run in R (Version x64-2.15.1; R Core Team (2014)) using TinnR as an graphic user interface [25]. The R programming code of the model is available from the corresponding author upon request. The relative importance of each risk or protective factor for the 'disease severity index' in the different age groups was determined by developing a regression model with STATA/IC 12.0 for Windows [64-bit x86–64] (StataCorp LP, Texas, USA). In this step, the disease severity indices of all iterations except of the first 100 were analysed for their association with the presence of risk and protective factors, i.e. the impact of the risk and protective factors on the numeric values in each age category.

Results

Validation

The outcomes of various scenarios were plotted as line charts and compared with recently published data on the prevalence of *M. hyopneumoniae* infection in pigs at different age. When all protective factors were present ([P] = Positive; Vac[P], Acc[P], Suc[P]) and risk factors were absent ([N] = Negative; Con[N], Inf[N]), the percentage of finishing pigs susceptible to *M. hyopneumoniae* at the end of the fattening period was >85 % on average and the percentage of pigs, which had been infected during their growth period was <10 % (mean; evidenced by details in Table 2 and 'Additional file 1'). Mortality that can be observed in this scenario is attributed to 'baseline mortality', which is approx. 15 to 20 % from birth to slaughter [23]. The observation of less than 10 % potentially seropositive pigs (due to exposure to *M. hyopneumoniae* followed by latency until seroconversion = $I_a + I_c + R$) and the absence of biologically significant within-herd transmission in most simulations are consistent with findings of a recent study [26]. In the latter, no spread of the pathogen and no disease could be confirmed in well-managed pig herds. In such scenarios, all animals should be seronegative at the end of the fattening period, because of waning of maternally derived antibodies, waning of antibodies after vaccination and the absence of exposure to the pathogen. In contrast, nearly all susceptible pigs became exposed and subsequently infectious (Fig. 2), when all protective factors were absent (Vac[N], Acc[N], Suc[N]) and all risk factors were present (Con[P], Inf[P]). The 'disease severity' in this 'high risk' scenario (Fig. 3) was well in accordance with findings in the field, where herds with similar risk and protective factors show comparable results in terms of pathogen transmission [26]. In contrast, the 'disease severity' was negligible in the 'low risk' scenario. Details can be studied in a graph provided as 'Additional file 2'.

Sensitivity analysis

The estimation of the model outcomes was based on 1000 iterations, which was considered sufficient since the moving-average disease severity index (mean of last 100 values) was stable after this number of iterations. More details regarding the convergence of the outcome due to the necessity of stabilizing the effect of 'contact between fattening pigs of different age during restocking of compartments' are displayed in a graph, which is provided as 'Additional file 3'.

The sensitivity of the model to variation in the transition parameters β and ρ was assessed. The overall outcome "disease severity" was strongly influenced by the level of β, when simultaneously changed for all age groups by multiplying with values between 0.2 and 2 (Fig. 4), but not influenced by ρ, when simultaneously

Table 2 Numerical results of disease severity (number of pigs per day either acutely or chronically infectious and diseased divided by the number of all pigs per all days in the model, given in per cent) and heat map for 18 different scenarios of a compartmental mathematical model of within-herd transmission of *M. hyopneumoniae*

Scenario	Risk or protective factor					Suckling period	Nursery period	Growing period	Finishing period	Whole life time
						Disease Severity				
No.	Vac	Acc	Suc	Con	Inf	Median (%)	Median (%)	Median (%)	Median (%)	Median (%)
1	N	N	P	P	P	1	10	3	13	9
2	P	N	P	P	P	1	10	2	11	8
3	P	P	P	P	P	0	1	0	0	0
4	P	P	N	P	P	0	2	1	7	4
5	P	P	P	N	P	0	1	0	3	2
6	P	P	P	P	N	0	1	0	11	5
7	P	P	N	N	P	0	2	1	16	12
8	P	P	P	N	N	0	1	1	27	20
9	P	P	N	P	N	0	3	2	30	14
10	P	N	N	P	P	3	21	4	12	11
11	P	N	N	N	P	3	20	4	13	11
12	P	N	N	P	N	3	23	8	24	18
13	P	N	N	N	N	3	23	8	25	20
14	P	N	P	N	P	1	10	2	15	12
15	P	N	P	N	N	1	11	4	30	24
16	P	N	P	P	N	1	11	4	30	17
17	P	P	N	N	N	0	3	2	34	25
18	N	P	N	N	N	0	3	2	34	26

Vac (P): vaccination of suckling pigs against *M. hyopneumoniae*. (N): no vaccination
Acc (P): gilts have contact to living animals during their acclimatisation. (N): no contact to living animals
Suc (P): duration of suckling period is 21 days. (N): suckling period is extended to 28 days
Con (P): growers have no contact to finishing pigs during restocking of compartments. (N): contact between different age groups
Inf (P): pigs do not suffer from co-infections. (N) presence of co-infections
*Severity of disease is defined as the average proportion of days that each pig is acute or chronic infectious during a particular period (e.g. only nursery period. only fattening period or whole life time)

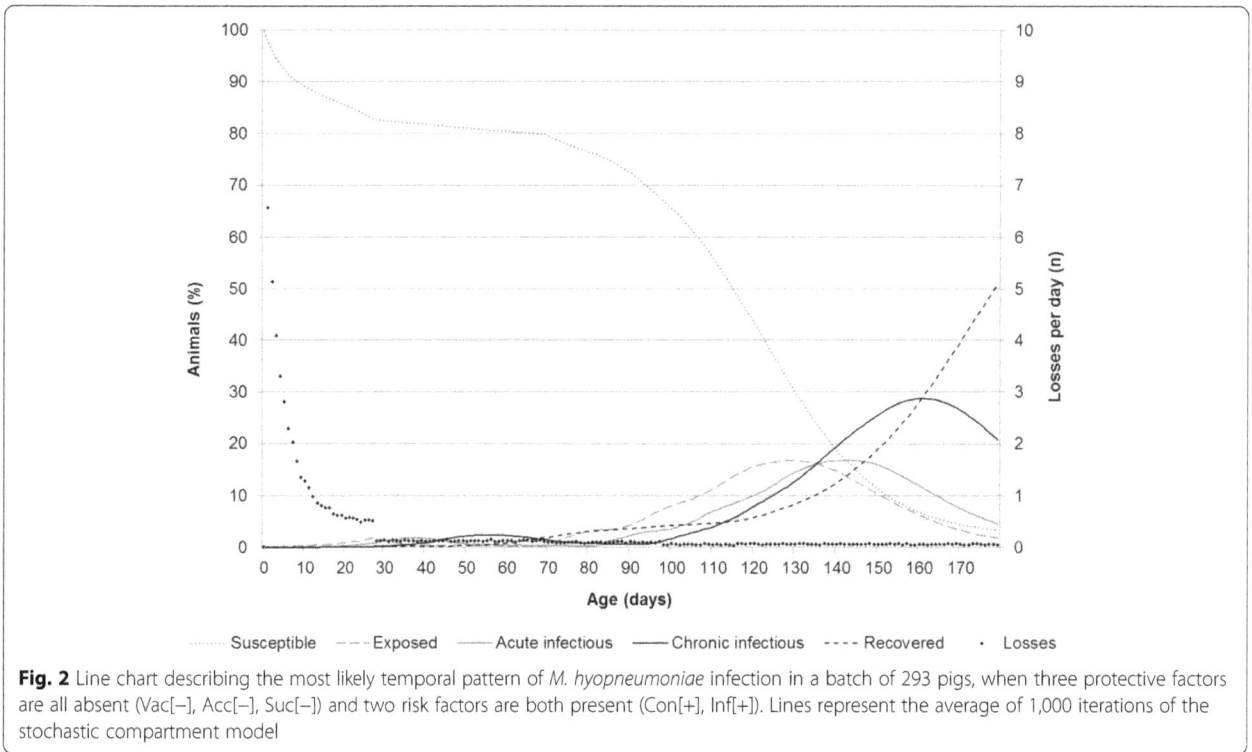

Fig. 2 Line chart describing the most likely temporal pattern of *M. hyopneumoniae* infection in a batch of 293 pigs, when three protective factors are all absent (Vac[–], Acc[–], Suc[–]) and two risk factors are both present (Con[+], Inf[+]). Lines represent the average of 1,000 iterations of the stochastic compartment model

changed for all groups with factors ranging from 0.2 to 2 (Fig. 5).

Impact of different factors

Overall, 18 different scenarios reflecting different combinations of risk and protective factors were tested (Table 2). Actually, the number of possible scenarios would have been 32 ($n = 2^f$ with f = number of factors; $n = 2^5 = 32$), but taking into account that in more than 70 % of pig herds in Europe vaccination against *M. hyopneumoniae* is routinely applied to suckling pigs [2], it was

decided to use only two scenarios without vaccination. As a result, the number of scenarios dropped from 32 to 18 ($n = 2^4$ [all scenarios with vaccination] + 2 [specific scenarios without vaccination]).

The lowest 'disease severity' was observed under scenario #3, where gilts are in contact with live animals during their acclimatisation, piglets suckle for 21 days and are vaccinated against *M. hyopneumoniae*, fattening pigs do not have contact with other age groups during (re-)stocking of compartments and are not suffering from co-infections. Under this scenario, pigs become

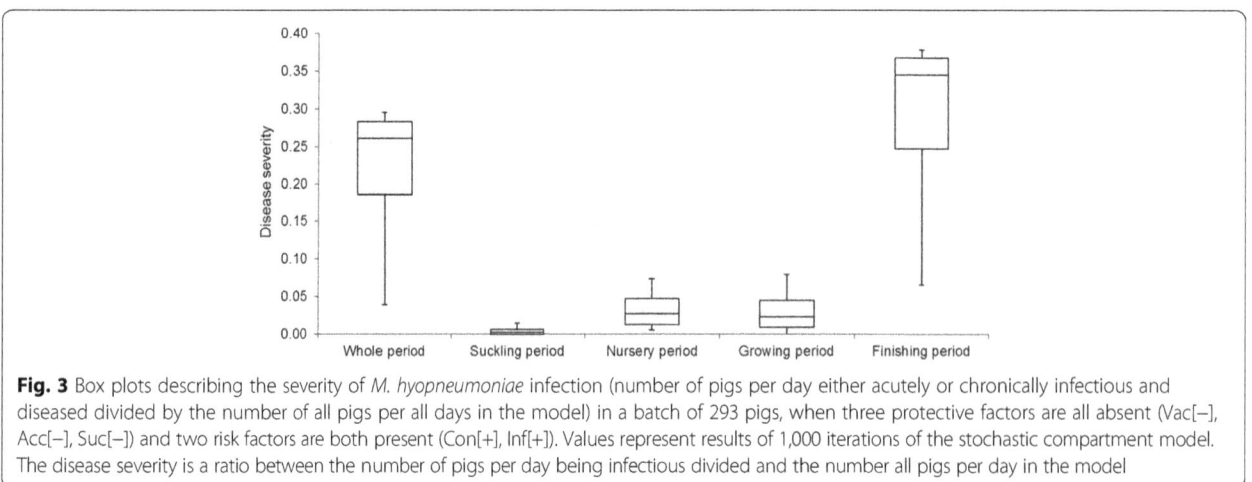

Fig. 3 Box plots describing the severity of *M. hyopneumoniae* infection (number of pigs per day either acutely or chronically infectious and diseased divided by the number of all pigs per all days in the model) in a batch of 293 pigs, when three protective factors are all absent (Vac[–], Acc[–], Suc[–]) and two risk factors are both present (Con[+], Inf[+]). Values represent results of 1,000 iterations of the stochastic compartment model. The disease severity is a ratio between the number of pigs per day being infectious divided and the number all pigs per day in the model

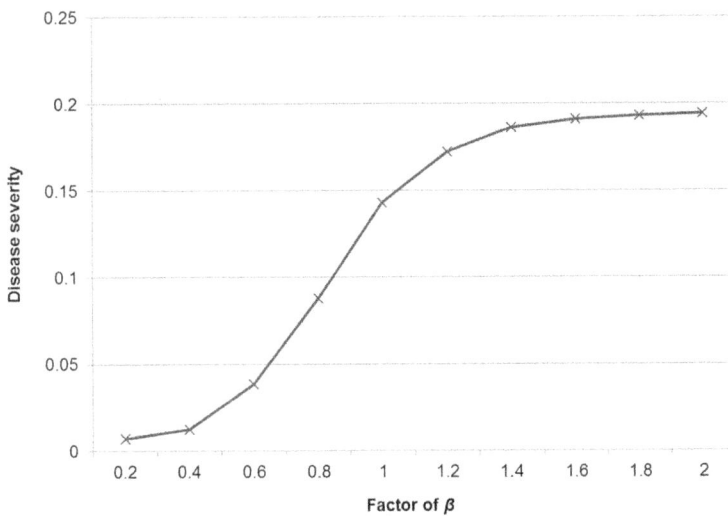

Fig. 4 Evaluation of the sensitivity of the outcome variable (disease severity = number of pigs per day either acutely or chronically infectious and diseased divided by the number of all pigs per all days in the model) to variation in the transition parameter β, when simultaneously changed for all age groups by multiplication with a factor between 0.2 and 2

either acutely or chronically diseased and infectious for 0.3 % of their lifetime as determined by estimated 'disease days' and 'pig days', i.e. the 'disease severity'. In 35.4 % of all simulations of scenario #3 no spread of infection was observed among suckling pigs (Fig. 6). Corresponding figures for nursery, growing and finishing pigs were 2.4 %, 53.0 % and 65.8 %, respectively.

The highest 'disease severity' over the whole period was observed in scenario #18. In this scenario gilts do have contact with live animals during their acclimatisation, but

suckling pigs are weaned first after 28 days and do not receive vaccination against *M. hyopneumoniae*, fattening pigs have contact with pigs of other ages during (re-)stocking of compartments and pigs are suffering from co-infections. Pigs in this scenario become diseased and either acute or chronic infectious for 26.1 % of their lifetime (Table 2). In 7.6 % of all simulations, there is no transmission of the infection in suckling pigs. Among growing and finishing pigs, this was the case in 1.1 % of all simulations (Fig. 6).

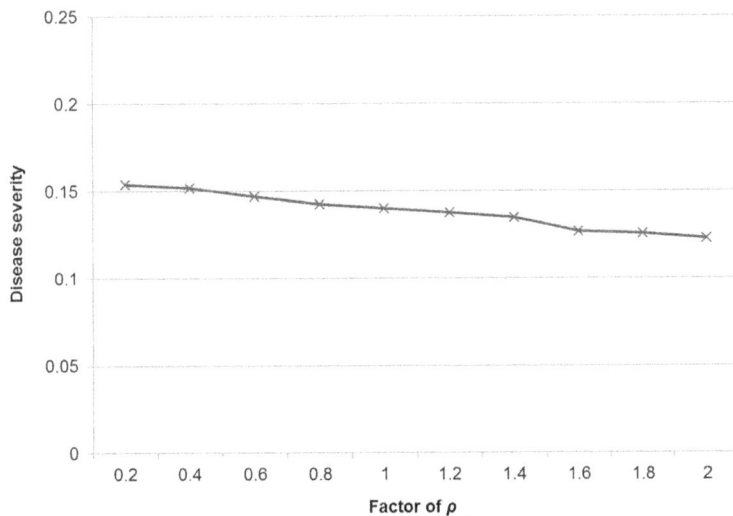

Fig. 5 Evaluation of the sensitivity of the outcome variable (disease severity = number of pigs per day either acutely or chronically infectious and diseased divided by the number of all pigs per all days in the model) to variation in the transition parameter ρ, when simultaneously changed for all age groups by multiplication with a factor between 0.2 and 2

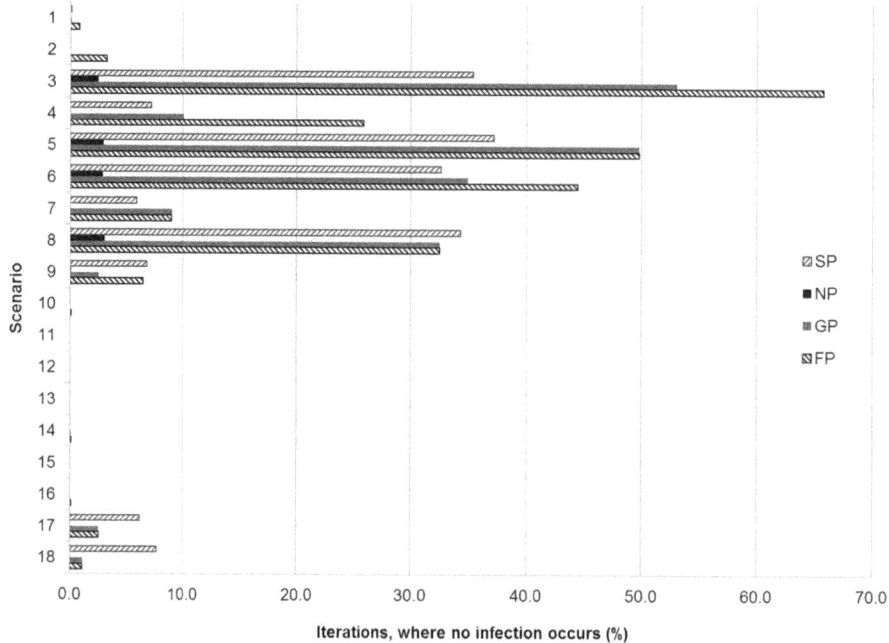

Fig. 6 Summary of simulations that did not lead to transmission of infection in 18 scenarios of a compartmental mathematical model of within-herd transmission of *M. hyopneumoniae* (SP = suckling pigs; NP = nursery pigs; GP = growing pigs; FP = finishing pigs)

When analysing the detailed results of the different scenarios (Table 2), it was observed that scenario #3 revealed the lowest disease severity in all age groups. In contrast, the highest values for 'disease severity' in each particular age group were distributed among two scenarios per age group (#12, #13, #17 and #18).

Multinomial regression analysis was performed in order to compare 'disease severity' over the whole lifetime of pigs for the different scenarios (Table 2) with the value of scenario #3 as a baseline. Significant differences were observed for all scenarios, when compared to #3 ($p < 0.001$).

Suckling pigs
In scenario #12, suckling pigs were either acutely or chronically diseased and infectious during 2.6 % of their time, this being slightly more than suckling pigs in scenarios #10, #11 and #13. These four scenarios were the only ones, where gilts did not have contact with live animals during their acclimatisation and the suckling period was 28 days compared with 21 days in other scenarios.

Nursery and growing pigs
In scenarios #12 and #13 comparably high values for 'disease severity' in nursery and growing pigs were found with highest figures being 23.0 % and 8.4 %, respectively. In both scenarios gilts had no contact with live animals during their acclimatisation and the suckling period was 28 days compared with 21 days, and co-infections were present.

Finishing pigs
The oldest age group was most affected in terms of 'disease severity', when gilts had contact with live animals during their acclimatisation and the suckling period was 28 days compared with 21 days and pigs were not vaccinated against *M. hyopneumoniae* and co-infections were present, and growing and/or finishing pigs had contact with pigs of other age groups during (re-) stocking of compartments (scenario #18). These finishing pigs demonstrated an average of 34.4 % of 'diseased days'.

The results of the logistic regression showed that vaccination of suckling pigs was influential for 'disease severity' in growing and fattening pigs, but not in suckling and nursery pigs (Fig. 7). Lack of contact between gilts and other live pigs during the acclimatisation significantly influenced the 'disease severity' in suckling pigs and less in growing and finishing pigs. The length of the suckling period equally affected the severity of the disease in all age groups with nursery pigs demonstrating the strongest association. The contact between finishing pigs and pigs of other age groups (i.e. growing pigs or finishing pigs in another compartment) influenced the course of infection among finishing pigs, but not among pigs of other age groups. Finally, the presence of co-infections was associated with higher values for 'disease severity' in growing and fattening pigs, but not in other age groups.

When analysing the impact of single risk or protective factors, the whole setting of the particular scenario needs to be considered. For example, the impact of co-

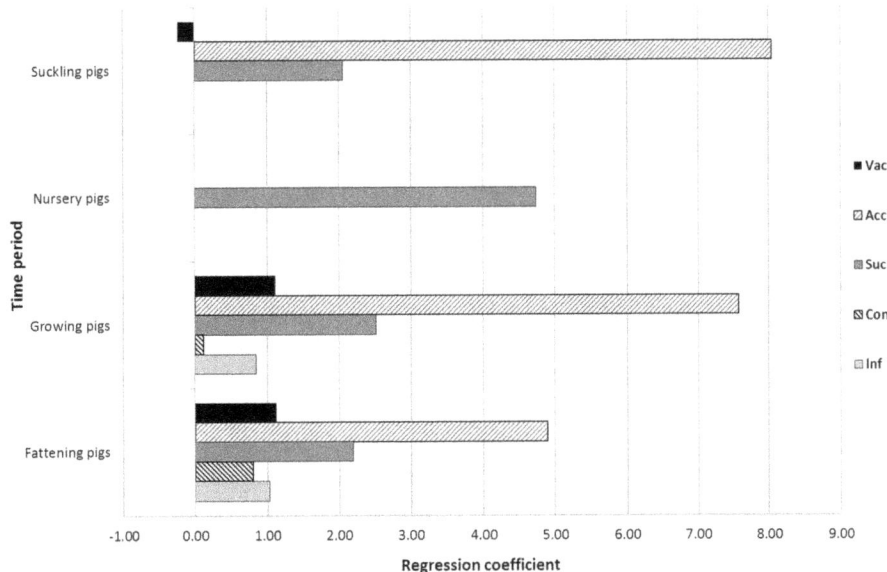

Fig. 7 Regression coefficients describing the impact of different risk and protective factors on the 'disease severity' in a compartmental mathematical model of within-herd transmission of *M. hyopneumoniae* (SP = suckling pigs; NP = nursery pigs; GP = growing pigs; FP = finishing pigs; Con & Inf for SP and NP have been dropped from the model due to *P* > 0.05)

infections on the overall disease severity for the whole lifetime was more significant when vaccines were applied to piglets, acclimatisation was performed, suckling period was only 21 days, and contact between fattening pigs of different age was possible (Vac[P], Acc[P], Suc[P], Con[N]). With this setting, the disease severity was 0.02 in case of co-infections being absent (scenario #5) and 0.20 in case of co-infections being present (scenario #8), which reflects a 10-times increase. In a slightly different setting where acclimatisation is not performed properly but everything else is identical (scenario #14 vs. #15) the disease severity elevates from 0.12 without co-infections to 0.24 with co-infections, which is 'only' a 2-times increase.

Noteworthy, a reduction of disease severity from particular scenarios is reached by introducing a risk factor instead of eliminating. For example, in scenario #17 vaccination is applied to piglets and gilts have contact to live animals during acclimatisation, though ending up with a disease severity score of 0.25 for the whole lifetime. When skipping the acclimatisation (scenario #13) the disease severity score will be reduced by 20 % to 0.20 for the whole lifetime. This effect is due to an 'earlier' spread of the infection, which leads to more recovered and, thereby, no longer susceptible animals in the fattening units.

Discussion

A stochastic compartmental model of within-herd transmission of *M. hyopneumoniae* was developed and used to assess the impact of different risk and protective

factors and to compare potential control measures. The results showed that appropriate gilt acclimatisation, short suckling period and maintenance of all-in-all-out procedure in all steps of production are the most important management factors for reducing within-herd transmission of *M. hyopneumoniae*. Farmers and veterinarians can carefully use this model and specifically the table with the outcomes of different scenarios to explore the most crucial points in a particular pig herd, where frequent transmission of *M. hyopneumoniae* occurs.

The flexible model described in this study can be adapted to assess the transmission of the pathogen in different herd management systems, e.g. variation in the duration of suckling period, contact between pigs of different age etc. Therefore, the model – considering the specific conditions - can be used in different industry settings, and can help to investigate the impact of control measures in different production systems. In order to facilitate such wider use of the model, the open source software 'R' was used as software platform for coding and simulations. The entire R code is available from the authors on request.

Some assumptions, like random mixing of all animals in each batch, might deviate results of the model from the reality, but they had to be made with regard of simplicity. The R code in its current form requires already a significant amount of computing power and would no longer run on a standard personal computer in less than 24 h, when including more steps of modelling, e.g. contact structure considering different litters of suckling pigs, etc.

Moreover to this simplification, the model has been parameterised by considering default production values from Germany (e.g. baseline mortality in particular age categories, etc.) and thus is limited to similar industry settings. It cannot be ruled out that in extremely different settings, e.g. backyard farming in Asia, the outcomes of this model do not apply and request a careful interpretation. This also applies to transition parameters calculated from other studies. There is always a specific (farm) setting, i.e. management, behind the outcome, that can have an impact on the data and thereby could have influence our assumptions, e.g. the β for each age group, which was calculated from observed increases of prevalence in a longitudinal study [13]. Similar, the experts might have over- or underestimated the multiplying factor for β when asked for the impact of co-infections on this figure. Finally, the model does neither account for multiple infections with several strain of *M. hyopneumoniae* nor for virulence of the one or more strains in particularly infected herds. Infections with more than one strain have been reported [34] and also virulence might vary significantly [1], but lack of detailed information about impact on parameters and a tremendous increase of computing power needed to account for these factors in the model precluded further consideration. It is assumed that in herds infected with a low virulent strain, all effects will be smaller, whereas in a herd infected with a high virulent strain all effects might be more sever. The same applies to the potential number of strains.

The model described here is complementary to an earlier study [35]. The latter focused on the veterinarian's view on the severity of EP and how this view changes with the increased availability of consistent scientific evidence, whereas our model focuses on the course of infection and the impact of intervention strategies. There is no direct link between the two models and it remains questionable, whether there is an option to establish such an interface, because the aim and scope of both models are quite diverse.

Validation and model sensitivity

The model was tested for internal and external validity. No 'unexpected' model behaviour was observed, and all outcomes, especially when testing and analysing 'extreme scenarios', were consistent with published data and were biologically sound. Similar attempts of model validation, i.e. comparison of data and evaluation of biological soundness, have been described previously for other models estimating the transmission of PRRSv [17] and *Salmonella typhimurium* [18] in pig herds.

Instead of a deterministic model, a stochastic approach was chosen in order to account for biologically occurring variation in pig populations and the course of *M.*

hyopneumoniae infection. In the early stages of the epidemic, single exposed pigs might die by chance (e.g. crashed by the mother dam) prior to transmitting the pathogen to a pen-mate, thereby leading to extinction of transmission. This variation of the course of infection is consistent with reports about different infection and disease pathogenesis patterns [33]. The stochastic approach chosen here also accounts for variation that can occur between herds.

The model was analysed for its sensitivity to assumptions in transition parameters. This was conducted to better assess model robustness and to better understand the course of *M. hyopneumoniae* infection in the model population. This sensitivity analysis focused on the most important parameters of the model only, as has been done in other published studies [18, 36]. Specifically, the transition parameter β was selected for sensitivity analysis, because it is hypothesised that most of the 'risk factors' influence this parameter and, thus, knowledge of its sensitivity towards changes is of greatest importance. Moreover, the transition parameter ρ was subjected to a specific sensitivity analysis, because its values were based on expert opinion rather than published literature. No other transition parameters were considered in the sensitivity analysis, as it was felt that a focussed analysis would then have been very difficult given the likely increased variation in output values.

Impact of different risk and protective factors

Overall, 18 scenarios based on the combination of five different risk and protective factors were analysed in this study. Based on the outcome of the iterations within each of the 18 scenarios, it was confirmed that gilts are the most influential factor for *M. hyopneumoniae* infection levels in suckling pigs. This is reflected in the percentage of iterations without any spread of infection, which was high in all scenarios, where gilts were assumed to have been subjected to appropriate acclimatisation with contact to other live pigs (scenarios 3–9 and 17–18). This observation regarding gilt acclimatisation was further confirmed by the results of the regression analysis, where the acclimatisation of gilts was the most important risk factor for a high 'disease severity score' among suckling, growing and finishing pigs. Similar importance of gilts for the course of the infection has been described in other studies determining the prevalence of *M. hyopneumoniae* in suckling pigs and corresponding risk factors, respectively [27, 37]. The hypothesis of young breeding animals being the main source of shedding of *M. hyopneumoniae* in sow herds is underlined by the observation that prevalence of the infection is significantly higher in those herds, where no acclimatisation for replacement boars (i.e. teaser boars) is undertaken [8].

The length of the suckling period was the most important factor with regard to *M. hyopneumoniae* infection in nursery pigs in our model. In longitudinal studies it was shown that the prevalence of *M. hyopneumoniae* infections increases during the suckling period in both sows [22] and suckling pigs [38]. Taking this into account the reason for the success of 'segregated early weaning' in order to create pig populations free of *M. hyopneumoniae* [39] becomes apparent. Especially during the first days *post-partum* the likelihood of transmitting the pathogen from sows to their offspring seems to be very low, whereas there is an exponential increase of the chance towards the end of the three to five week period of suckling. Subsequently there is no further transmission between piglets, since infected piglets are now in the incubation period. Thus, the number of nursery pigs infected is mainly driven by infection through their dams.

Considering the overall impact on the disease, the all-in-all-out principle is the most important measure for preventing the transmission of *M. hyopneumoniae* in closed pig herds. The importance of separating age groups has been described numerous times [2, 3, 40]. The feedback, i.e. increasing infection pressure, was modelled as a random contact between the oldest finishing pigs and a group of growing pigs at any point in time during their production stage. On the particular day of contact, the likelihood for the growing pigs to become exposed (i.e. force of infection) was not only influenced by the number of growing pigs in I_a and I_c, but also by the number of fattening pigs in I_a and I_c. The effect of these scenario characteristics is long term, significantly higher than the short-term effect among the first batch of growing pigs. This could explain, why after reaching a steady state of 'high transmission rates followed by acute and chronic infectiousness followed by high transmission in the next contact batch there is such a huge impact of the break achieved by the all-in-all-out risk management approach. These findings appear to be biologically sound and consistent with observations made for other pathogens, giving confidence in the model structure and its outputs [17, 18].

The observation that 'vaccination' had only marginal impact on the disease may be attributed to the limits of current vaccines against *M. hyopneumoniae*. They neither prevent from infection, nor do protect the animals 100 % from disease, when applied very early in pigs' life [15]. Moreover, only the aspect of reduction in the transmission rate was considered in the model, whereas a potential shortening of the time of being infectious could not be taken into account due to a lack of detailed information. The same facts apply to maternally derived immunity comprised by cells and specific antibodies that piglets receive from their dam. It is possible that both influence the infectious process by reducing clinical expression of EP in such piglets and thereby reducing the infectious period for the same animals. However, the effect is supposed being marginal, no robust data is available and therefore, this has not been considered in the model.

Conclusion

The output produced by this stochastic compartmental mathematical model of within-herd transmission of *M. hyopneumoniae* allows comparison of different prevention programmes and strategies for controlling EP. The identified intervention measures, namely appropriate acclimatisation of gilts, short suckling period and implementation of the all-in-all-out approach, will result in reduction of prevalence and, thus in improved pig health and welfare as well as a considerable reduction in antimicrobial usage. If combined with economic calculations, the model can provide a practical tool for informing decisions for specific herds.

Additional files

Additional file 1: Line diagram of animals per compartment. Line diagram describing the most likely course of a *M. hyopneumoniae* infection in a batch of 293 pigs, when three protective factors are all present (Vac[P], Acc[P], Suc[P]) and two risk factors are both absent (Con[N], Inf[N]). Lines represent the average of 1,000 iterations of the stochastic compartment model. (TIF 178 kb)

Additional file 2: Box plot of disease secerity. Box plots describing the severity of a M. hyopneumoniae infection in a batch of 293 pigs, when three protective factors are all present (Vac[P], Acc[P], Suc[P]) and two risk factors are both absent (Con[N], Inf[N]). Values represent results of 1,000 iterations of the stochastic compartment model. (TIF 67 kb)

Additional file 3: Diagram showing convergence of the outcome variable. Evaluation of the convergence of the outcome variable (disease severity) for an example scenario after several iterations with randomly selected input parameters for the binomially distributed elements (i.e. probability of transition between compartments). (TIF 300 kb)

Competing interest

The authors have no financial or personal relationship with people or organisations that could inappropriately influence or bias the content of this paper.

Authors' contributions

HN, BW and DUP drafted and designed the study. HN and GF developed the model with input from BW and KDCS. GF assisted HN with performing statistical analysis. HN and KDCS drafted the manuscript. BW and GF critically revised the manuscript and all authors read and approved the final manuscript.

Acknowledgments

This research was supported by a Marie Curie Intra European Fellowship within the 7th European Community Framework Programme (Grant number PIEF-GA-2010-274091).

Author details

[1]Veterinary Epidemiology, Economics and Public Health Group, Royal Veterinary College London, Hawkshead Lane, Hatfield, Hertfordshire AL97TA, UK. [2]Clinic for Swine, Vetsuisse Faculty, University of Berne, Bremgartenstrasse 109a, 3012 Bern, Switzerland. [3]International Livestock Research Institute, Addis Ababa, Ethiopia.

References

1. Vicca J, Stakenborg T, Maes D, Butaye P, Peeters J, de Kruif A, et al. Evaluation of virulence of Mycoplasma hyopneumoniae field isolates. Vet Microbiol. 2003;97:177–90.
2. Maes D, Segales J, Meyns T, Sibila M, Pieters M, Haesebrouck F. Control of Mycoplasma hyopneumoniae infections in pigs. Vet Microbiol. 2008;126:297–309.
3. Sibila M, Pieters M, Molitor T, Maes D, Haesebrouck F, Segales J. Current perspectives on the diagnosis and epidemiology of Mycoplasma hyopneumoniae infection. Vet J. 2009;181:221–31.
4. Maes D, Verdonck M, Deluyker H, de Kruif A. Enzootic pneumonia in pigs. Vet Quart. 1996;18:104–9.
5. Marois C, Le Carrou J, Kobisch M, Gautier-Bouchardon AV. Isolation of Mycoplasma hyopneumoniae from different sampling sites in experimentally infected and contact SPF piglets. Vet Microbiol. 2007;120:96–104.
6. Kobisch M. Mycoplasma diseases in pigs - old diseases still causing trouble. In: Cargill C, McOrist S, editors. Congress of the International Pig Veterinary Society. Melbourne: Causal Productions Pty Ltd; 2000. p. 5.
7. Ostanello F, Dottori M, Gusmara C, Leotti G, Sala V. Pneumonia disease assessment using a slaughterhouse lung-scoring method. J Vet Med A Physiol Pathol Clin Med. 2007;54:70–5.
8. Grosse Beilage E, Rohde N, Krieter J. Seroprevalence and risk factors associated with seropositivity in sows from 67 herds in north-west Germany infected with Mycoplasma hyopneumoniae. Prev Vet Med. 2009;88:255–63.
9. Steenhard NR, Jungersen G, Kokotovic B, Beshah E, Dawson HD, Urban Jr JF, et al. Ascaris suum infection negatively affects the response to a Mycoplasma hyopneumoniae vaccination and subsequent challenge infection in pigs. Vaccine. 2009;27:5161–9.
10. Nathues H, Kubiak R, Tegeler R, grosse Beilage E. Occurrence of Mycoplasma hyopneumoniae infections in suckling and nursery pigs in a region of high pig density. Vet Rec. 2010;166:194–8.
11. Sibila M, Nofrarias M, Lopez-Soria S, Segales J, Riera P, Llopart D, et al. Exploratory field study on Mycoplasma hyopneumoniae infection in suckling pigs. Vet Microbiol. 2007;121:352–6.
12. Villareal I, Vranckx K, Duchateau L, Pasmans F, Haesebrouck F, Jensen JC, et al. Early Mycoplasma hyopneumoniae infections in European suckling pigs in herds with respiratory problems: detection rate and risk factors. Vet Med. 2010;55:318–24.
13. Sibila M, Nofrarias M, Lopez-Soria S, Segales J, Valero O, Espinal A, et al. Chronological study of Mycoplasma hyopneumoniae infection, seroconversion and associated lung lesions in vaccinated and non-vaccinated pigs. Vet Microbiol. 2007;122:97–107.
14. Jensen CS, Ersboll AK, Nielsen JP. A meta-analysis comparing the effect of vaccines against Mycoplasma hyopneumoniae on daily weight gain in pigs. Prev Vet Med. 2002;54:265–78.
15. Haesebrouck F, Pasmans F, Chiers K, Maes D, Ducatelle R, Decostere A. Efficacy of vaccines against bacterial diseases in swine: what can we expect? Vet Microbiol. 2004;100:255–68.
16. Porphyre T, Giotis ES, Lloyd DH, Stark KD. A metapopulation model to assess the capacity of spread of meticillin-resistant Staphylococcus aureus ST398 in humans. PLoS One. 2012;7:e47504.
17. Evans CM, Medley GF, Creasey SJ, Green LE. A stochastic mathematical model of the within-herd transmission dynamics of Porcine Reproductive and Respiratory Syndrome Virus (PRRSV): fade-out and persistence. Prev Vet Med. 2010;93:248–57.
18. Ivanek R, Snary EL, Cook AJ, Grohn YT. A mathematical model for the transmission of Salmonella Typhimurium within a grower-finisher pig herd in Great Britain. J Food Prot. 2004;67:2403–9.
19. Hone J. A mathematical model of detection and dynamics of porcine transmissible gastroenteritis. Epidemiol Infect. 1994;113:187–97.
20. Goodwin RF, Pomeroy AP, Whittlestone P. Characterization of Mycoplasma suipneumonia: a mycoplasma causing enzootic pneumonia of pigs. J Hyg. 1967;65:85–96.
21. Kobisch M, Blanchard B, Le Potier MF. Mycoplasma hyopneumoniae infection in pigs: duration of the disease and resistance to reinfection. Vet Res. 1993;24:67–77.
22. Nathues H, Doehring S, Woeste H, Fahrion AS, Doherr MG, grosse Beilage E. Individual risk factors for Mycoplasma hyopneumoniae infections in suckling pigs at the age of weaning. Acta Vet Scand. 2013;55:44.
23. Gatzka EM, Schulz K, Ingwersen J, (ZDS) Z der DS e. V. Schweineproduktion. Alfter-Impekoven, Germany: Druckerei Martin Roesberg; 2011.
24. Casellas J, Noguera JL, Varona L, Sanchez A, Arque M, Piedrafita J. Viability of Iberian x Meishan F2 newborn pigs. II. Survival analysis up to weaning. J Anim Sci. 2004;82:1925–30.
25. Faria JC. Resources of Tinn-R GUI/Editor for R Environment. Ilheus, Brasil: UESC; 2011.
26. Nathues H, Chang YM, Wieland B, Rechter G, Spergser J, Rosengarten R, Kreienbrock L, grosse Beilage E. Herd-Level Risk Factors for the Seropositivity to Mycoplasma hyopneumoniae and the Occurrence of Enzootic Pneumonia Among Fattening Pigs in Areas of Endemic Infection and High Pig Density. Transbound Emerg Dis. 2014;61(4):316-28. doi: 10.1111/tbed.12033. Epub 2012 Dec 2
27. Nathues H, Woeste H, Doehring S, Fahrion AS, Doherr MG, grosse Beilage E. Herd specific risk factors for Mycoplasma hyopneumoniae infections in suckling pigs at the age of weaning. Acta Vet Scand. 2013;55:30.
28. Chae C. Vaccinating pigs against Mycoplasma hyopneumoniae infection: failure to prevent transmission. Vet J. 2011;188:7–8.
29. Meyns T, Dewulf J, de Kruif A, Calus D, Haesebrouck F, Maes D. Comparison of transmission of Mycoplasma hyopneumoniae in vaccinated and non-vaccinated populations. Vaccine. 2006;24:7081–6.
30. Meyns T, Maes D, Dewulf J, Vicca J, Haesebrouck F, de Kruif A. Quantification of the spread of Mycoplasma hyopneumoniae in nursery pigs using transmission experiments. Prev Vet Med. 2004;66:265–75.
31. Villarreal I, Vranckx K, Calus D, Pasmans F, Haesebrouck F, Maes D. Effect of challenge of pigs previously immunised with inactivated vaccines containing homologous and heterologous Mycoplasma hyopneumoniae strains. BMC Vet Res. 2012;8:2.
32. Nathues H, Strutzberg-Minder K, Kreienbrock L, Grosse Beilage E. [Possibilities and limits of serological diagnosis in pig stocks in the case of Mycoplasma hyopneumoniae infection]. Dtsch Tierarztl Wochenschr. 2006;113:448–52.
33. Sibila M, Calsamiglia M, Vidal D, Badiella L, Aldaz A, Jensen JC. Dynamics of Mycoplasma hyopneumoniae infection in 12 farms with different production systems. Can J Vet Res. 2004;68:12–8.
34. Nathues H, grosse Beilage E, Kreienbrock L, Rosengarten R, Spergser J. RAPD and VNTR analyses demonstrate genotypic heterogeneity of Mycoplasma hyopneumoniae isolates from pigs housed in a region with high pig density. Vet Microbiol. 2011;152:338–45.
35. Otto L, Kristensen CS. A biological network describing infection with Mycoplasma hyopneumoniae in swine herds. Prev Vet Med. 2004;66:141–61.
36. Andraud M, Grasland B, Durand B, Cariolet R, Jestin A, Madec F, et al. Modelling the time-dependent transmission rate for porcine circovirus type 2 (PCV2) in pigs using data from serial transmission experiments. J R Soc Interface. 2009;6:39–50.
37. Calsamiglia M, Pijoan C. Colonisation state and colostral immunity to Mycoplasma hyopneumoniae of different parity sows. Vet Rec. 2000;146:530–2.
38. Sibila M, Mentaberre G, Boadella M, Huerta E, Casas-Diaz E, Vicente J, Gortazar C, Marco I, Lavin S, Segales J. Serological, pathological and polymerase chain reaction studies on Mycoplasma hyopneumoniae infection in the wild boar. Vet Microbiol. 2007;97–107.
39. Wallgren P, Sahlander P, Hassleback G, Heldmer E. Control of infections with Mycoplasma hyopneumoniae in swine herds by disrupting the chain of infection, disinfection of buildings and strategic medical treatment. Zentralbl Vet B. 1993;40:157–69.
40. Stark KD. Epidemiological investigation of the influence of environmental risk factors on respiratory diseases in swine–a literature review. Vet J. 2000;159:37–56.
41. Villarreal I, Meyns T, Dewulf J, Vranckx K, Calus D, Pasmans F, et al. The effect of vaccination on the transmission of Mycoplasma hyopneumoniae in pigs under field conditions. Vet J. 2011;188:48–52.
42. Sorensen V, Ahrens P, Barfod K, Feenstra AA, Feld NC, Friis NF, et al. Mycoplasma hyopneumoniae infection in pigs: duration of the disease and evaluation of four diagnostic assays. Vet Microbiol. 1997;54:23–34.

15

Randomised controlled field study to evaluate the efficacy and clinical safety of a single 8 mg/kg injectable dose of marbofloxacin compared with one or two doses of 7.5 mg/kg injectable enrofloxacin for the treatment of *Actinobacillus pleuropneumoniae* infections in growing-fattening pigs in Europe

Erik Grandemange[1]* [iD], Pierre-Alexandre Perrin[1], Dejean Cvejic[2], Miriam Haas[2], Tim Rowan[3] and Klaus Hellmann[2]

Abstract

Background: Acute outbreaks of *Actinobacillus pleuropneumoniae* (APP) require rapid, effective, parenteral antimicrobial treatment. The efficacy and safety of a single, short-acting, high dose of marbofloxacin (Forcyl® swine 160 mg/mL) compared with 1 or 2 doses of 7.5 mg/kg enrofloxacin in APP outbreaks in European farms was studied.

Methods: A controlled, randomised block, blinded, multicentre, field study was conducted on four farms with acute respiratory disease associated with APP. Animals with clinical signs of respiratory disease were allocated similarly to intramuscular treatments of either a single dose 8 mg/kg marbofloxacin on day 0 or, 7.5 mg/kg enrofloxacin (Baytril 1nject®) on day 0 and again on day 2, if clinical signs had not improved.

Results: The results were similar for intention to treat (242 pigs) and per protocol populations (239 pigs). On day 0, all pigs had pyrexia (means, 40.6 °C), moderate to severe clinical signs (depression, cough, dyspnoea). Following treatment, animals improved rapidly and on day 7, clinical signs were absent or mild in all pigs and mean temperatures for each treatment were <39.5 °C ($P > 0.05$). The primary efficacy criterion, animals cured, for marbofloxacin and enrofloxacin was 81.8 and 81.4% on day 7, and 84.2 and 82.2% on day 21, respectively. Results for cure, respiratory disease removals and mortalities, and relapses were compared using confidence intervals and confirmed that marbofloxacin was non-inferior to enrofloxacin ($P > 0.05$). There were no significant treatment differences in live weight gains, adverse events and injection site reactions (<2.5% animals) ($P > 0.05$). Significantly more animals developed concurrent disorders in the enrofloxacin (7.5%) than marbofloxacin (0.0%) group ($P < 0.01$). On day 0, the MIC_{90} values of APP for marbofloxacin and enrofloxacin were 0.06 μg/mL for APP, less than the clinical breakpoints.

(Continued on next page)

* Correspondence: erik.grandemange@vetoquinol.com
[1]Vetoquinol SA, Research and Development Centre, B.P. 189, 70204 Lure Cedex, France
Full list of author information is available at the end of the article

(Continued from previous page)

Conclusions: Marbofloxacin (single dose of 8 mg/kg) and enrofloxacin (1 or 2 doses of 7.5 mg/kg) were clinically safe and effective in the treatment of clinical respiratory disease associated predominantly with APP in four European commercial, fattening pig herds.

Keywords: Marbofloxacin, Enrofloxacin, Respiratory disease, Efficacy, *Actinobacillus pleuropneumoniae*, Minimum inhibitory concentration

Background

Respiratory infections are a common cause of morbidity and mortality in growing-fattening pigs [1, 2]. Even on well-managed pig farms with effective prevention systems, pigs may become infected with bacterial pathogens requiring antimicrobial treatment. Common porcine, bacterial respiratory pathogens include *Actinobacillus pleuropneumoniae* (APP), *Pasteurella multocida* (PM), *Haemophilus parasuis*, *Mycoplasma hyopneumoniae* and *Bordetella bronchiseptica* [2, 3]. APP is found worldwide and is an important pathogen of pigs. Clinical signs are most common in pigs less than 6 months of age and include acute, life-threatening, pleuropneumonia with coughing, fever and lethargy. At post mortem lesions there may be necrotic and haemorrhagic lung lesions with lung tissue sequestration and fibrotic pleuritis and pericarditis. Infected but clinically healthy animals carrying the pathogen are an important source of the infection [1–3]. Reduced production efficiency including decreased daily weight gain, reduced feed conversion, carcass trimming and condemnation, and costs and time for intensive animal treatment [1, 2] may be associated with APP infections.

The treatment of acute APP infections is essential to ensure animal welfare and will contribute to minimising adverse economic effects. Selection of an antimicrobial treatment by a field veterinarian, animal owner or farm staff requires consideration of efficacy, dosage regimen and formulation based on the product label including precautions to minimise the potential for resistance development [2, 3]. Minimising use of antimicrobials is widely recognised as important to restricting the development of antimicrobial resistance and this favours the treatment of individual, clinically affected animals rather than administration through feed or water involving treatment of an entire group of pigs containing the clinically affected animals. Furthermore, for acutely diseased pigs that are unlikely to eat and perhaps drink in severe cases it is essential to administer antimicrobials to individual animals, for example by parenteral injection. An individual animal treatment which only requires a single administration is desirable to minimise animal handling and to facilitate compliance with the recommended dosing regimen by farm staff. However, many antimicrobial treatments require at least daily administration for three or more days [2, 4, 5].

The fluoroquinolone antimicrobials are unusual in that their safety and concentration-dependent mode of action facilitates the use of a single, short-acting, high dose to provide both good efficacy and to minimise resistance development in target pathogens such as APP [6, 7]. Analysis based on antimicrobial pharmacokinetics (PK) in growing-fattening pigs and on pharmacodynamics (PD), using both minimum inhibitory concentrations (MIC) and mutation prevention concentrations (MPC) of representative field isolates of APP, PM and *H. parasuis* has provided a strong rationale for field use of a single, IM dose of 8 mg/kg marbofloxacin in the treatment of acute actinobacillosis and which is also unlikely to favour resistance development in the target pathogens [8–12]. However, fluoroquinolones are classified as critically important antimicrobials for human health and in order to minimise resistance development their veterinary use should be reserved for the treatment of clinical conditions which have responded poorly, or are expected to respond poorly to other classes of antimicrobials. Wherever possible, use of a fluoroquinolone product should only occur when based on relevant epidemiological data and susceptibility testing (preferably specific to the affected herd), and after consideration of alternatives, local antimicrobial usage policies and the absence of an alternative and effective non-critically important antimicrobial [13–15]. Improvements to husbandry practices and vaccination should also be considered to reduce the risk of future disease outbreaks [14].

The use of studies with negative (untreated) controls to evaluate efficacy of antimicrobials is limited for ethical and animal welfare reasons. A well-controlled, in vivo study based on an aerosol challenge infection of APP in pigs showed that a single IM dose of 8 mg/kg marbofloaxcin was at least as effective as a positive control of conventional daily dosing for three days with enrofloxacin (2.5 mg/kg/ day; total dosage 7.5 mg/kg/animal) and superior to a negative, saline control treatment (clinical cures 6 days after infection were 91, 83 and 9%, respectively) [16]. The study reported here was to determine whether or not similar efficacy of a single 8 mg/kg dose of marbofloxacin would be obtained under field conditions of natural outbreaks of APP clinical disease in pigs. Some preliminary results of the study were presented previously [17].

Methods

The study treatments are shown in Table 1. The distribution of animals to study sites (farms) and treatment groups, and clinical scores and rectal temperatures before treatment on day 0 (per protocol population) are shown in Table 2. The distribution by farm of bacterial pathogens isolated before treatment on day 0 from lower respiratory tract lesions and bronchoalveolar lavage samples, and ranges of minimum inhibitory concentrations (MIC) of marbofloxacin and enrofloxacin are shown in Table 3.

Herd description, study animals, management

Pig fattening units on each of four farms (two in each of Germany (G) and Hungary (H)) were selected for the study based on history of swine respiratory disease (SRD) associated with APP confirmed by necropsy and bacteriology in the previous three months. Three of the farms (HA, HB, GA) included breeding and fattening pig units, and one farm (GB) was of fattening pigs only. Within each farm, pigs were obtained from a single source. Pig population sizes for each farm were 1600, 6500, 9500 and 13,000 for farms GB, GA, HB, and HA, respectively. Study animals were housed on fully (HB, GA, GB) or partially (HA) slatted floors with negative pressure ventilation and, in three farms (HA, HB GA), temperature controlled environments. Commercial feed was given either *ad libitum* (HA, HB, GB) or restricted (GA) as meal (GA, GB) or pellets (HA, HB)), and water by nipple drinkers. Breeds were Hungarian Large White x Hungarian Landrace x Duroc (HA), European hybrid (HB), BHZP Viktoria and BHZP Naima (GA) and Topigs (GB). Routine vaccinations were used on each farm, including for prevention of the following infections: PCV2 and *Mycoplasma hyopneumoniae* (HA, HB, GB) and PRRSV (HA, GA, GB). A total of 242 fattening, male (mostly castrates) and female pigs, weighing 25 to 94 kg live weight, and between 15 and 20 weeks of age were enrolled in the study.

Administration of vaccines was completed at least 3 weeks before first treatment (day 0); administration of anti-inflammatory and other antimicrobial products was not permitted in the study and for 7 days (or 21 days for long-acting products) prior to day 0.

Study design

The objectives of the study were to determine the clinical efficacy and clinical safety under field conditions of IM administration of a single dose of 8 mg/kg marbofloxacin (160 mg/mL, Forcyl® Swine, Vetoquinol SA, France) compared with one or two IM administrations of 7.5 mg/kg enrofloxacin (100 mg/mL, Baytril 1Inject®, Bayer Vital GmbH, Germany) against naturally-occurring respiratory disease associated principally with APP in pigs on commercial farms in Europe. The control product, enrofloxacin was chosen as a reference or control product as it, like marbofloxacin is a second generation fluoroquinolone and has similar pharmacokinetic properties, is indicated for the treatment of APP in pigs and may be used for single dose therapy. It should be noted that the dosage regimen for enrofloxacin in the treatment of SRD in the study was according to the previous summary of product characteristics, and that this has since changed to a single dose of 7.5 mg/kg only and the current summary of product characteristics does not refer to administration of a second dose [13]. The study design was a positive controlled, randomised and blocked, blinded, multicentre, clinical field study with natural infection. The experimental and treatment unit was the individual animal. There were four farms in the study and the study was designed and powered to compare the treatments using the combined data from the four farms (Table 2). The distribution and sensitivity range of the isolates from the lower respiratory tract were also similar between farms on day 0 (Table 3). The study was not designed, and did not have power to make conclusions based on any apparent differences in results between farms and such difference may be confounded with other, uncontrolled variables (e.g. housing, diet, management and genotype).

Study day 0 was defined individually for each animal as the day it first met the clinical criteria for treatment and was first administered either the investigational veterinary product, marbofloxacin, or the positive control product, enrofloxacin. The primary efficacy criterion was animals cured clinically on day 7 and the power of the study was based on this criterion. A minimum of 112 clinically affected, per protocol animals were required for each treatment group to provide statistical power of 80% and a non-inferiority margin of 0.15 (15 percentage points) based on known efficacy of approximately 80%

Table 1 Study treatment groups (dosages and duration of treatments are as recommended in product data sheets at the time of the study)

Treatment group (Active ingredient)	Route of administration	Dosage mg/kg	Duration of treatment	Day(s) of observation	Number of animals[a]
Marbofloxacin	IM	8	Once on day 0 only	0, 1, 2, 3, 7, 21	122
Enrofloxacin	IM	7.5	Once on day 0 & on day 2 if clinical signs had not improved	0, 1, 2, 3, 7, 21	120

[a]Intention to treat populations

Table 2 Distribution of animals by farm and treatment group, and homogeneity of clinical scores and rectal temperatures before treatment on day 0 (per protocol population)

| | Farm site | Marbofloxacin (T1) | | | | Enrofloxacin (T2) | | | | T1 vs. T2 |
		Total no. animals	Mild	Moderate	Severe	Total no. animals	Mild	Moderate	Severe	P value[a]
Respiratory scores % [n][b]	GA	36	0.0 [0]	97.2 [35]	2.8 [1]	35	0.0 [0]	100 [35]	0.0 [0]	0.324
	GB	35	0.0 [0]	82.9 [29]	17.1 [6]	35	68.6 [24]	31.4 [11]	0.0 [0]	0.166
	HA	24	0.0 [0]	100 [24]	0.0 [0]	24	0.0 [0]	100 [24]	0.0 [0]	nc
	HB	26	0.0 [0]	100 [26]	0.0 [0]	24	0.0 [0]	95.8 [23]	4.2 [1]	0.298
	Combined	121	0.0 [0]	94.2 [114]	5.8 [7]	118	0.0 [0]	89.8 [106]	10.2 [12]	0.193
Depression scores % [n][b]	GA	36	97.2 [35]	2.8 [1]	0.0 [0]	35	97.1 [34]	2.9 [1]	0.0 [0]	0.984
	GB	35	85.7 [30]	11.4 [4]	2.9 [1]	35	85.7 [30]	14.3 [5]	0.0 [0]	0.961
	HA	24	70.8 [17]	29.2 [7]	0.0 [0]	24	83.3 [20]	16.7 [4]	0.0 [0]	0.308
	HB	26	100 [0]	0.0 [0]	0.0 [0]	24	95.8 [23]	4.2 [1]	0.0 [0]	0.298
	Combined	121	89.3 [108]	9.9 [12]	0.8 [1]	118	90.7 [107]	9.3 [11]	0.0 [0]	0.647
Rectal temperatures °C	GA	36		40.4 (0.047)		35		40.4 (0.049)		0.702
	GB	35		40.6 (0.068)		35		40.6 (0.069)		0.556
	HA	24		40.6 (0.114)		24		40.4 (0.060)		0.737
	HB	26		40.7 (0.077)		24		40.9 (0.091)		0.240
	Combined	121		40.6 (0.037)		118		40.6 (0.034)		0.603

Farm site: Country identification *G* Germany, *H* Hungary. A and B indicate different farms within country

Numbers of animals and percentages refer to the per protocol populations. Animals euthanised prior to study for diagnostic purposes are excluded from these populations

[a]For respiration and depression scores, p values are from Mantel-Haenszel mean score for each site separately and on Cochran-Mantel-Haenszel mean score statistic for combined

[b]Refer to Clinical examinations for details of scoring. [n] number of animals. nc Not calculated

Rectal temperatures shown as mean (standard error). For rectal temperatures, p values are based on Wilcoxon rank sum statistic for each site separately and on the extended Mantel-Haenszel statistic for combined

for the control product, an anticipated placebo or self-cure response of 46% [18] and a 5% significance level. Animals were enrolled according to pre-defined inclusion and exclusion criteria and were allocated equally to each treatment group on day 0. On day 0, animals were injected IM with the either marbofloxacin or enrofloxacin on either the right hand side (farms HA and HB) or the left hand side (farms GA and GB) of the neck. For the enrofloxacin treatment group only, a second administration approximately 48 h later was permitted if clinical signs had not improved, as assessed by the blinded examining veterinarian using the same pre-defined criteria as applied on day 0.

The study was conducted according to good clinical practice [19] by four, separate investigators with independent monitoring by a contract research organisation (Klifovet AG, Germany). To facilitate quality and consistency across the study sites or farms, all staff received specific training for the study including, as appropriate necropsy examinations, sample collection and clinical examination scoring. The conduct of the study was monitored at all stages by an appointed individual that was independent of the investigators and veterinarians, and responsible for overseeing the clinical study and ensuring that it was conducted, recorded, and reported in accordance with the study protocol, standard operating procedures, Good Clinical Practice and the applicable regulatory requirements. This included on-site inspections during necropsies, product administration and clinical examinations. There were different investigators, examining veterinarians and dispensers for each farm. The investigators and examining veterinarians could be the same individual and were specialised veterinary pig practitioners, experienced in both clinical and post mortem examinations. The treatments were administered by the dispensers (the individual farm veterinarians) following a pre-established randomisation plan. The study was blinded by using different personnel: All personnel making clinical, post mortem and laboratory examinations, and decisions to treat (including any decision to administer a second treatment of enrofloxacin) or to withdraw animals from the study were blinded (and remained blinded until the end of the study) to the allocation of animals to treatment; different, unblinded personnel were used for administration of treatments. A single, centralised laboratory was used for all microbiological isolation and PCR analyses (University of Veterinary Medicine, Hannover, Germany) and another laboratory (Vetoquinol SA, Lure , France) was used for all determinations of MIC. All laboratory staff were blinded. The in vivo phase of the study was conducted between November 2013 and April

Table 3 Distribution by farm of bacterial pathogens isolated before treatment on day 0 from lower respiratory tract lesions and bronchoalveolar lavage samples, and ranges of minimum inhibitory concentrations (MIC) of marbofloxacin and enrofloxacin

		MIC range (µg/mL)		
	Farm site	Marbofloxacin	Enrofloxacin	n
A. pleuropneumoniae	GA	0.03–0.06	0.06–0.12	9
	GB	0.03–0.25	0.03–0.25	9
	HA	0.06–0.12	0.06–0.12	18
	HB	0.03–0.06	0.03–0.06	25
H. somnus	GA	–	–	0
	GB	0.015	0.008	1
	HA	–	–	0
	HB	0.03	0.03	1
P. multocida	GA	–	–	0
	GB	0.015	0.008	1
	HA	0.015–0.03	0.008	7
	HB	–	–	0
B. bronchiseptica	GA	0.5	0.5	4
	GB	0.25–0.5	0.25–0.5	4
	HA	–	–	0
	HB	0.25	0.5	1

Farm site: Country identification G Germany, H Hungary. A and B indicate different farms within country
MIC concentrations ranges (µg/mL) of the antimicrobial for which all of the isolates were inhibited
n total number of isolates from lung/lower respiratory tract and bronchoalveolar lavage, combined, for which MIC was determined

2014. Statistical analyses, accountability of marbofloxacin and enrofloxacin use, and quality assurance procedures were conducted by independent staff.

Variables for efficacy and safety assessments
Clinical examinations and live weights
Animals were examined by the blinded, examining veterinarians on days 0, 1, 2, 3, 7 and 21. Rectal temperatures and clinical assessments (scores) of respiratory signs, depression and injection site reactions were recorded. For an animal to be enrolled on day 0, it was required to have a temperature of ≥40.2 °C, and a minimum of moderate respiratory signs and moderate depression as determined by the blinded examining veterinarian. Respiratory signs were assessed as normal, mild (mild dyspnoea and/or cough, little or no nasal discharge), moderate (moderate dyspnoea with multiple episodes of coughing within a few minutes and nasal discharge) or severe (coughing, nasal discharge, and gasping or open mouthed breathing and/or cyanosis). Signs of depression was assessed as absent, mild (slight depression, active but not fully alert, reduced appetite), moderate (obvious depression, responded only after stimulation, head down, anorexia) or severe (not eating, no response

to stimulation, unable to stand, and moribund). Animals showing severe respiratory signs or severe depression were considered for immediate euthanasia. Normal rectal temperature was defined as ≤40 °C based on preliminary clinical examinations and rectal temperature recordings of pigs at each farm prior to the APP outbreaks. Injection site reactions were recorded as reddening, swelling, induration and pain on palpation.

The primary and secondary efficacy criteria were animals cured on day 7 and day 21, respectively. Cure was defined as normal rectal temperature (≤40 °C) and absence of clinical signs of depression and absence of respiratory signs. Any animals removed from the study was assigned a reason for removal and if appropriate necropsied. Animals removed because of SRD before day 7 were counted as not cured. Animals removed from the study were either given alternative treatment or euthanised for animal welfare reasons.

Live weights of animals were recorded on days 0 and 21.

Post mortem and laboratory examinations
The aetiology of each SRD outbreak was established by necropsy of pigs within 1 h of euthanasia (or natural mortality) of up to 10 pigs per farm in the 24 h before first treatment administration. These pigs were not part of the intention to treat population; all other pigs on each farm that met the inclusion criteria on a single day (i.e. day 0 which was a calendar date specific to each farm) were included in this population. Each pig selected for necropsy had clinical signs of SRD. The numbers of pigs selected for necropsy (and the numbers of live animals enrolled in the study) for farms GA, GB, HA and HB were 4 (and 71), 10 (and 70), 6 (and 50), and 10 (and 51), respectively. To assist the rapid and consistent collection of samples for bacteriology, necropsies were performed to a standard procedure on each farm in a designated area. In addition, necropsies were made from days 1 to 21 on five animals either removed from the study and euthanised on welfare grounds or after natural mortality. Broncho-alveolar lavage samples (BAL) [20] for bacteriology were collected from another 36 pigs (maximum of 10 animals / farm) before treatment on day –1 or 0 and again from the same animals on day 7. Nasal swabs (single nostril, approximately 10 cm deep) were collected on days 0 and 7 from all live animals that were not sampled by BAL.

A total of 369 bacterial isolates (APP, *B. bronchiseptica*, *H. parasuis* and PM), were obtained either from lungs at necropsy or, from live animals by BAL or nasal swabbing and were identified by culture and PCR [21–27]. The isolates were used for MICs determinations by standard, broth microdilution, procedures of Vetoquinol laboratories (with adherence to the Clinical and Laboratory Standards Institute (CLSI) guidelines [28–30]) except for *H. parasuis* where veterinary fastidious medium was used as described for APP in the CLSI standard VET01-A4 [28]. The MIC determinations included standard reference (quality control) strains of *Staphylococcus aureus* ATCC 29213 and *Escherichia coli* ATCC 25922, and sterility and growth controls on each plate. The MICs of the quality control strains were within the CLSI quality control ranges. Where 10 or more isolates of a bacterial species were available, the MIC_{50} and MIC_{90} values (concentration of antimicrobial required to inhibit 50 and 90%, respectively, of a population of isolates of the same species) were calculated and then rounded up to the next value in standard antimicrobial sensitivity test dilution series [31].

On farms HA and GA only, blood samples for serology were collected from 10 pigs selected randomly from within the per protocol populations on day 0 and these pigs were resampled on day 21. These samples were not an integral part of the study and were collected to assist in the diagnosis of possible intercurrent disease if it should have arisen during the study. Samples were analysed for seroconversion to PRRS virus (ELISA; PRRS X3 Ab test, IDEXX), PCV-2 virus (Capture-ELISA; INgezim Circovirus IgM/IgG, INGENASA) and Influenza A virus (H1N1, H1N2, H3N2, H1N1 haemagglutination test, IDT Biologika).

Statistical analyses

The intention to treat population of animals was a total of 242 (Table 1) and of these, three animals were excluded from the per protocol population because of concomitant disorders not related to SRD which did not allow the animals to continue in the study as other treatments were required that were not compliant with the protocol. The per protocol population was a total of 239 animals (Tables 2 and 4). Safety evaluations used all of the 242 animals that were enrolled in the study on day 0 (intention to treat population) and the per protocol population of 239 animals was used for efficacy evaluations. Homogeneity criteria of per protocol populations on day 0 for age, sex, weight, respiratory and depression scores, and rectal temperature were confirmed to be similar between treatments ($P > 0.05$). Animals in each treatment group were mixed together within each pen on each farm and the individual animal was the experimental unit. Comparisons of animals cured clinically on days 7 and 21, were made by non-inferiority analyses for marbofloxacin compared with enrofloxacin and the null hypothesis was rejected if the lower bound of the 95% confidence interval was greater than 0.15 (corresponding to a 15% difference in percentages of animals cured; Fisher's exact test, two-tailed). Animals removed because of SRD before day 7 were counted as not cured. Non-inferiority analyses were also used for comparisons between treatments of animals that were (i) mortalities

or removed for SRD, and (ii) relapsed with SRD from days 8 to 21 inclusive. Cochran-Mantel-Haenszel chi-squared statistics (adjusted where appropriate for farm) and confidence intervals (CI) were used to confirm similarity of treatment groups before treatment administration on day 0, and following treatment to compare differences in respiratory and depression scores between treatment groups. Reductions in rectal temperatures from day 0 to day 7 were compared by repeated measures of analysis of variance and 95% confidence limits for least squared means. Live weights, adjusted for day 0 values, were compared by analysis of variance. Percentages of animals in each treatment group with concurrent disorders, injection site reactions, adverse events (any observation in animals that was unfavourable and unintended and occurred after the use of an investigational veterinary or control product, whether or not considered to be product related) and suspected adverse drug reactions were compared using Fisher's exact test. Statistical significance of difference was obtained when $P < 0.05$ (two-tailed). Data was validated by the double data entry method. All statistical calculations were performed using SAS® 9.3 software programmes (SAS Institute Inc, Cary, North Carolina, USA).

Ethical and animal welfare approvals

The study was a clinical field trial conducted using naturally occurring cases of SRD, treated with approved veterinary prescription products and was conducted under detailed and direct veterinary supervision. The study was reviewed and approved by an ethical and animal welfare committee (Klifovet reference number: 01449-009-1). The owners of the farms in the study gave their written informed consent. The study was conducted according to European regulatory requirements and in compliance with German and Hungarian drug and animal welfare legislation, and with European Medicines Agency guidelines for demonstration of efficacy of veterinary medicinal products containing antimicrobial substances and for statistical principles in veterinary clinical trials [32, 33]. Animals were excluded or removed from the field trial if the severity of the clinical signs indicated, in the view of the attending veterinarians, that euthanasia (or withdrawal from the study) was most appropriate. Animals intended for treatment and removed from the study are reported in the results.

Results

The clinical results are shown in Table 4. The study comprised four outbreaks of APP, one from each of the four farms, and each outbreak of APP was the first that occurred on each farm beginning from November 2013. For the marbofloxacin and enrofloxacin treatments, there were 122 and 120 pigs in the intention to treat

Table 4 Clinical efficacy and safety results for marbofloxacin and enrofloxacin in the treatment of APP associated respiratory disease in fattening pigs

		Marbofloxacin				Enrofloxacin				CI of treatment difference
		Absent	Mild	Moderate	Severe	Absent	Mild	Moderate	Severe	
Respiratory scores % [n][a]	Day 0	0.0 [0]	0.0 [0]	94.2 [114]	5.8 [7]	0.0 [0]	0.0 [0]	89.8 [106]	10.2 [12]	
	Day 2	43.0 [52]	53.7 [65]	2.5 [3]	0.8 [1]	46.2 [54]	49.6 [58]	4.3 [5]	0.0 [0]	
	Day 3	68.6 [83]	28.1 [34]	3.3 [4]	0 [0]	65.8 [77]	32.5 [38]	1.7 [2]	0 [0]	
	Day 7	94.2 [113]	5.8 [7]	0.0 [0]	0.0 [0]	93.2 [109]	6.8 [8]	0.0 [0]	0.0 [0]	
	Day 21	94.7 [108]	3.5 [4]	1.8 [2]	0.0 [0]	95.7 [110]	4.3 [5]	0.0 [0]	0.0 [0]	
Depression scores % [n][a]	Day 0	0.0 [0]	89.3 [108]	9.9 [12]	0.8 [1]	0.0 [0]	90.7 [107]	9.3 [11]	0.0 [0]	
	Day 2	59.5 [72]	38.0 [46]	2.5 [3]	0.0 [0]	59.8 [70]	40.2 [47]	0.0 [0]	0.0 [0]	
	Day 3	80.2 [97]	18.2 [22]	1.7 [2]	0 [0]	80.3 [94]	19.7 [23]	0 [0]	0 [0]	
	Day 7	90.8 [109]	9.2 [11]	0.0 [0]	0.0 [0]	92.3 [108]	7.7 [9]	0.0 [0]	0.0 [0]	
	Day 21	97.4 [111]	2.6 [3]	0.0 [0]	0.0 [0]	97.4 [112]	2.6 [3]	0.0 [0]	0.0 [0]	
Rectal temperatures °C	Day 0	40.6 (0.41) [121]				40.6 (0.40) [118]				
	Day 2	39.6 (0.42) [121]				39.7 (0.36) [117]				−0.05; 0.15
	Day 3	39.6 (0.49) [121]				39.6 (0.56) [117]				−0.016; 0.11
	Day 7	39.4 (0.52) [120]				39.4 (0.51) [117]				−0.12; 0.14
	Day 21	39.4 (0.43) [114]				39.5 (0.42) [115]				0.01; 0.23
Retreatment % animals[b]	Day 2	n/a				17.8 [21]				
Clinical cure % animals[b]	Day 7	81.8 [99]				81.4 [96]				−9.37; 10.29
	Day 21	84.2 [101]				82.2 [97]				−7.54; 11.47
SRD removals & mortalities %[b]	Days 0–21	5.0 [6]				2.5 [3]				−7.22; 2.38
SRD relapses % animals[b]	Days 8–21	0.0 [0]				1.0 [1]				−0.99; 3.07
Adverse events % animals (CI)[c]		4.1 [5]				6.7 [8]				−3.1; 8.3
Injection site reactions % animals[c]		2.4 [3]				1.6 [2]				
Concurrent disorders % animals[c]		0.0[d] [0]				7.5[e] [9]				
Live weight gain kg	Days 0–21	19.81 (5.06) [114]				20.05 (7.03) [115]				−0.026; 0.109
No. animals: Intention to treat[c]	Day 0	122				120				
No. animals: Per protocol[b]	Day 7	121				118				

Results are for the overall study which included 4 farms and are shown as mean (standard deviation) unless indicated otherwise; *CI* confidence interval

[a]Refer to Clinical examinations for detailed description of individual scores. [n] number of animals

[b]Indicated efficacy data percentages are based on per protocol populations. Note that percentages for respiratory and depression scores, and rectal temperatures are based on numbers of animals in a treatment group on a given day, [n]

[c]Indicated safety data percentages are based on intention to treat populations. There were no suspected adverse drug reactions

[d,e]values in a row are significantly different. *n/a* Not applicable

Animals euthanised prior to study for diagnostic purposes are excluded from each of the populations

populations, and 121 and 118 pigs in the per protocol populations, respectively. Three animals were removed from the study prior to treatment administration on day 0 for reasons not related to SRD (one pig allocated to each of the treatment groups died during blood sampling and one pig allocated to the enrofloxacin group was euthanised for welfare reasons and at necropsy had extensive pulmonary haemorrhages). Of 36 pigs (up to 10 pigs per farm) examined by necropsy prior to treatment administration, 30 had both gross lesions of pleuropneumonia and moderate to heavy growth of APP on culture (pure cultures on NAD supplemented blood agar, confirmed by PCR; serotypes 2 (farms HB, GA,

GB) and 7 (HA)). Six of the 36 animals did not have typical lesions and samples were not collected for bacteriology from these animals.

The outbreaks of APP were acute and 100% of enrolled pigs on day 0 showed moderate to severe respiratory clinical signs and, moderate signs of depression in each of the treatment groups ($P > 0.05$; one animal on day 0 was unintentionally included with severe depression). On day 0, all enrolled animals were pyrexic with mean rectal temperatures of 40.6 °C in both treatment groups ($P > 0.05$). Following antimicrobial treatment on day 0, there were rapid clinical responses in both treatment groups ($P > 0.05$) and by day 2 there were marked reductions in the prevalence and severity of pigs with moderate or severe respiratory signs and/or depression, and mean rectal temperatures were reduced to 39.6 and 39.7 °C for the marbofloxain and enrofloxacin groups, respectively ($P > 0.05$). However, on day 2, 21 animals (17.8%) in the enrofloxacin group distributed across three of the farms (HA, HB and GA) were assessed by the blinded examining veterinarians to still have clinical signs that had not improved (i.e. signs were the same or of greater severity than on day 0) and therefore, following the recommendations of the previous Summary of Product Characteristics, a second administration of enrofloxacin was given to these animals. (Note that the dosage regimen for enrofloxacin in the treatment of SRD is now for a single dose of 7.5 mg/kg only) [13]. In the marbofloxacin group on day 2, one animal (0.8%) showed severe respiratory signs but it did not have signs of depression and was allowed to continue in the study (without additional treatment) by the blinded examining veterinarian. Overall in each of the treatment groups, animals continued to improve compared with day 0 and by one week after treatment, the percentages of animals with either no respiratory signs and/or no depression were >90% and mean rectal temperatures were normal ($P > 0.05$).

Efficacy as indicated by clinical cure on day 7 was apparent in 99 (81.8%) and 96 (81.4%) of animals in the per protocol marbofloxacin and enrofloxacin groups, respectively. Results for both treatment groups were consistent and similar between the per protocol and intention to treat analyses. The difference in percentages of animals cured on day 7 for marbofloxacin – enrofloxacin were +0.4% for the per protocol population and +1.8% for the intention to treat population. Non-inferiority of marbofloxacin compared with enrofloxacin was shown, and the mean cure rates on day 7 were similar ($P > 0.05$). Inferiority, the null hypothesis, would have been rejected if the lower bound of the 95% confidence interval of the difference in the percentage of animals cured on day 7 was greater than –15%. At the end of the study, day 21, the clinical cure for marbofloxacin was 84.2% and non-inferior to that for enrofloxacin, 82.2% ($P > 0.05$). From day 0 to day 7, and from day 8 to day 21 the SRD removals and mortalities, and relapses of animals in each treatment were similar and non-inferior for marbofloxacin compared with enrofloxacin ($P > 0.05$).

Serological assays on the blood samples collected on days 0 and 21 from samples of pigs in the per protocol populations on farms GA and HA found no evidence of seroconversion to PRRSV, PCV2 or swine influenza viruses. This suggests that there were no clinical disease outbreaks of these viral infections in the three-week study period on farms GA and HA.

Adverse events in the present study occurred similarly in the marbofloxacin and enrofloxacin groups (4.1 and 6.7%, respectively; $P > 0.05$) and were considered by the each of the investigators as unlikely to have been related to the antimicrobial treatments (i.e. there were no suspected adverse drug reactions attributed to either marbofloxacin or enrofloxacin). Adverse events included inflammation of the pinna associated with ear tagging, death associated with blood sampling, diarrhoea and lameness. Injection site reactions of limited swelling and, or pain of short duration (<3 days) occurred in 2.46 and 1.67% of the marbofloxacin and enrofloxacin groups, respectively ($P > 0.05$). Concurrent disorders (lameness, diarrhoea, swollen leg, abscess, hernia, tail bite and haematoma) beginning after enrolment on day 0 were observed in 9 or 7.5% of animals in the enrofloxacin group (3, 1, 5 and 0 animals for farms GA, GB, HA and HB, respectively) significantly more than 0% in the marbofloxacin group ($P < 0.01$). In the marbofloxacin and enrofloxacin groups, the mean live weights on day 0, 56.3 and 55.5 kg, respectively, and the mean live weight gains from day 0 to day 21, 19.81 and 20.05 kg, respectively, were similar ($P > 0.05$).

The MIC and susceptibility results for isolates obtained from the four farms in the study are shown in Tables 3 and 5. Determination of MICs for marbofloxacin and enrofloxacin were successfully made on a total of 361 and 352 isolates, respectively. The majority of the isolates were from day 0 (pre-treatment) and day 7, and comprised 66 APP, 50 PM, 20 H. parasuis and 230 B. bronchiseptica isolates. Sixty-four APP isolates, eight PM, two H. parasuis and 22 B. bronchiseptica isolates were from lung and BAL samples; the remaining isolates were from nasal swabs. Sixty-one isolates of APP were obtained on day 0, and, following treatment, no APP were isolated on day 7 by BAL; five APP isolates were obtained from lungs at necropsy of animals removed from the study on days 1 and 15. The MIC90 values for the 66 APP isolates were 0.06 µg/mL for marbofloxacin and enrofloxacin. Clinical susceptibility breakpoints for APP and PM have been published by CLSI for enrofloxacin [29] and by CASFM (Comité de l'antibiogramme de la société Française de Microbiologie) for marbofloxacin [30]. All of the APP isolates were susceptible to both marbofloxacin and enrofloxacin (clinical breakpoint ≤0.25 µg/mL; resistance ≥1 µg/mL for enrofloxacin and 1 and 2 µg/mL respectively for marbofloxacin). Thirty-two isolates of PM were obtained on day 0 and the MIC90 values were 0.03 and 0.015 µg/mL for marbofloxacin and enrofloxacin, respectively. As for APP, all of the PM isolates were also susceptible to both antimicrobials (clinical breakpoint ≤0.25 µg/mL; resistance ≥1 µg/mL for enrofloxacin and 1 and 2 µg/mL respectively for marbofloxacin). On day 7, 18 PM isolates were obtained, each with similar or lower MICs to those on day 0. Comparable data for breakpoints of H. parasuis, and B. bronchiseptica have not been published.

Table 5 Bacterial pathogens isolated on days 0 and 7 from lower respiratory tract lesions, bronchoalveolar lavage and nasal swabs, minimum inhibitory concentrations (MIC) and susceptibilities to marbofloxacin and enrofloxacin

		Marbofloxacin					Enrofloxacin				
		MIC range	MIC_{50}	MIC_{90}	S%	n	MIC range	MIC_{50}	MIC_{90}	S%	n
A. pleuropneumoniae	Day 0	0.03–0.12	0.06	0.06	100	61	0.015–0.12	0.06	0.06	100	61
	Day 7	nc	nc	nc	nc	0	nc	nc	nc	nc	0
H. parasuis	Day 0	0.25–2.0	0.015	0.06	n/a	18	0.004–1.0	0.015	0.03	n/a	13
	Day 7	0.015	nc	nc	n/a	2	0.008	nc	nc	n/a	2
P. multocida	Day 0	0.008–0.03	0.015	0.03	100	32	0.004–0.015	0.008	0.015	100	32
	Day 7	0.008–0.03	0.015	0.03	100	18	0.008–0.015	0.008	0.008	100	18
B. bronchiseptica	Day 0	0.25–1.0	0.5	0.5	n/a	92	0.25–0.5	0.5	0.5	n/a	92
	Day 7	0.25–0.5	0.5	0.5	n/a	138	0.25–1.0	0.5	0.5	n/a	134

MIC_{50}, MIC_{90}, lowest concentrations (μg/mL) of the antimicrobial for which 50 and 90% of the isolates were inhibited, respectively; n, total number of isolates from lung/lower respiratory tract, bronchoalveolar lavage and nasal swabs, combined, for which MIC was determined; n/a susceptibility data not available; nc, not calculated for <10 isolates; S, percentage of isolates within a species that were susceptible to the antimicrobial based on European susceptibility monitoring and where available CLSI breakpoints [28, 29, 38]

Discussion

In the present study, the clinical efficacies of marbofloxacin and enrofloxacin were similar and were characterised by rapid reductions in clinical signs and pyrexia as indicated by marked reductions in individual clinical signs two days after treatment and, by day 7, clinical signs were absent or mild in all pigs and mean temperatures for each treatment group were <39.5 °C. However, reductions in rectal temperatures (which may occur in the absence of resolution of clinical signs) were not considered alone and were interpreted in conjunction with clinical signs when determining clinical cure. The analysis of the primary efficacy criterion, percentage of animals with clinical cure at day 7, confirmed the efficacy of the antimicrobials in the treatment of SRD and actinobacillosis and the non-inferiority of marbofloxacin compared with the reference antimicrobial, enrofloxacin. Clinical cures for each antimicrobial on days 7 and 21 were similar, (81-84%) and the percentages of animals (3.5–5.0%) that either relapsed after day 7 or where removed at any time from the study for SRD reasons were also similar.

Comparison of these efficacy results with those of previous studies should be made circumspectly because of likely differences in, for example, aetiology, animals, environment, antimicrobial sensitivity of the pathogens, clinical severity at time of treatment and efficacy criteria. This makes it difficult to reach conclusions regarding the relative efficacy of different antimicrobial classes in the treatment of APP and SRD. The results of this study suggest when there is no non-critical alternative antimicrobial available and relevant epidemiological and sensitivity results are supportive, that use of one of the injectable fluroquinolones, marbofloxacin or enrofloxacin may be anticipated to provide efficacy in pigs with acute clinical APP. The efficacy results in the present multicentre study for the treatment of SRD associated predominantly with APP were comparable to the results obtained in other field studies. For example, in an outbreak of SRD and actinobacillosis treated with amoxicillin (7 mg/kg/day) or marbofloxacin (2 mg/kg/day) each administered daily for 3–5 days the clinical cures on day 5 were 68 and 74.5%, and relapses to day 21 of 11.9 and 17.2%, respectively [34]. In that study, each of the dosage regimes facilitated time-dependent bacterial killing which, it is now known is appropriate for amoxicillin but is less effective when used for fluroquinolones that are more effective when given in higher doses to facilitate concentration-dependent bacterial killing [6, 7]. In this field study, dosage regimens appropriate for concentration-dependent bacterial killing were administered. For both marbofloxacin and enrofloxacin, efficacy was assessed based on clinical efficacy rather than on post-treatment bacteriology. In two, single-centre, studies conducted in USA on SRD in pigs with mixed infections of APP, PM, H. parasuis and Streptococcus suis, the efficacy 4 days after treatment with a single dose of enrofloxacin 7.5 mg/kg was 33.0 and 89.7%; however, details of mortalities and subsequent relapses were not given [35]. In another report of six field studies conducted to a common protocol in five geographically separate centres in USA and Canada, the overall efficacies for treatment of SRD by tulathromycin and ceftiofur were 70.6 and 64.4%, respectively, and the efficacies for treatment of SRD predominantly associated with APP were, in Iowa, 68.2 and 79.5%, respectively, and in Nebraska, 81.3 and 77.1%, respectively [18]. In another multicentre, field study of outbreaks of SRD conducted on farms in Germany, France, UK and Netherlands, in which the efficacy criterion was animals successfully completing the study 10 days after treatment, efficacy was 82% in tulathromycin-treated pigs and 68.4% in pigs treated with either tiamulin or florfenicol [36].

In this study, necropsies of clinically affected pigs were conducted immediately prior to beginning treatment on each affected farm and showed gross pathologic lesions of diffuse fibrinous pneumonia, typical of acute actinobacillosis. The principal and numerically predominant pathogen isolated from lung tissues at necropsy was APP as confirmed by PCR. Based on the bacteriology of the lung and BAL samples, it is possible that some of the individual cases of actinobacillosis were complicated by secondary, concurrent infections of PM, *H. parasuis* and/or *B. bronchiseptica*. In pigs, successful isolation of pathogens associated with active pneumonia from BAL and nasal samples varies between bacterial species and, particularly for APP the frequency of isolation tends to be low [20, 37]. In the present study, distribution of APP isolates at inclusion indicated that lung sampling at necropsy was the most accurate technique to isolate this pathogen compared with BAL and nasal swab (Fig. 1). There were large differences in APP isolation frequency between the sampling methods suggesting that sampling of the upper airways in pigs may not allow the correct identification of the causal pathogen(s) of lower respiratory tract bacterial infections and thus potentially misleading the choice of antimicrobial for treatment.

The MIC_{90} values for APP isolated from the necropsy and BAL samples was 0.06 μg/mL for each of the antimicrobials and were similar to those reported in an European antimicrobial susceptibility monitoring survey of isolates collected from untreated clinical cases in 2002–2006 [38]. This and other reports [39, 40] suggest that there had been little or no change in susceptibility of APP European field isolates to marbofloxacin and enrofloxacin between 1994 and 2009. Comparison of the MIC values of marbofloxacin and enrofloxacin

determined in the present study with the values in the European survey for APP and PM indicated that all of the isolates of these species would have been susceptible to both of the antimicrobials. In vitro, APP is typically susceptible to a wide range of antimicrobials including fluoroquinolones although there is increasing resistance to penicillins, tetracylines and trimethoprim-sulphonamides [2, 38–40] and normally these or other non-critical antimicrobials should be used in preference to fluoroquinolones and consistent with antimicrobial usage policies and product labels [14, 15].

The variability in PK parameters between animals and the variability in PD parameters (e.g. MIC) within populations of microorganism may influence efficacy and the potential for resistance development in the target pathogen. Simulations of this variability in PK-PD have been used to evaluate marbofloxacin in the treatment of APP infections in nursery and fattening pigs, and showed that a single dose of 8 mg/kg would provide robust efficacy and minimise resistance development in APP with MICs of 0.03–0.12 μg/mL [9, 10] which are comparable to the APP MIC range reported here.

Limitations of this multicentre clinical trial include the following. The number of individual farms, four was small and may not represent a wider diversity of naturally occurring SRD outbreaks with differences in pathogens, environment, husbandry, pig genotypes and timing of treatment interventions. The individual farm outbreaks of disease were not on their own large enough to enable evaluation of farm (or outbreak) by treatment interactions. The primary efficacy variable (cure on day 7) was based on discontinuous and subjective clinical scores whereas preferably it would use a larger number of independent, continuous and objective variables.

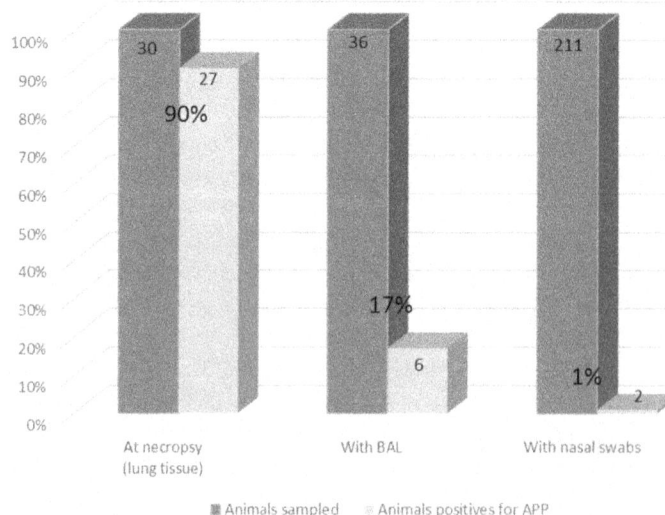

Fig. 1 Percentage of APP isolation from different sampling sites at inclusion to the study

Pyrexia as measured by rectal temperatures is an objective and continuous variable however on its own it may be misleading as pyrexia may resolve without cure necessarily having occurred. This study used a positive control whereas scientifically a negative control study may be preferred however, this would be expected to raise ethical and animal welfare concerns. The efficacy cure rates observed in this and other published studies may not be replicated exactly under different clinical conditions.

Conclusions

Marbofloxacin treatment as a single IM dose of 8 mg/kg was clinically safe and clinically effective in the treatment of respiratory disease associated predominantly with APP in four European commercial, fattening pig herds. Enrofloxacin given either as 1 or 2 doses of 7.5 mg/kg was also safe and effective.

Abbreviations
APP: *Actinobacillus pleuropneumoniae*; BAL: Bronchoalveolar lavage; CLSI: Clinical and Laboratory Standards Institute; CP: Control product; IVP: Investigational veterinary product; MIC_{50}: MIC_{90}, lowest concentrations (µg/mL) of the antimicrobial for which 50 and 90% of the isolates were inhibited, respectively; MPC: Mutant prevention concentration; PD: Pharmacodynamics; PK: Pharmacokinetics; PM: *Pasteurella multocida*; SRD: Swine respiratory disease

Acknowledgements
The pig farmers, their staff and veterinarians are gratefully acknowledged for their support throughout the study. Statistical analyses by P. Klein, dsh statistical services, Pfaffenhofen, Germany; Microbiology by J. Verspohl and M. Homuth, University of Hannover, Germany and F. El Garch, Vetoquinol SA, France.

Funding
This study was financially supported by Vetoquinol SA as part of the work required for approval by the Agencies of European countries for marketing authorisation of Forcyl® for use in swine.

Authors' contributions
All authors contributed to the design of the study and interpretation of results. DC and MH managed and monitored the study. All authors read and approved the final manuscript.

Authors' information
K. Hellmann is managing director, Klivovet AG.

Competing interests
The authors declare that they have no competing interests.

Author details
[1]Vetoquinol SA, Research and Development Centre, B.P. 189, 70204 Lure Cedex, France. [2]Klifovet AG, Geyerspergerstr 27, D-80689 Munich, Germany. [3]Rowdix Ltd, Folly Hall, Cawton, York YO62 4LW, UK.

References
1. Done S, White M. Porcine respiratory disease and complexes: the story to date. In Pract. 2003;25:410–4.
2. Gottschalk M. Actinobacillosis. In: Zimmermann JF, Karriker LA, Ramirez A, Schwartz KJ, Stevenson GW, editors. Diseases of Swine. 10th ed. Ames: Wiley-Blackwell, John Wiley Inc; 2012. p. 653–69.
3. Rycroft AN, Garside LH. Actinobacillus species and their role in animal disease. Vet J. 2000;159:18–36.
4. Kahn CM, Line S, editors. The Merck Veterinary Manual. 10th ed. Whitehouse Station: Merck & Co Inc; 2010. p. 1351–7.
5. Friendship RM. Antimicrobial drug use in swine. In: Giguere S, Prescott JF, Baggot JD, Walker RD, Dowling PM, editors. Antimicrobial Therapy in Veterinary Medicine. 4th ed. Iowa: Blackwell Publishing; 2006. p. 535–43.
6. Ahmad I, Huang L, Hao H, Sanders P, Yuan Z. Application of PK/PD modelling in veterinary field: dose optimisation and drug resistance prediction. Biomed Res Int. 2016. doi:10.1155/2016/5465678.
7. Walker RD, Dowling PM. Fluoroquinolones. In: Giguere S, Prescott JF, Baggot JD, Walker RD, Dowling PM, editors. Antimicrobial Therapy in Veterinary Medicine. 4th ed. Iowa: Blackwell Publishing; 2006. p. 263–84.
8. Martinez M, Silley P. Antimicrobial drug resistance. In: Cunningham F, Elliot J, Lees P, editors. Comparative and Veterinary Pharmacology. Handbook for Experimental Pharmacology 199. Berlin: Springer-Verlag; 2010. p. 227–64.
9. Zumbusch HJ, Perrin PA. Employment of the PK/PD analysis to marbofloxacin in order to predict clinical/bacteriological outcomes and for the determination of the daily exposure of treated animals. Tierarztl Umsch. 2014;69:511–21.
10. Vilalta C, Giboin H, Schneider M, El Garch F, Fraile L. Pharmacokinetic/pharmacodynamic evaluation of marbofloxacin in the treatment of Haemophilus parasuis and Actinobacillus pleuropneumoniae infections in nursery and fattener pigs using Monte Carlo simulations. J Vet Pharmacol Ther. 2014;37:542–9.
11. Schneider M, Paulin A, Dron F, Woehrlé F. Pharmacokinetics of marbofloxacin in pigs after intravenous and intramuscular administration of a single dose of 8 mg/kg: dose proportionality, influence of the age of the animals and urinary elimination. J Vet Pharmacol Ther. 2014;37:523–30.
12. Schneider M, Galland D, Giboin H, Woehrlé F. Pharmacokinetic/pharmacodynamic testing of marbofloxacin administered as a single injection for the treatment of porcine respiratory disease. Noordwijkerhout: EAVPT congress; 2012. p. 192.
13. Summary of Product Characteristics: Baytril 1nject 100 mg/ml Injektionslösung für Rinder und Schweine. Heads of Medicines Agencies, Europe. http://mri.medagencies.org/download/AT_V_0007_002_FinalSPC.pdf.
14. EMA. EMA/CVMP. CVMP strategy on antimicrobials 2011–2015 (EMA/CVMP/287420/2010). London: European Medicines Agency; 2010.
15. European Union. Guidelines for the prudent use of antimicrobials in veterinary medicine (Commission Notice 2015/C 299/04; 3.2). Off J Eur Union. 2015;58.
16. Hoeltig D, Rohde J, Brunner B, Hellmann K, Grandemange R, Waldmann KH. Efficacy of one-shot marbofloxacin treatment on development of porcine pleuropneumonia. Proc 24th International Pig Veterinary Society, Dublin, Ireland; 2016. p. 180.
17. Grandemange E, Perrin P-A, Cvejic D, Haas D, Hellmann K. Field evaluation of the efficacy and safety of Forcyl® in the treatment of swine respiratory disease in naturally infected pigs. Proc. 7th European Symposium on Porcine Health Medicine, Nantes, France; 2015. p. 153.
18. Nutsch RG, Hart FJ, Rooney KA, Weigel DJ, Kilgore WR, Skogerboe TL. Efficacy of tulathromycin injectable solution for the treatment of naturally occurring swine respiratory disease. Vet Ther. 2005;6:214–24.
19. Veterinary International Cooperation on Harmonisation of Technical Requirements for Registration. Good Clinical Practice, VICH GL9 (GCP) June

2000. http://vichsec.org/guidelines/pharmaceuticals/pharma-efficacy/good-clinical-practice.html.

20. Moorkamp L, Nathues H, Spergser J, Tegeler R, Beilage EG. Detection of respiratory pathogens in porcine lung tissue and lavage fluid. Vet J. 2008;175:273–5.

21. Boudewijn C, Baele M, Opsomer G, de Kruif A, Decostere A, Haesebrouck F. tRNA-intergenic spacer PCR for the identification of Pasteurella and Mannheimia spp. Vet Microbiol. 2004;98:251–60.

22. Christensen H, Angen Ø, Elmerdahl Olsen J, Bisgaard M. Revised description and classification of atypical isolates of Pasteurella multocida from bovine lungs based on genotypic characterization to include variants previously classified as biovar 2 of Pasteurella canis and Pasteurella avium. Microbiology. 2004;150:1757–67.

23. Sachse K, Frey J. PCR detection of microbial pathogens, detection, identification, and subtyping of actinobacillus pleuropneumoniae. In: Methods in molecular biology. 2003. p. 87 ff.

24. Dongyou L, Lawrencea ML, Austin FW. Specific PCR identification of Pasteurella multocida based on putative transcriptional regulator genes. J Microbiol Methods. 2004;58:263–7.

25. Oliveira S, Galina L, Pijoan C. Development of a PCR test to diagnose Haemophilus parasuis infections. J Vet Diagn Invest. 2001;13:495–501.

26. Sneath PHA, Stevens M. Actinobacillus rossii sp. nov., Actinobacillus seminis Spa nov., noma rev., Pastewella bettii sp. nov., Pasteurella lymphangitidis sp. nova, Pastewella mairi sp. nova, and Pasteurella tvehalosi Spa nova. Int J Syst Bacteriol. 1990;40:148–53.

27. Bisping W, Amtsberg G. Farbatlas zur Diagnose bakterieller Infektionserreger der Tiere. Berlin: Paul Parey Verlag; 1988. p. 154.

28. Clinical and Laboratory Standards Institute (CLSI). Performance Standards for Antimicrobial disk and dilution susceptibility test for bacteria isolated from animals; Approved standard. 4th ed. Wayne: CLSI; 2013.

29. Clinical and Laboratory Standards Institute (CLSI). Performance Standards for Antimicrobial disk and dilution susceptibility test for bacteria isolated from animals; second information supplement. Wayne: CLSI; 2013.

30. Comité de l'antibiogramme de la société Française de Microbiologie (CA-SFM). Antibiogramme vétérinaire du CA-SFM, Recommandations 2013. Paris: SFM.

31. Schwarz S, Silley P, Simjee S, Woodford N, van Duijkeren E, Johnson AP, Gaastra W. Editorial: assessing the antimicrobial susceptibility of bacteria obtained from animals. J Antimicrob Chemother. 2010;65:601–4.

32. EMA. EMEA/CVMP. Guideline for demonstration of efficacy for veterinary medicinal use containing antimicrobials substances (EMEA/CVMP/627/01-Final). London: The European Agency for the evaluation of Medicinal Products; 2001. http://www.ema.europa.eu/docs/en_GB/document_library/Scientific_guideline/2009/10/WC500004492.pdf.

33. EMA. EMEA/CVMP. Guideline on statistical principles for veterinary clinical trials (EMEA/CVMP/81976/2010). London: The European Agency for the evaluation of Medicinal Products; 2012. http://www.ema.europa.eu/docs/en_GB/document_library/Scientific_guideline/2012/01/WC500120834.pdf .

34. Thomas E, Grandemange E, Pommier P, Wessel-Robert S, Davot JL. Field evaluation of efficacy and tolerance of a 2% marbofloxacin injectable solution for the treatment of respiratory disease in fattening pigs. Vet Q. 2000;22:131–5.

35. US Food and Drug Administration. Freedom of Information Summary Baytril 100 Enrofloxacin Injectable Solution Swine. NADA 141–068 March 14, 2008. http://www.fda.gov/downloads/AnimalVeterinary/Products/ApprovedAnimalDrugProducts/FOIADrugSummaries/ucm116772.pdf. Accessed 31 Mar 2016.

36. Nanjiana IA, McKelvie J, Benchaoui HA, Godinho KS, Sherington J, Sunderland SJ, Weatherely AJ, Rowan TG. Evaluation of therapeutic activity of tulathromycin against swine respiratory disease on farms in Europe. Vet Ther. 2005;6:203–13.

37. Palzer A, Ritzmann M, Wolf G, Heinritzi K. Associations between pathogens in healthy pigs and pigs with pneumonia. Vet Rec. 2008;162:267–71.

38. De Jong A, Thomas V, Simjee S, Moyaert H, El Garch F, Maher K, Morrisey I, Butty P, Klein U, Marion H, Rigaut D, Valle M. Antimicrobial susceptibility monitoring of respiratory tract pathogens isolated from diseased cattle and pigs across Europe: The Vetpath Study. Vet Microbiol. 2014;172:202–15.

39. Vanni M, Merenda M, Barigazzi G, Garbarino C, Luppi A, Tognetti R, Intorre L. Antimicrobial resistance of Actinobacillus pleuropneumoniae isolated from swine. Vet Microbiol. 2012;156:172–7.

40. Giboin H, Kroemer S, Galland D, El Garch F, Woerhle F. Long term European epidemiologic survey of sensitivity to antimicrobials of bacteria isolated from reproductive, respiratory or digestive diseases in pigs (1998–2009). Proc 4th European Symposium on Porcine Health Medicine, Bruges, Belgium; 2012. p. 132 (P041).

16

Evaluation of the relationship between the biosecurity status, production parameters, herd characteristics and antimicrobial usage in farrow-to-finish pig production in four EU countries

Merel Postma[1*], Annette Backhans[2,3], Lucie Collineau[4,5], Svenja Loesken[6], Marie Sjölund[2,3], Catherine Belloc[5], Ulf Emanuelson[3], Elisabeth grosse Beilage[6], Elisabeth Okholm Nielsen[7], Katharina D. C. Stärk[4], Jeroen Dewulf[1] and on behalf of the MINAPIG consortium

Abstract

Background: High antimicrobial usage and the threat of antimicrobial resistance highlighted the need for reduced antimicrobial usage in pig production. Prevention of disease however, is necessary to obtain a reduced need for antimicrobial treatment. This study aimed at assessing possible associations between the biosecurity level, antimicrobial usage and farm and production characteristics in order to advice on best practices for a low antimicrobial usage and maximum animal health and production.

A cross-sectional study was conducted in 227 farrow-to-finish pig herds in Belgium, France, Germany and Sweden between December 2012 and December 2013. Associations between biosecurity status, antimicrobial usage, and production parameters were evaluated with multivariable general linear models, according to an assumed causal pathway.

Results: The results showed that higher antimicrobial usage in sows tended to be associated with higher antimicrobial usage from birth until slaughter ($p = 0.06$). The antimicrobial usage from birth until slaughter was positively associated with the number of pathogens vaccinated against ($p < 0.01$). A shorter farrowing rhythm ($p < 0.01$) and a younger weaning age ($p = 0.06$) tended to be also associated with a higher antimicrobial usage from birth until slaughter whereas a better external biosecurity ($p < 0.01$) was related with a lower antimicrobial usage from birth until slaughter.

Conclusion: Management practices such as weaning age and biosecurity measures may be important factors indirectly impacting on antimicrobial usage. We therefore promote a holistic approach when assessing the potential to reduce the need for antimicrobial treatments.

Keywords: Antimicrobial usage, Biosecurity, Production parameters, Pig production, Causal path

* Correspondence: merel.postma@ugent.be
[1]Veterinary Epidemiology Unit, Department of Reproduction, Obstetrics and Herd Health, Faculty of Veterinary Medicine, Ghent University, Salisburylaan 133, 9820 Merelbeke, Belgium
Full list of author information is available at the end of the article

Background

In many countries of the European Union (EU) pig production is amongst one of the highest using sectors of antimicrobial (AM) agents in animal production as reported in detail for some EU countries [1–3]. After the discovery of penicillin by Fleming in 1928 and its subsequent usage around world war II antimicrobials became very important in the curing of bacterial infections in both humans and animals. Unfortunately however, bacteria are capable of developing resistance mechanisms against the antimicrobials used, either by genetic mutations or by taking up resistance genes from other bacteria [4]. This resistance selection is mainly triggered by the use of antimicrobials (Callens B.F., Boyen F., Berge A.C., Chantziaras. I., Haesebrouck F., Dewulf J., Epidemiology of acquired antimicrobial resistance in bacteria from food-producing animals, submitted). EU countries with a high antimicrobial usage (AMU) rank also high in their resistance levels [5]. Therefore, reduced and prudent antimicrobial usage in animals became of high interest in recent years, mainly due to the public health threat of antimicrobial resistance (AMR) development and possible transmission from the animal to the human population [6-9]. The first efforts in some EU countries show that a reduced usage of antimicrobials results in reduction of resistance levels as well [3, 10], which is the main focus of the international fight against antimicrobial resistance in animal production [11].

To be able to reduce antimicrobial usage, it is important to ensure healthier animals and therefore reduce the necessity for antimicrobial treatment. Some authors have suggested a broad range of possible alternatives [12–14], for example the increased use of vaccines to make animals less sensitive to infections [15–18] or an improved management and increased biosecurity level [19, 20]. However, several of these suggested alternatives are based upon clinical observations or rational deduction rather than quantitative observations making them prone to critics due to insufficient scientific bases of their efficacy for the replacement of antimicrobials.

Therefore, a good insight in the associations between preventive measures, management factors, production parameters, biosecurity status and antimicrobial usage is of critical importance to better understand the value of the different alternatives and to help herd advisors and farmers in the optimization of their farm management. Knowing whether such associations exist provides researchers, farmers, herd advisors (e.g. veterinarian, feed advisor, climate specialist) and policy makers with potential tools to improve herd production combined with reduced necessity of antimicrobial products.

This study aimed at studying and visualizing associations between management characteristics, production parameters, biosecurity status and antimicrobial usage data from four EU countries. The results of this study will be used by the MINAPIG consortium to study the implementation of high biosecurity, vaccines and herd health management measures as potential drivers for reduced antimicrobial usage in pig production.

Methods
Herd selection

This study was performed in four EU countries with a medium to highly intensive pig production [21]; Belgium, France, Germany and Sweden. Per country the aim was to include 60 farrow-to-finish herds with ≥ 100 sows and ≥ 500 finishers. For Belgium an email list of pig farmers who subscribed to a newsletter issued by the faculty of veterinary medicine of Ghent University was used to select the herds based on willingness to participate. Only the Dutch speaking part of Belgium, Flanders, which represents 90 % of pig production in Belgium [22], was included in the study due to logistic reasons. Herds in the north-western part of France, representing 75 % of the country's pig production, were randomly selected from a database of the Institute for pig and pork industry. In Germany the herds were selected from consultancy circles and with veterinarians' input in the three regions with the largest pig production, Niedersachsen, Nordrhein-Westfalen and Mecklenburg-Vorpommern (64 % of total German production) [23]. A request for participation by their herd veterinarian or a consortium partner was used to reach the 60 participating pig farmers in Sweden.

Finally in Belgium 52 herds participated in this retrospective study and in the other three countries there were 60 participants. For five Belgian herds the information on the antimicrobial usage was not complete, resulting in a total of 47 herds used in the analyses for Belgium and a total of 227 herds in the study. Our criterion of including herds with ≥100 sows had to be lowered to ≥70 sows to reach the maximum of participating herds. Three Belgian herds, six French herds and one Swedish herd had a number of sows between 70 and 100.

Herd visit

A strict protocol was used to visit and interview the participating herds, guaranteeing a similar collection and entry of data over the countries. Interviewers received a training to standardize the method for data collection. Furthermore, the participating herds were visited by one veterinarian/researcher in Belgium, one in France and one in Germany and by two veterinarians/researchers or a veterinarian from the Swedish Animal Health Service ($n = 15$) in Sweden. Agreement between the project partners on the completeness and accuracy of the herd visit protocol was reached by consultation, discussion and consensus.

Herds were visited once on a convenient day in the period between December 2012 and December 2013. A farm inspection in combination with the completion of the questionnaire was performed by the interviewer during the herd visit. The collected herd management and technical parameter information corresponded to the year preceding the herd visit.

Data collection

Technical parameters (e.g. number of weaned piglets per sow per year (WSY)) and herd management characteristics (e.g. farrowing rhythm) were collected, together with information on the biosecurity status of the herd using the risk-based scoring system Biocheck.UGent™ (www.Biocheck.UGent.be). The technical parameters were collected from the herd management system if available or by interviewing the farmer.

The farrowing rhythm refers to the interval, expressed in weeks, between the birth of two batches of piglets. In this study this ranged between a 1-week system and a 5-week system for Belgium, France and Germany, while in Sweden systems with a farrowing rhythm of over 5-weeks were also used. The latter were coded for analysis as >5-week systems. The number of weaned piglets per sow per year was calculated as the number of litters per year times the number of live-born piglets per sow minus the mortality until weaning. The weaning age was expressed as the average duration, in days, from the birth of a piglet until it was weaned. The number of pathogens vaccinated against was created by summing up all vaccinations used in a herd, either for sows, boars, gilts or piglets on the date of the herd visit, except the vaccine used for immune-castration of male animals. For combination vaccines every single pathogen they have activity against was accounted for separately. Anti-inflammatory, anti-coccidial and zinc-oxide usage was expressed as being applied yes or no. A more detailed description of the other variables mentioned in Table 1, such as the gender and education level, can be found in [19]. The questionnaire can be obtained upon request from the first author.

Biosecurity quantification

The biosecurity status of the participating farms was quantified by using the risk-based tool Biocheck.UGent™ [24]. This assessment tool makes comparison of the biosecurity status of herds within and between countries possible by returning 109, mainly dichotomous and trichotomous, questions into a score from 0 to 100 for both external and internal biosecurity, where zero means absolute lack of any biosecurity measures and 100 means declaration of full application of all assessed biosecurity measures. The Biocheck.UGent™ consists of 6 subcategories for internal biosecurity (1. disease management, 2. farrowing and suckling period, 3. nursing unit, 4. fattening unit, 5. measures between compartments, 6.

working lines) and 6 for external biosecurity (1. purchase of breeding pigs, 2. purchase of piglets, 3. artificial insemination, 4. transport of animals, 5. feed and water supply, 6. removal of manure and dead animals). The Biocheck.UGent™ system is described in more detail in Laanen et al. [20, 25], Backhans et al. [26] and Postma et al. [19] in which it has shown to be a comprehensive, repeatable scoring system with a predictive and discriminating validity.

Antimicrobial usage quantification

Information on the antimicrobial usage for the preceding year in Belgium, Germany and Sweden, and the last batch in France, was collected at in point in time. Invoices from the veterinarian and feed company combined with information from the farmer were used in Belgium. In France this information came from the journal of treatment of and interview with the farmer. While in Germany the delivery and treatment forms from the prescribing veterinarian were used. In Sweden paper copies derived from treatment records, which are mandatory and inspected by the county administration board, were used.

From the collected information the product name including details such as formulation and concentration, amount purchased/used and the animal category in which it was used were registered. If the animal category in which the product was used was not explicitly mentioned on the invoice, the farmer was asked to provide more information.

Herd level antimicrobial usage data were used to calculate the "treatment incidence" (TI) per herd and age category by the formula described below and as described and used before in several publications [1, 20, 27, 28].

$$TI = \frac{\text{Total amount of activesubstance administered (mg)}}{DDDA\left(\frac{mg}{kg}\right) * \text{number of days at risk} * \text{kg animal at risk}} * 1000 \text{ pigs at risk}$$

The TI is a technical unit of measurement that quantifies how many animals out of a theoretical group of 1000 animals received daily an AM treatment. Or, if one animal would live for a theoretical period of 1000 days, how many of these days it would have been treated with an antimicrobial. Divided by 10 this gives the percentage of the lifespan an average animal on this herd was treated with a daily dose of antimicrobials. Combined TI's were calculated for sows, gilts and boars (TI Breeding) and over a standardized period at risk of 200 days for the lifespan of a pig from birth until slaughter (TI 200). The 200 days, as the standard duration between birth and slaughter, was agreed upon based on consensus between the project partners from the participating countries. This TI 200 days makes it easier to

Table 1 Results of univariable and multivariable general linear regression models

Outcome variable	Risk factor	N	Country corrected univariable			Country corrected multivariable	
			β-coefficient	p-value	Adjusted R²	β-coefficient	p-value
LOG TI Breeding	TI 200	227	<0.01	<0.01	0.148	<0.01	**0.01**
	Internal biosecurity	227	0.22	0.36	0.073		
	External biosecurity	227	0.51	0.08	0.083		
	Years experience	221	−0.07	0.81	0.071		
	Pathogens vaccinated	227	2.35	0.14	0.079		
	# sows	227	0.01	0.33	0.074		
	# employees	221	0.43	0.78	0.066		
	Gender	214		0.60	0.071		
	Male	137	3.14	0.60			
	Female	77	Ref.	Ref.			
	Education	210		0.11	0.082		
	Lower	84	−15.47	0.05			
	Higher	84	−15.77	0.06			
	University	42	Ref.	Ref.			
	Farrowing rhythm (cat)	219		0.76	0.060		
	>5	18	−0.81	0.95			
	5	20	2.76	0.82			
	4	48	−1.34	0.89			
	3	80	4.33	0.62			
	2	21	14.94	0.20			
	1	32	Ref.	Ref.			
LOG TI 200	TI Breeding	227	<0.01	**<0.01**	0.332	<0.01	**<0.01**
	Internal biosecurity	227	−0.01	0.11	0.325		
	External biosecurity	227	−0.02	**0.01**	0.353	−0.03	**<0.01**
	Weaning age	216	−0.05	**0.05**	0.335	−0.05	0.06
	Years experience	221	<0.01	0.28	0.324		
	Pathogens vaccinated	227	0.18	**<0.01**	0.355	0.14	**<0.01**
	# sows	227	<0.01	**0.01**	0.346		
	# employees	221	0.05	0.32	0.315		
	Gender	214		0.51	0.313		
	Male	137	0.11	0.51			
	Female	77	Ref.	Ref.			
	Education	210		0.39	0.331		
	Lower	84	0.07	0.77			
	Higher	84	0.28	0.24			
	University	42	Ref.	Ref.			
	Zinc oxide	205		0.29	0.310		
	Yes	39	0.25	0.29			
	No	166	Ref.	Ref.			
	Anti-inflammatory weaners	227		**0.05**	0.338		
	Yes	71	0.37	0.05			
	No	156	Ref.	Ref.			

Table 1 Results of univariable and multivariable general linear regression models *(Continued)*

Outcome	Factor	N	Univar. estimate	Univar. *p*	R²	Multivar. estimate	Multivar. *p*
	Anti-coccidial	214		0.10	0.313		
	Yes	90	0.28	0.10			
	No	124	Ref.	Ref.			
	Farrowing rhythm	219		**<0.01**	0.360		**<0.01**
	>5	18	−0.78	0.05		−0.88	**0.02**
	5	20	−1.15	<0.01		−1.10	**<0.01**
	4	48	−0.51	0.07		−0.44	0.11
	3	80	−0.38	0.12		−0.21	0.42
	2	21	0.10	0.75		−0.06	0.85
	1	32	Ref.	Ref.		Ref.	Ref.
Number of weaned piglets per sow per year (WSY)	Years experience	217	−0.02	0.27	0.354		
	External biosecurity	223	0.05	**<0.01**	0.362		
	Internal biosecurity	223	0.03	0.06	0.349		
	Weaning age	212	−0.17	**<0.01**	0.367	−0.19	**<0.01**
	Pathogens vaccinated	223	0.18	0.06	0.349		
	Mortality until weaning	222	−0.18	**<0.01**	0.423	−0.21	**<0.01**
	#sows	223	<0.01	**<0.01**	0.391		
	#employees	217	0.22	**0.02**	0.359		
	TI Breeding	223	0.01	**<0.01**	0.362	0.01	0.06
	TI 200	223	<0.01	0.71	0.339		
	Anti-inflammatory sucklers	223					
	Yes	122	0.43	0.39	0.340		
	No	105	Ref.	Ref.			
	Anti-inflammatory weaners	223					
	Yes	71	0.57	0.13	0.345		
	No	156	Ref.	Ref.			
	Anti-inflammatory sows	215					
	Yes	217	1.18	0.49	0.343		
	No	2	Ref.	Ref.			
	Anti-coccidial	211					
	Yes	90	0.08	0.82	0.337		
	No	124	Ref.	Ref.			
	Zinc oxide	201					
	Yes	39	0.86	0.06	0.363		
	No	166	Ref.	Ref.			
	Country * Weaning age						**0.02**
	Belgium * Weaning age					−0.20	0.18
	France * Weaning age					0.21	**0.04**
	Germany * Weaning age					0.15	0.18
	Sweden * Weaning age					Ref.	Ref.

LOG log transformation. Light gray values in the univariable model indicate that these factors were not significant (*p* < 0.20) in the univariable model. In the multivariable model p-values which are significant with *p* < 0.05 are black and bold, 0.05 < *p* < 0.10 are black and *p* > 0.10 are light gray. Significant interactions are listed where applicable. All models were corrected for the country effect by adding country in the model as a fixed variable. Only relevant variables are listed compare the usage over countries, since the period at risk is standardized between these countries. For sows the period at risk was set to 1 year.

To be able to compare the usage over countries a standardised assumed weight at treatment was set for the different age categories; suckling piglet = 2 kg, weaner = 7 kg, finisher = 35 kg, sow = 220 kg. Furthermore, to be able to compare the different products and their concentrations within similar antimicrobial classes used in the different countries, a consensus defined daily dose animal (DDDA) per antimicrobial class, including consensus long acting factors, were established. The procedure used to come to these consensus DDDAs was extensively described in Postma et al. [29].

Data processing

A LOG transformation of the data for the number of sows as an outcome variable (data not shown) in the regression models was needed to correct for the right skewedness of this variable.

Outcomes for TI 200 and TI breeding were also LOG transformed using SPSS statistics 22 (IBM), after adding one to the original outcome to adjust for zero values in the data.

Biocheck.UGent™ is a webbased scoring system using Limesurvey.

Statistical analysis

Initially all possible causal routes linking antimicrobial usage, biosecurity status, herd characteristics and technical parameters (e.g. number of sows, WSY, average daily weigh gain (ADG, g/day), mortalities (%)) were identified based on logical reasoning with the main focus on parameters influencing the antimicrobial usage or the ones being influenced by the antimicrobial usage. Subsequently each of the identified possible associations was assessed using a regression model with the specific predictor always in combination with country as a second predictor variable to account for country specific characteristics.

All associations that showed a univariable p-value of < 0.20 were retained for the multivariable analysis. The multivariable general linear model was constructed using the stepwise backward selection procedure, including testing of two-way interactions of significant main effects. Confounding effects were evaluated during the modelling process by checking changes in parameter estimates. The association in the multivariable linear regression model was considered significant if $p < 0.05$ and a p-value between 0.05 and 0.10 was considered nearly significant and relevant to describe. Normal probability tests and plots were examined to check whether the assumptions of normality and homoscedasticity of residuals were fulfilled.

All statistical analyses were performed using SPSS statistics 22 (IBM). All tested variables can be found in Table 1.

Results
Farm characteristics

A 3-week farrowing rhythm system was most commonly used (80/227 herds). Followed by a 4 week system (48/227), a 1-week system (32/227), a 2-week system (21/227), a 5-week system (20/227) and a >5-week system (18/227). The mean weaning age was highest in Sweden (35 days) and lowest in Belgium (23.5 days). The mean number of piglets weaned per sow per year was comparable in Belgium (27.2, SD = 2.6), France (26.5, SD = 2.3) and Germany (27.4, SD = 2.3), but lower in Sweden (23.2, SD = 2.3). In Belgium, France and Germany the number of pathogens vaccinated against had a median of 7, while in Sweden this was 4. Out of 227 herds, 71 reported to use anti-inflammatory products in the weaners, while 90 out of 227 used anti-coccidial products in the suckling piglets.

Other herd characteristics of interest were described in more detail in the publication of Postma et al. [19].

Biosecurity status

The external biosecurity level (65.5, range 43–93) was overall higher compared to the internal biosecurity level (55.7, range 6–88). External biosecurity was highest in Germany (70.2) and lowest in France (59.4), while the internal biosecurity level was highest in Sweden (58.8) and lowest in Belgium (50.3). In Postma et al. [19] results of the biosecurity quantification in the herds in the four participating countries and the link with production characteristics were described in detail. Since five Belgian herds were lacking information on antimicrobial usage they were removed from analysis in this study, resulting in slightly different results compared to the ones published in Postma et al. [19].

Antimicrobial usage

Average antimicrobial usage in the breeding animals (23.0) was lower compared to the usage from birth until slaughter (TI 200) in the growing pigs (128.3). For both the TI 200 days (Sweden = 22.7; Germany = 242.8) and the TI breeding animals (Sweden = 10.9, Germany = 42.0) Sweden was the lowest using country and Germany the highest.

The quantification of the antimicrobial usage and the results in the four countries is described in detail in Sjölund et al. (Sjölund M., Postma M., Collineau L., Lösken S., Backhans A., Belloc C., Emanuelson, U., Große Beilage, E., Stärk, K. D. C., Dewulf, J., Quantitative and qualitative antimicrobial usage patterns in farrow-to-finish pig herds in Belgium, France, Germany and Sweden, submitted).

Associations between antimicrobial usage, biosecurity level and farm characteristics

The country corrected univariable analysis resulted in retaining several variables related with the antimicrobial usage or with each other (Table 1). The associations that remained significant in the multivariable models are shown in the causal path in Fig. 1.

The multivariable model for the LOG TI Breeding, corrected for the country effect showed significant associations with the LOG TI 200 ($p < 0.01$). A higher antimicrobial usage in the breeders was associated with a higher antimicrobial usage in the growing pigs (LOG TI 200).

The LOG TI Breeders was positively associated with the number of WSY ($p = 0.06$), meaning that farms with a higher antimicrobial usage in the breeding animals on average weaned slightly more piglets, however, the ß-value was low.

For the LOG TI 200 the multivariable model showed, after correction for a possible country effect, three variables that were directly associated with the antimicrobial usage from birth until slaughter and one that was nearly significant.

The LOG TI 200 was associated with the weaning age ($p = 0.06$); herds with a higher weaning age showed a

lower TI 200. A significant ($p < 0.01$) lower TI 200 was observed for 5-week or >5-week systems in comparison to 1-week system. Also for 2-, 3- and 4-week systems a non-significant trend towards a lower TI 200 was observed in comparison to a one week system. Herds with a higher score on their external biosecurity status also showed a lower TI 200 ($p < 0.01$). While herds vaccinating against more pathogens showed a higher TI 200 ($p < 0.01$).

It should be noted that parameters such as the internal biosecurity level, number of sows or employees, gender of the responsible person in the farrowing unit, the education level of the responsible person or the use of products like zinc oxide were not retained in any of the multivariable models associated with antimicrobial usage. The level of antimicrobial usage furthermore was not significantly associated with production parameters such as the ADG or the mortality until weaning.

Discussion

By showing associations between a higher level of biosecurity, a longer farrowing rhythm or weaning at an older age and a reduced antimicrobial usage the aim of this study was met and the results of this paper have the potential to advise on best practices.

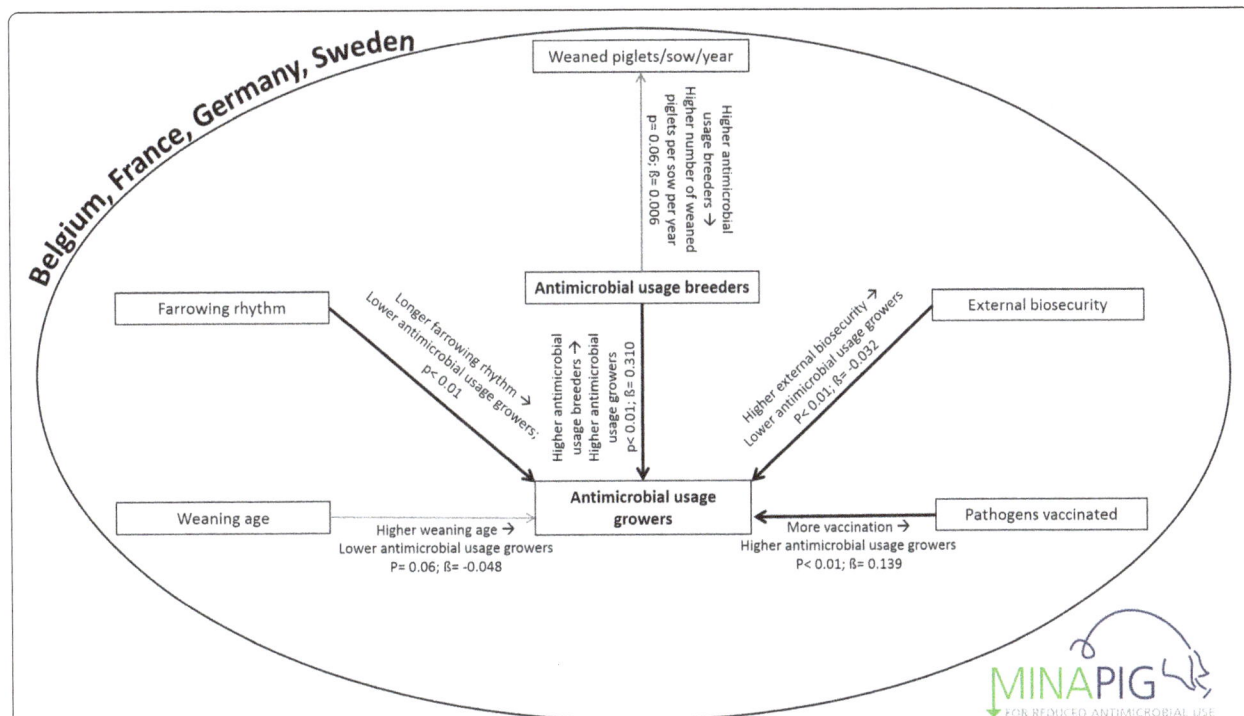

Fig. 1 Causal pathway associations for TI 200 days and TI Breeding. Causal pathway with statistically significant associations in the multivariable models for the TI 200 days and the TI Breeding associated with production, management or biosecurity variables. TI = treatment incidence (antimicrobial usage quantification), WSY = number of weaned piglets per sow per year. Black lines represent the result of a multivariable linear regression analysis based on data from 4 EU countries. The light gray line indicates $0.05 < p < 0.10$. The p-values and β-values correspond to the multivariable model. All models were corrected for the country effect by placing country as a fixed variable in the model, hence the circle around the figure

Associations between antimicrobial usage, biosecurity level and farm characteristics

To overcome national differences in cultures, habits, regulations, pig production structure, disease prevalence and other external factors all models were corrected for country by adding country as a fixed factor in all models. The obtained association are therefore corrected for the country effect and interaction with country was tested as well.

In Fig. 1 the causal pathway shows an association ($p = 0.06$) between the TI Breeding and the number of weaned piglets (WSY). Improved piglet survival might be the result of a more active presence in the farrowing unit by the farmer during the farrowing period, which is the most likely period of antimicrobial treatment for sows. When better attention is paid during the farrowing process piglet survival might improve, resulting in more weaned piglets per sow per year [30, 31]. Another possible explanation for the positive association between the TI Breeding and the WSY could be the increase in the farrowing index due to a positive effect of the antimicrobial usage in the reduced incidence of mastitis and endometritis problems in the sows. A healthy sow might also nurse her piglets better, resulting in a more optimal transmission of maternal antibodies. Although we assumed in the causal pathway that treatment of breeders could have an effect on the number of weaned piglets per sow per year, it may also be possible that in fact the association could be reversed and that high productive sows are more sensitive to diseases and require more antimicrobial treatments, in which case the higher productivity would lead to a higher TI Breeding. Other unmeasured factors might have also influenced this outcome. In all cases we should keep in mind that the association we found was only minor, with a low ß-coefficient and should therefore not be used as an excuse to increase antimicrobial usage in breeding animals. Furthermore, antimicrobial usage in the sow was recently negative associated with the bacterial gut flora and antimicrobial resistance levels of the piglet [32].

The link between the level of usage in the breeding animals with the level of usage in pigs from birth to slaughter was expected, as a high overall disease pressure in a herd may explain the high usage in both breeding animals and the animals from birth until slaughter. A limited number of herds concentrated the majority of antimicrobial treatments and a certain attitude/behaviour of the farmer towards regular usage of medicines might be another explanation for the association between usage in breeding animals and growers [33].

Vaccines are used to improve the immunity status of the animals which should result in a reduced risk for animals to become diseased and subsequently leading to a reduced need for antimicrobial treatment. Therefore vaccines are often suggested as a suitable alternative for antimicrobial use [10, 12, 34–37]. This is an apparent contradiction with the observed positive association between the number of pathogens vaccinated against and the TI 200 in the present study, although this was also observed by Temtem et al. [38]. This association might be due to a high disease pressure on these herds which has not (yet) been brought under control through vaccination, due to insufficient detection of disease, or it might again be an indication of a certain attitude of the farmer and/or his veterinarian, i.e. using/prescribing a lot of veterinary medicinal products as an insurance against disease [33, 39]. This association could be further explored by looking at vaccination details, disease pressure and antimicrobial treatment indications.

The association we found between the weaning age ($p = 0.06$) and TI 200 suggests that a higher weaning age results in healthier, more robust animals who have a reduced necessity for antimicrobials. This is in agreement with the idea that stronger animals, for example when weaned at a later age, are also more likely to have better coping abilities against possible (pathogenic) threats [40, 41].

For the farrowing rhythm we found that a 5-week and ≥ 5-week system were significantly associated with a lower antimicrobial usage. Also for 2-, 3- and 4-week systems a non-significant trend towards a lower TI 200 was observed in comparison to a one week system. We did furthermore see that the herds with a 3-week system had on average a higher weaning age, while for example a 4-week system had lower average weaning ages in Belgium, France and Germany [19]. However, since both variables were included in the multivariable model this indirect effect was already accounted for and the single effects of the farrowing rhythm and the weaning age on the TI 200 both hold strong. One explanation for the lower TI 200 in longer farrowing rhythms might be that a longer period in-between two batches guarantees a better separation between the age groups and allows for more cleaning and disinfection time, resulting in less risk of transmission of pathogens between them. For example Nathues et al. [42] showed that piglets within a herd with a 3-week system were less likely to be infected with *Mycoplasma hyopneumoniae* compared to a 2-week system. His findings did not hold true for a 4-week system, but more pathogens and factors most likely influence our finding and not only *M. hyopneumoniae*, resulting in a positive effect in general for the longer farrowing rhythms.

Both the better results related to a longer farrowing rhythm and even more important the finding that a higher weaning age lead to a lower TI 200 might be of great relevance in future advising of pig farmers to reduce their antimicrobial usage. Further research should investigate this association in more detail and determine whether this trend can be confirmed. If so, it would be possible to reduce antimicrobial usage by developing more strict regulation and legislation on the weaning age.

A last important finding was the association between the level of external biosecurity and the TI 200 ($p < 0.01$). External biosecurity controls the risk of entrance and exit of pathogens into a herd. Introduction of pathogens from an outside source poses the largest risk for disease onset in pig production [24, 43–45]. When we would be able to reduce this risk it is also likely that less antimicrobials would be needed [46, 47]. Moreover, external and internal biosecurity are shown to be highly correlated to each other [19]. Due to this association internal biosecurity improvement might also have an effect on the antimicrobial usage from birth until slaughter. Laanen et al. [20] showed this association between internal biosecurity and TI in her study performed in Belgium in 2009–2010. Since improvement of the internal biosecurity level could be a rather simple intervention (e.g. strict hygiene protocols, correct use of working lines) at herd level, this might be an important consideration in the reduction of antimicrobial usage.

We should also stress that no significant positive associations were found between a higher usage and better production results such as ADG or mortality, as also supported by a paper of van der Fels-Klerx et al. [48]. Although it is sometimes suggested that the use of antimicrobials results in heavier pigs, as also stimulated in earlier years by the use of antimicrobial growth promotors in the feed, we did not find a significant link in this study. In the EU the use of antimicrobial growth promotors in feed was banned since 2006 [49]. The use of zinc oxide also showed no association with antimicrobial usage, although often it is promoted as an alternative in the reduction of antimicrobial usage [12, 50]. Unknown however, was how long the herds already used zinc oxide and whether this could already have affected their antimicrobial usage. Improved health of the pigs might result in a better ADG and lower mortality, however, no significant direct association between these and the antimicrobial usage were found and most likely more factors were of importance in the herds' ADG and mortality results. Results suggest that administering antimicrobials did not improve technical results.

Future studies should try to confirm the above presented findings so that they could be validated as successful actions in the reduction of antimicrobial usage.

Study design and limitations

Only a limited number of studies have investigated the associations between production parameters, other herd characteristics and antimicrobial usage [20]. A recent review of Aarestrup [10] emphasizes the need for research on effects of interventions. The current study attempts to provide a first overview of the associations between production parameters, preventive measures such as high biosecurity status and vaccination level and herd and management characteristics with the level of antimicrobial usage. Knowledge on these associations might be used as input for future intervention studies.

We should however, be aware that this study is likely influenced by the fact that the participating farmers resembled the better end of the population since their selection was based on willingness to participate (except in France where random sampling was used, by selecting herds from the database of Institute for pig and pork industry including on average 53 % of herds located in North-West France with >49 sows) and interest in the topic, resulting in a selection bias. Variability between researchers was minimized by providing all interviewers with the same training in execution of the questionnaire form, however, it might have caused some random noise as well. In France information on antimicrobial usage was collected from the last batch whereas for the other countries the year preceding the herd visit was used. This could have led to a limited bias due to difference in disease prevalence in combination with seasonal influences. Recall bias was considered to be of minimal importance since the majority of collected information was checked using visual inspection and/or documentation. We should also stress that the obtained associations were the result of a cross-sectional study design, not allowing to make direct causal conclusions. By designing the causal pathway however, we tried to give a clear overview of obtained associations.

Conclusions

This cross-sectional study on 227 pig herds in Belgium, France, Germany and Sweden showed that the antimicrobial usage in breeding animals tends to be positively associated with the number of weaned piglets per sow per year and the antimicrobial usage from birth to slaughter (TI 200) in growing pigs. The TI 200 was shown to be lower in herds with a farrowing rhythm ≥5-weeks, a higher biosecurity status and tended to be lower with weaning of the piglets at an older age. Policy makers, herd advisors and farmers should benefit from this knowledge in order to reduce the antimicrobial usage on pig herds.

Abbreviations

ADG: average daily weight gain; AM: antimicrobial; AMR: antimicrobial resistance; AMU: antimicrobial usage; DDDA: defined daily dose animal; EU: European Union; LOG: logaritmic; TI: treatment incidence; WSY: number of weaned piglets per sow per year.

Competing interests

Boehringer Ingelheim is partner in the MINAPIG consortium, however, they did not participate in the study design nor in the collection, analysis and interpretation of data, nor in the decision to submit the manuscript for publication. The same applies to the funding party EMIDA ERA-NET. None of the authors has any financial or personal relationships that could inappropriately influence or bias the content of the paper.

Authors' contributions

MP carried out the study in Belgium, participated in and prepared protocols for the study design performed statistical analysis and drafted the manuscript. AB and MS, LC and CB, SL and EgB performed the collecting of data in Sweden, France and Germany respectively and participated in the study design and analysis. EON helped in the study design and draft of the manuscript. UE and JD participated in the study design and statistical analysis and helped to draft the manuscript. KS coordinated and helped in the study design. All authors read and approved the final manuscript.

Acknowledgements

The MINAPIG consortium would like to thank all participating farmers, their employees and herd veterinarians for their cooperation. The authors would also like to thank the other MINAPIG consortium partners for their help in developing the protocol for this study.
Members of the MINAPIG consortium in alphabetical order: Margit Andreasen, Boehringer Ingelheim, Denmark; Annette Backhans, SLU, Sweden; Catherine Belloc, ONIRIS, France; Lucie Collineau, SAFOSO, Switzerland; Jeroen Dewulf, Ghent University, Belgium; Ulf Emanuelson, SLU, Sweden; Elisabeth grosse Beilage, TiHo Hannover, Germany; Bernd Grosse Liesner, Boehringer Ingelheim, Germany; Christian Alexander Körk, Boehringer Ingelheim, Germany; Ann Lindberg, SVA, Sweden; Svenja Lösken, TiHo Hannover, Germany; Merel Postma, Ghent University, Belgium; Hugo Seemer, Boehringer Ingelheim, Germany; Marie Sjölund, SVA and SLU, Sweden; Katharina Stärk, SAFOSO, Switzerland; Vivianne Visschers, ETHZ, Switzerland. MINAPIG project: Evaluation of alternative strategies for raising pigs with minimal antimicrobial usage: Opportunities and constraints. More information can be found at www.minapig.eu.

Prior presentation of data

Preliminary results of this study were presented at the Minapig pre-conference preceding the 7th European Symposium of Porcine Health Management, Nantes, 22nd – 24th April 2015.

Funding

This project was part of the European MINAPIG project (Evaluation of alternative strategies for raising pigs with minimal antimicrobial usage): Opportunities and constraints, http://www.minapig.eu), which was funded by the ERA-NET programme EMIDA (EMIDA19)[1] and by the participating national funding agencies.

Author details

[1]Veterinary Epidemiology Unit, Department of Reproduction, Obstetrics and Herd Health, Faculty of Veterinary Medicine, Ghent University, Salisburylaan 133, 9820 Merelbeke, Belgium. [2]Department of Animal Health and Antimicrobial Strategies, National Veterinary Institute, SVA, SE-751 89 Uppsala, Sweden. [3]Department of Clinical Sciences, Swedish University of Agricultural Sciences, P.O. Box 7054SE-750 07 Uppsala, Sweden. [4]SAFOSO AG, Waldeggstrasse 1, CH-3097 Liebefeld, Switzerland. [5]UMR1300 BioEpAR, LUNAM Université, Oniris, INRA, BP40706, F-44307 Nantes, France. [6]Field Station for Epidemiology, University of Veterinary Medicine Hannover, Büscheler Straße 9, D-49456 Bakum, Germany. [7]Danish Agriculture and Food Council, Axeltorv 3, DK-1609 Copenhagen V, Denmark.

References

1. Callens B, Persoons D, Maes D, Laanen M, Postma M, Boyen F, et al. Prophylactic and metaphylactic antimicrobial use in Belgian fattening pig herds. Prev Vet Med. 2012;106:53–62.

2. Filippitzi M, Callens B, Pardon B, Persoons D, Dewulf J. Antimicrobial use in pigs, broilers and veal calves. Vlaams Diergeneeskundig Tijdschrift. 2014; 83(5):215–24.

3. MARAN, van Geijlswijk IM, Jacobs J, Heederik D, Wagenaar JA, Mouton JW. MARAN 2013 - Monitoring of Antimicrobial Resistance and Antibiotic Usage in Animals in the Netherlands in 2013. Bilthoven, the Netherlands: Central Veterinary Institute of Wageningen University and Research Centre in collaboration with the Food and Consumer Product Safety Authority (NVWA) and the National Institue for Public Health and the Environment (RIVM); 2014. http://wageningenur.nl/upload_mm/d/c/3/9e6f26a2-4a19-4042-9fb0-e32921d8bdee_NethMap-MARAN2014.pdf.

4. World Health Organization. Antimicrobial resistance - http://www.who.int/mediacentre/factsheets/fs194/en/: World Health Organization; 2015. Contract No.: Fact sheet No 194.

5. Chantziaras I, Boyen F, Callens B, Dewulf J. Correlation between veterinary antimicrobial use and antimicrobial resistance in food-producing anmls: a report on seven countries. Journal of Antimicrobial Chemotherapy. 2013;69(3):827–34.

6. European Food Safety Authority (EFSA), European Centre for Disease Prevention and Control (ECDC). EU summary report on antimicrobial resistance in zoonotic and indicator bacteria from humans, animals and food in 2013. Parma, Italy; 2015. Contract No.: 4036. http://ecdc.europa.eu/en/publications/Publications/antimicrobial-resistance-zoonotic-bacteria-humans-animals-food-EU-summary-report-2013.pdf

7. Wegener HC, editor. Antbiotic resistance: Linking human and animal health - Improving food safety through a one health approach: worshhop summary. Institute of Medicine. Washington, DC, USA: The National Academies Press; 2012.

8. Delia G. Review of evidence on antimicrobial resistance and animal agriculture in developing countries. United Kingdom: International Livestock Research Institute; 2015.

9. Dorado-García A, Dohmen W, Bos MEH, Verstappen KM, Houben M, Wagenaar JA, et al. Dose–response Relationship between Antimicrobial Drugs and Livestock-Associated MRSA in Pig Farming. Emerg Infect Dis. 2015;21(6):950–9. doi:10.3201/eid2106.140706.

10. Aarestrup FM. The livestock reservoir for antimicrobial resistance: a personal view on changing patterns of risks, effects of interventions and the way forward. Philosophical transactions B. 2015;370(20140085). doi:10.1098/rstb.2014.0085.

11. European Commission. Communication from the Commission to the European Parliament and the Council - Action plan against the rising threats from Antimicrobial Resistance - http://ec.europa.eu/dgs/health_consumer/docs/communication_amr_2011_748_en.pdf. Brussels, Belgium; 2011 Contract No.: 748.

12. Postma M, Stärk KDC, Sjölund M, Backhans A, Beilage EG, Lösken S, et al. Alternatives to the use of antimicrobial agents in pig production: A multi-country expert-ranking of perceived effectiveness, feasibility and return on investment. Prev Vet Med. 2015;118(4):457–66. doi:http://dx.doi.org/10.1016/j.prevetmed.2015.01.010.

13. Seal BS, Lillehoj HS, Donovan DM, Gay CG. Alternatives to antibiotics: a symposium on the challenges and solutions for animal production. Anim Health Res Rev. 2013;14(1):78–87.

14. Cheng G, Hao H, Xie S, Wang X, Dai M, Huang L et al. Antibiotic Alternatives: The Substitution of Antibiotics in Animal Husbandry? Frontiers in Microbiology. 2014;5. doi:10.3389/fmicb.2014.00217.

15. Adam M, editor. A meta-analysis on field experiences with vaccination against ileitis showing a reduction on antibiotic use. 8th International Symposium on the Epidemiology and Control of Foodborne Pathogens in Pork (SafePork); 2009 30 September - 2 October 2009. Quebec City, Canada; 2009.

16. Bak H, Rathkjen PH. Reduced use of antimicrobials after vaccination of pigs against porcine proliferative enteropathy in a Danish SPF herd. Acta Vet Scand. 2009;51:1.

17. Brockhoff E, Cunningham G, Misutka C. A retrospective analysis of a high health commercial pig production system showing improved production and reduced antibiotic use after implementation of a PCV2 vaccination. 8th International Symposium on the Epidemiology and Control of Foodborne Pathogens in Pork (SafePork); 2009 30 September - 2 October 2009. Quebec City, Canada; 2009.

18. Aerts R, Wertenbroek N, editors. Implementing PCV2 vaccination resulting in reduction of antibiotic use on Dutch farrow-to-finish farm. 9th International Symposium on the Epidemiology and Control of Foodborne Pathogens in Pork (SafePork); 2011 19–22 June 2011. Maastricht, The Netherlands; 2011.

19. Postma M, Backhans A, Collineau L, Loesken S, Sjölund M, Belloc C, et al. The biosecurity status and its associations with production and management characteristics in farrow-to-finish pig herds. Animal. 2016; 10(03):478–89. doi:10.1017/S1751731115002487.

20. Laanen M, Persoons D, Ribbens S, de Jong E, Callen B, Strubbe M, et al. Relationship between biosecurity and production/antimicrobial treatment characteristics in pig herds. The Veterinary Journal. 2013;198(2):508–12.

21. Marquer P, Rabade T, Forti R. Statistics in focus: Pig farming sector - statistical portrait. Contract No.: KS-SF-14-015-EN-N; 2014. http://ec.europa.eu/eurostat/statistics-explained/index.php/Pig_farming_sector_-_statistical_portrait_2014.

22. VILT. VLaams Infocentrum Land- en Tuinbouw. Belgische veestapel groeit verder aan. Brussels, Belgium: VILT; 2010. Retrieved on 14 December 2014.

23. Statistisches Bundesamt. Land- und Forstwirtschaft, Fischerei - Viehhaltung der Betriebe Agrarstrukturerhebung - 2013. Wiesbaden, Germany: Contract No.: Fachserie 3 Reihe 2.1.3; 2014.

24. Ghent University. In: Biocheck.UGent,. Retrieved on 10 March 2015, www.biocheck.ugent.be, Ghent University, Faculty of Veterinary Medicine, Department of Reproduction Obstetrics and Herd Health, Veterinary Epidemiology Unit, Merelbeke, Belgium. 2010. www.biocheck.ugent.be.

25. Laanen M, Beek J, Ribbens S, Vangroenweghe F, Maes D, Dewulf J. Biosecurity on pig herds: development of an on-line scoring system and the results of the first 99 participating herds. Vlaams Diergeneeskundig Tijdschrift. 2010;79(4):302–6.

26. Backhans A, Sjölund M, Lindberg A, Emanuelson U. Biosecurity level and health management practices in 60 Swedish farrow-to-finish herds. Acta Vet Scand. 2015;57(1):14. doi:10.1186/s13028-015-0103-5.

27. Timmerman T, Dewulf J, Catry B, Feyen B, Opsomer G, de Kruif A, et al. Quantification and evaluation of antimicrobial drug use in group treatments for fattening pigs in Belgium. Prev Vet Med. 2006;74(4):251–63.

28. Sjölund M, Backhans A, Greko C, Emanuelson U, Lindberg A. Antimicrobial usage in 60 Swedish farrow-to-finish pig herds. Prev Vet Med. 2015;121(3–4): 257–64. doi:http://dx.doi.org/10.1016/j.prevetmed.2015.07.005.

29. Postma M, Sjölund M, Collineau L, Lösken S, Stärk KDC, Dewulf J. Assigning defined daily doses animal: a European multi-country experience for antimicrobial products authorized for usage in pigs. Journal of Antimicrobial Chemotherapy. 2015;70(1):294–302. doi:10.1093/jac/dku347.

30. Kraeling R, Webel S. Current strategies for reproductive management of gilts and sows in North America. Journal of Animal Science and Biotechnology. 2015;6(1):3.

31. Kirkden RD, Broom DM, Andersen ILINVITEDREVIEW. Piglet mortality: Management solutions. J Anim Sci. 2013;91(7):3361–89. doi:10.2527/jas.2012-5637.

32. Callens B, Faes C, Maes D, Catry B, Boyen F, Francoys D, et al. Presence of Antimicrobial Resistance and Antimicrobial Use in Sows Are Risk Factors for Antimicrobial Resistance in Their Offspring. Microb Drug Resist. 2014;21(1): 50–8. doi:10.1089/mdr.2014.0037.

33. Visschers VHM, Backhans A, Collineau L, Iten D, Loesken S, Postma M, et al. Perceptions of antimicrobial usage, antimicrobial resistance and policy measures to reduce antimicrobial usage in convenient samples of Belgian, French, German, Swedish and Swiss pig farmers. Prev Vet Med. 2015;119 (1–2):10–20. doi:http://dx.doi.org/10.1016/j.prevetmed.2015.01.018.

34. McEwen SA, Fedorka-Cray PJ. Antimicrobial use and resistance in animals. Clin Infect Dis. 2002;34((Supplement 3):S93–106. doi:10.1086/340246.

35. Andrew P, Volker G, den Hurk SvDL-v. Veterinary vaccines: alternatives to antibiotics? Anim Health Res Rev. 2008;9 (Special Issue 02):187–99. doi:10.1017/S1466252308001606.

36. Allen HK, Levine UY, Looft T, Bandrick M, Casey TA. Treatment, promotion, commotion: antibiotic alternatives in food-producing animals. Trends Microbiol. 2013;21(3):114–9. doi:http://dx.doi.org/10.1016/j.tim.2012.11.001.

37. Allen HK, Trachsel J, Looft T, Casey TA. Finding alternatives to antibiotics. Ann N Y Acad Sci. 2014;1323(1):91–100. doi:10.1111/nyas.12468.

38. Temtem C, Alban L, Pedersen KS, Nielsen LR. Associations between vaccination and the antimicrobial consumption in danish pig herds, 2013. Porto, Portugal: 11th SafePork conference; 2015.

39. Speksnijder DC, Jaarsma ADC, van der Gugten AC, Verheij TJM, Wagenaar JA. Determinants Associated with Veterinary Antimicrobial Prescribing in Farm Animals in the Netherlands: A Qualitative Study. Zoonoses Public Health. 2015;62:39–51. doi:10.1111/zph.12168.

40. The Pig Site. Maximum productivity. In: Pig health. http://www.thepigsite.com/pighealth/article/306/maximum-productivity/. Accessed 2015/06/24.

41. Thomson JR, Friendship RM. Immunology. In: Zimmermann JJ, Karriker LA, Ramirez A, Schwartz KJ, Stevenson GW, editors. Diseases of swine. 10th ed. Chichester, West Sussex, United Kingdom: Wiley-Blackwell; 2012. p. 749.

42. Nathues H, Woeste H, Doehring S, Fahrion AS, Doherr MG, Beilage E. Herd specific risk factors for Mycoplasma hyopneumoniae infections in suckling pigs at the age of weaning. Acta Vet Scand. 2013;55(1):30. doi:10.1186/1751-0147-55-30.

43. Lambert M-È, Arsenault J, Poljak Z, D'Allaire S. Epidemiological investigations in regard to porcine reproductive and respiratory syndrome (PRRS) in Quebec, Canada. Part 2: Prevalence and risk factors in breeding sites. Prev Vet Med. 2012;104(1–2):84–93. doi:http://dx.doi.org/10.1016/j.prevetmed.2011.11.002.

44. Lewerin SS, Österberg J, Alenius S, Elvander M, Fellström C, Tråvén M, et al. Risk assessment as a tool for improving external biosecurity at farm level. BMC Vet Res. 2015;11:171. doi:10.1186/s12917-015-0477-7.

45. Ribbens S, Dewulf J, Koenen F, Mintiens K, de Kruif A, Maes D. ype and frequency of contacts between Belgian pig herds. Prev Vet Med. 2009;88(1): 57–66. doi:http://dx.doi.org/10.1016/j.prevetmed.2008.08.002.

46. European Commission. A new Animal Health Strategy for the European Union (2007–2003) where "Prevention is better than cure". Luxembourg, Luxembourg: Office for Official Publications of the European Communities; 2007. Report No.: COM 539 (2007) final Contract No.: ISBN 978-92-79-06722-8.

47. European Commission. Communication from the Commission to the European Parliament and the Council - Action plan against the rising threats from Antimicrobial Resistance. COM (2011) 748. In: AMR Road map - Action no 10. Brussels, Belgium: European Commission; 2011. http://ec.europa.eu/dgs/health_consumer/docs/road-map-amr_en.pdf. COM (2011) 748 - AMR Road map - Action no 10.

48. van der Fels-Klerx HJ, Puister-Jansen LF, van Asselt ED, Burgers SLGE. Farm factors associated with the use of antibiotics in pig production. J Anim Sci. 2011;89(6):1922–9. doi:10.2527/jas.2010-3046.

49. European commission. Ban on antibiotics as growth promoters in animal feed enters into effect. Brussels, Belgium: European Commission; 2005.

50. Wierup M. The Swedish Experience of the 1986 Year Ban of Antimicrobial Growth Promoters, with Special Reference to Animal Health, Disease Prevention, Productivity, and Usage of Antimicrobials. Microb Drug Resist. 2001;7(2):183–90. doi:http://dx.doi.org/10.1089/10766290152045066.

Field evaluation of piglet vaccination with a *Mycoplasma hyopneumoniae* bacterin as compared to a ready-to-use product including porcine circovirus 2 and *M. hyopneumoniae* in a conventional French farrow-to-finish farm

Didier Duivon[1*], Isabelle Corrégé[2], Anne Hémonic[2], Martial Rigaut[1], David Roudaut[1] and Rika Jolie[3]

Abstract

Background: A controlled randomized trial was performed on a well-managed conventional French 180-sow farm. The trial compared the growth performances of piglets vaccinated at weaning (single shot) either with a commercial monovalent *Mycoplasma hyopneumoniae* bacterin vaccine or with a commercial bivalent vaccine (Porcilis® PCV M Hyo) against *M. hyopneumoniae* and porcine circovirus 2 (PCV2). The farm's porcine reproductive and respiratory syndrome status was stable, and most diseases (enzootic pneumonia, atrophic rhinitis, post-weaning multisystemic wasting syndrome) were controlled by routine vaccination.

Results: During the post-weaning phase, the growth performances of the piglets vaccinated with the bivalent vaccine were not significantly different from those vaccinated with the monovalent vaccine. However, during the fattening phase the group vaccinated with the bivalent vaccine had a significantly improved ADG (+34 g/d, $p = 0.047$), resulting in a 5-day earlier shipment to slaughter. The group also had a shorter and lower PCV2 load in serum during the fattening period, and an improved lung lesions score. In both groups, three pigs died during the peak PCV2 viraemia (16–23 weeks of age). Immunohistochemistry of the lymph nodes showed that in the group vaccinated with the bivalent vaccine, none of these pigs had PCV2-like lesions, while 2 out of the 3 from the other group did. Results suggest that the added PCV2 valence in the vaccination protocol helps countering the negative impact of subclinical PCV2 infection on growth. The calculated return on investment of the added PCV2 vaccine valence was €1.7 extra revenue per slaughtered pig (€ 39 additional revenue per sow and per year), despite the fact that the cost of the bivalent vaccine was higher than the monovalent *M. hyopneumoniae* vaccine.

Conclusion: In this healthy conventional sow farm, the combined *M. hyopneumoniae* and PCV2 vaccination was efficacious, convenient to administer and profitable.

Keywords: PCV2, *Mycoplasma hyopneumoniae*, Vaccine, Randomized controlled field trial

* Correspondence: didier.duivon@merck.com
[1]MSD Santé Animale, 7, rue Olivier de Serres - Angers Technopole, C.S. 17144, 49071 Beaucouzé cedex, France
Full list of author information is available at the end of the article

Background

Subclinical Porcine Circovirus type 2 (PCV2) infection is reported to be the most common form of PCV2 infection worldwide [1]. The only observed manifestation associated with this subclinical infection is a decreased average daily gain. Its diagnostic relies on the individual pig: absence of overt clinical signs, no or minimal histopathological lesions in tissues (mainly lymphoid) and low amount of PCV2 in few (lymphoid) tissues [1]. Since the availability of commercial PCV2 vaccines, veterinary practitioners have observed an improvement of growth performances, even in herds with no overt clinical signs of PCV2-associated diseases. Such field observations have been reported in Canada [2], the UK [3], Spain [4], Germany [5] and Switzerland [6]. Information on the cost of this condition is scarce, although the British report concludes that, at farm level, the economic impact of PCV2 can be mainly attributed to subclinically PCV2-infected pigs [3].

The objective of this trial was to assess the impact on growth performance in pigs of PCV2 vaccination under French farming conditions. In Western France (Brittany), Porcine Respiratory Disease Complex (PRDC) has been extensively studied; its main infectious risk factors are *Mycoplasma hyopneumoniae*, Porcine Reproductive and Respiratory Syndrome Virus (PRRSV) and the Swine influenza virus (SIV) H1N1, while PCV2 is less frequently identified [7]. However, an Austrian study of over 254,000 slaughtered pigs demonstrated that finishers raised on farrow-to-finish farms and that had not been vaccinated against PCV2 were at significantly higher risk of presenting pneumonia post-mortem than vaccinated fatteners from finisher farms [8]. Interestingly, Austria and Brittany have similar pig farm size and production systems.

Methods

A field trial was carried out on a French 180-sow farrow-to-finish farm, managed by the French Pork and Pig Institute (IFIP, Brittany) in order to evaluate a commercial bivalent vaccine that includes PCV2 and *M. hyopneumoniae* (Porcilis® PCV M Hyo) at weaning, and to compare it to a commercial monovalent one-shot *M. hyopneumoniae* bacterin vaccine.

The farm

The farm was managed under a strict 7-week all-in all-out system. Its health status was favourable: no active PRRSV circulation (high-parity sows are the only seropositive animals in the herd) and low SIV circulation post-weaning. Both enzootic pneumonia and atrophic rhinitis were present. All these pathogens were controlled through vaccination; no in-feed antibiotic supplementation was provided to the piglets post-weaning. Previous lung scoring indicated an average score of 2.3 out of 28, based on the scoring system according to Madec [9]. Its zootechnical and reproductive parameters place the farm among the top third of French farrow-to-finish farms.[1]

Piglet preparation

In a 24-sow batch, the otherwise routinely administered PCV2 booster vaccination was omitted, in order to avoid masking the potential effect of piglet PCV2 vaccination by dam vaccination [6]. All piglets born on this farm are individually identified and are weaned at 28 days of age. All piglets from this batch were individually weighed on day 27.

Group allocation of piglets

Within each litter, piglets were paired accounting for weight and sex; when no pair was available within a litter, the dam's parity and litter size were taken into consideration when pairing piglets of different litters. Within each pair of piglets, the first piglet was randomly allocated to either vaccine group and the second was allocated to the other vaccine group: the bivalent Porcilis® PCV M Hyo (MycPCV group) or a monovalent *M. hyopneumoniae* bacterin vaccine (Myc group). Both vaccines are based on the same *M. hyopneumoniae* vaccine strain (strain J).

Room/pen housing

During the entire trial, piglets from different vaccination groups were never mixed in the same pen.

At post-weaning, vaccinated piglets were placed in two identical rooms of 6 pens each, with 20 piglets per pen. All pens were identical in design and equipment (with the exception of their symmetry for the corridor, see Fig. 1), with a freely accessible feed trough.

After 6 weeks in post-weaning, piglets were individually weighed and transferred to the 2 adjacent fattening units. Again, all pens were identical in design and equipment, with an automatic feeding station. However, to comply with EU animal welfare regulation on stocking density, each fattening pen could only contain 14 pigs. Due to this constraint, only 84 out of the 120 pairs of piglets could be transferred to the on-site fattening unit.

To gain access to the automatic feeder, pigs have to push a door which lighter pigs (<20 kg live-weight) are not strong enough to open. As a consequence, only the pairs of piglets for which both individuals weighed over 20 kg and were healthy were transferred to fattening.

Pigs that were not doing well (arthritis, hernia...) or single pigs (death of the other pig in the pair) were discarded.[2] Pigs entering the fattening rooms were sorted for weight (three weight classes, see Fig. 1). Each pen only contained piglets from the same treatment group; in each room, MycPCV and Myc pens were

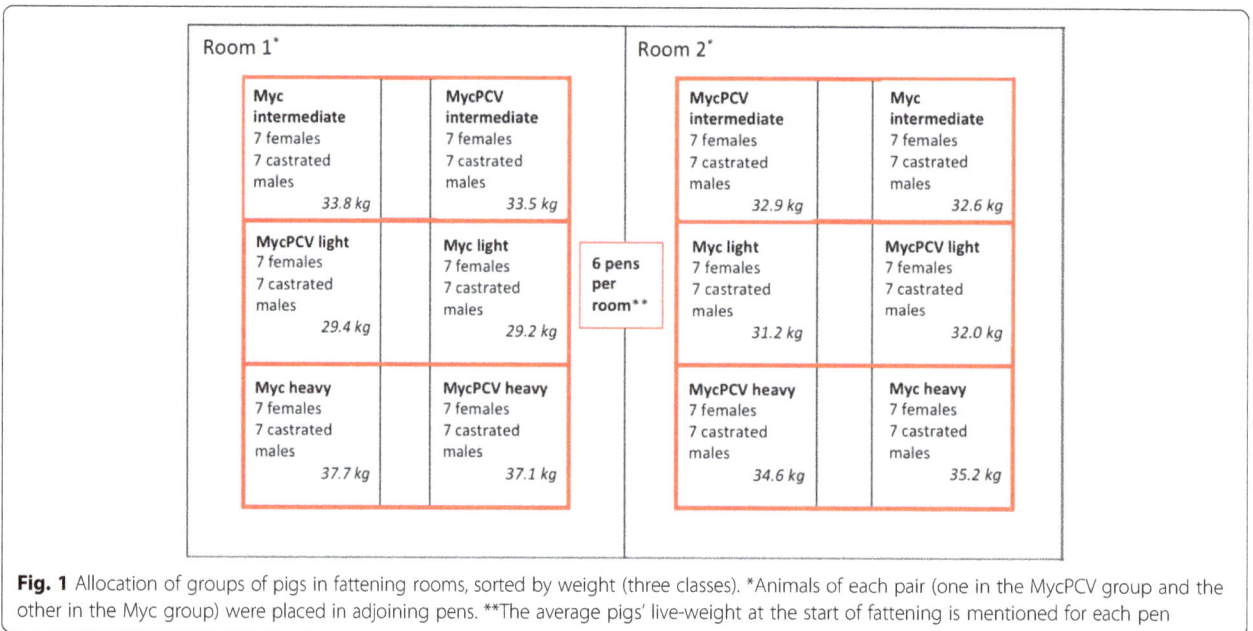

Fig. 1 Allocation of groups of pigs in fattening rooms, sorted by weight (three classes). *Animals of each pair (one in the MycPCV group and the other in the Myc group) were placed in adjoining pens. **The average pigs' live-weight at the start of fattening is mentioned for each pen

alternated. Automatic feeding stations recorded individual feed intake; feed was provided ad libitum.

All animals were individually weighed at regular intervals, starting 10 days after entering the fattening rooms to allow for adaptation to the automatic feeding system: at 14, 17, 20, 23 weeks of age and then every other week until slaughter.

Health monitoring

The animals were visited twice daily. All dead animals were removed from their pen for post-mortem examination. When the cause of death could not be ascribed to any other than a PCV2-related disease, mesenteric and inguinal lymph nodes were sampled, identified and frozen. Unthrifty pigs were humanely euthanized, and necropsied following the same protocol.

Blood was sampled from 18 pairs of pigs at 5 weeks of age, and from 12 pairs out of these 18 at 8 weeks of age. The same 12 pairs were repeatedly sampled at 12, 16, 20 and 23 weeks of age. Tests were performed at the Laboratory for Diagnostic Solutions Intervet Boxmeer, the Netherlands, with the IDEXX *M. hyo* Ab Test, the Alphalisa PCV type 2 (*M. hyopneumoniae* and PCV2 serology, respectively), and with an in-house quantitative PCR for PCV2 genome in serum (detection limit of $10^{2.9}$ genome copies per ml serum; quantification limit of $10^{3.4}$ genome copies per ml serum).

Lung checks

Lung checks were performed by the same operator, using the lung scoring system according to Madec [9].

Pathology

Frozen lymph node tissues were sent to the diagnostic laboratory (Labocea 22, Ploufragan, France). They were thawed and prepared for pathological examination. PCV2-like histopathological lesions were scored in compliance with current terminology [10].

Statistical analysis

Normality of variables was assessed with the Shapiro-Wilk test. A 5%-threshold was selected for the designation of a statistically significant difference. All statistical analyses were performed with SAS (SAS Institute Inc., Version 9.02). For fattening/finishing performances, the experimental unit was the pen. For clinical and pathological observation/scoring, the experimental unit was the individual pig. When a pig died, its paired piglet was also withdrawn from the data analyses.

Results

One hundred and twenty pairs of piglets (58 females, 62 castrated males) were vaccinated at 32 days of age. The body weight of the pigs at birth and weaning did not differ significantly between vaccine groups (variance analysis). The post-weaning average daily weight gain (ADG) did not differ significantly between the MycPCV (+511 g/d) and the Myc groups (+513 g/d, multifactorial variance analysis).

Out of the 84 pairs of piglets that entered the fattening rooms, 70 pairs made it to the slaughterhouse. The analysis of the performances was restricted to the data collected for these 140 pigs (see Table 1).

Pigs in the MycPCV group had an average + 34 g/d higher ADG over the fattening period than pigs in

Table 1 Performance of the 70 pairs of pigs that remained healthy over fattening

Variable	Myc group[a]				MycPCV group[b]				Difference	P value
	Average	Standard deviation	Mini	Maxi	Average	Standard deviation	Mini	Maxi		
Birth weight (kg)	1.5	0.3	0.9	3.0	1.6	0.3	0.8	2.4	0.0	>0.05
Weaning weight (kg)	9.0	1.4	5.3	12.7	9.0	1.4	6.0	12.5	0.0	>0.05
Weight at end of post-weaning (kg)	33.1	2.9	28.0	41.2	33.0	2.5	28.0	38.4	−0.1	>0.05
Post-weaning ADG (g/d)	512.8	56.7	375.5	653.0	511.1	49.6	395.7	634.0	−1.7	>0.05
Weight at start of fattening (kg)	37.2	3.4	30.2	46.6	36.4	3.3	28.4	43.5	−0.9	>0.05
Live-weight at slaughter (kg)	120.6	6.0	105.6	140.6	119.1	4.2	108.3	131.6	−1.5	>0.05
Fattening ADG (g/d)	850.5	85.3	615.9	1043.6	884.5	78.4	626.5	1023.9	33.9	=0.047
Fattening FCR	2.81	0.21	2.41	3.30	2.75	0.21	2.40	3.16	−0.06	>0.05
Age at slaughter (d)	182.5	11.6	161.0	198.0	177.7	9.5	161.0	198.0	−4.7	=0.049
Carcass yield[c]	0.8	0.0	0.7	0.8	0.8	0.0	0.7	0.8	0.0	>0.05
Lean %[c]	60.1	2.2	54.7	65.1	60.1	2.5	54.7	65.3	0.0	>0.05

[a]Six piglets from the Myc group died during fattening
[b]Ten piglets from the MycPCV group died during fattening. There was no statistical difference between the numbers of dead piglets in each group (exact Fischer test, $p > 0.05$)
[c]Data could be collected at slaughterhouse for 64 pairs of pigs

the Myc group; this difference was significant ($p = 0.047$). The feed conversion rate (FCR) and feed intake (data not shown) did not differ significantly between both groups over the fattening period (although the FCR was numerically lower in the MycPCV group, see Table 1).

Pigs in the MycPCV group were nearly 5 days younger at slaughter than Myc pigs ($p = 0.049$). After 186 days of age, 22 fatteners remained in the Myc group, while only 5 remained in the MycPCV group. Batch homogeneity was evaluated by comparing the distribution of the average, standard deviation and coefficient of variation of live-weights at first shipment to slaughter, the ages at

65 kg and slaughter age (data not shown). No significant difference in batch homogeneity was found, although slaughter age appeared to be more homogeneous in the MycPCV group (see Fig. 2). Carcase parameters did not differ significantly between groups (64 pairs evaluated).

M. hyopneumoniae antibody levels (S/P ratio) did not differ significantly between groups (non-parametric Mann-Whitney test), with the exception of 23 weeks of age (higher levels in MycPCV vs. Myc, $p < 0.05$), which might reflect a slower decay of post-vaccination *M. hyopneumoniae* antibody levels [11]. Both groups had otherwise similar serological profiles, with low antibody levels on weeks 5–8 (S/P ratio < 0.2, data not shown),

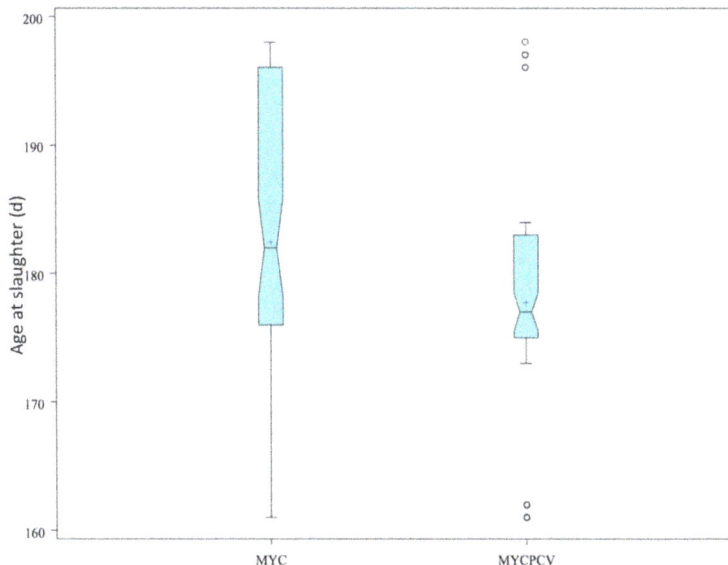

Fig. 2 Whiskers plot of the distribution of ages at slaughter for the 70 pairs of pigs

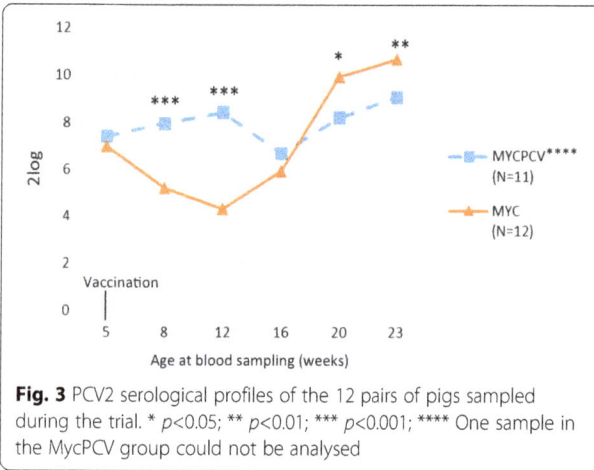

Fig. 3 PCV2 serological profiles of the 12 pairs of pigs sampled during the trial. * $p<0.05$; ** $p<0.01$; *** $p<0.001$; **** One sample in the MycPCV group could not be analysed

increasing levels on weeks 8–12 (peak S/P ratio at 0.4) at and a continuous decrease afterwards.

The PCV2 serological profiles differed greatly between groups (see Fig. 3). The Myc group piglets presented a clear decay in maternal PCV2 antibodies up to week 12. In both groups, the PCV2 genome could not be measured in the serum before week 12. A sharp increase in genomic serum loads was observed in week 16 in the Myc group (see Fig. 4), with a slow decline of the mean PCV2 genome load over the following weeks ($10^{5.2}$, $10^{5.6}$ and $10^{5.0}$ in weeks 16, 20 and 23 respectively). In contrast, pigs in the MycPCV group had significantly lower mean viraemia levels on weeks 16 and 20, and appeared to have cleared the infection by week 23 ($10^{1.7}$, $10^{2.0}$ and $10^{0.5}$ on weeks 16, 20 and 23 respectively). This difference is even more striking when comparing the areas under the curve (AUC) (normal distribution, Shapiro-Wilk test, $p = 0.4413$): 51.19 ± 13.33 in the Myc group and 16.70 ± 11.20 in the MycPCV group (Student t test, $p = 8.583 \, 10^{-7}$).

When the viremia results were obtained, the supervising veterinarian, in order to confirm whether the effect of PCV2 infection was observable in the tissues of the dead pigs (no overt clinical sign of PCV2-associated disease had been observed during the trial), sent the biological samples that had been stored in proper conditions (frozen) to the diagnostic laboratory. Three pigs in each group had died over the period of the PCV2 viremia peak (weeks 16–23). PCV2-like histopathological lesions, and PCV2 antigen in the lesions based on immunohistochemistry, were observed in the lymph nodes of 2 out of the 3 pigs from the Myc group that had died, while no such lesion/marking was observed in any of the 3 dead pigs from the MycPCV group (see Fig. 5).

Lung scoring was performed at the slaughterhouse for the 84 pairs of pigs. The average LLS was lower in the MycPCV group than in the Myc group (0.9 vs. 2.2, respectively), but this difference was not statistically significant ($p = 0.09$, non-parametric Wilcoxon test). However, the proportion of pigs with a LLS ≤ 4 was significantly higher in the MycPCV group than in the Myc group (94 vs. 84%, respectively, $p = 0.04$, Chi-2 test). In addition, no pig in the MycPCV group had a score over 7, whereas 10% of pigs in the Myc group did (see Fig. 6).

Discussion

The significant difference in ADG over fattening in the group vaccinated against both PCV2 and *M. hyopneumoniae*, as compared to the group vaccinated against *M. hyopneumoniae* alone is consistent with results of a recently published Spanish study on the efficacy of piglet PCV2 vaccination in farms with and without overt clinical signs of PCV2-associated diseases [4]. In both farms, ADG was significantly improved by vaccination during the fattening stage, but not over the post-weaning period. In a Canadian trial where only PCV2 vaccination

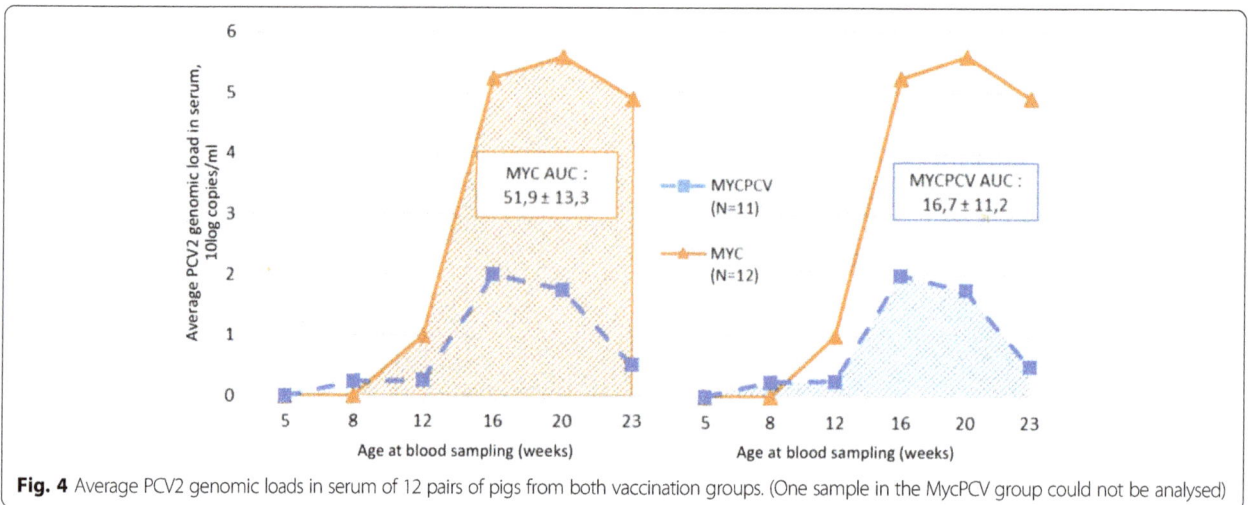

Fig. 4 Average PCV2 genomic loads in serum of 12 pairs of pigs from both vaccination groups. (One sample in the MycPCV group could not be analysed)

was performed at weaning (at 3 weeks of age, against placebo), ADG was found to be greater ($p < 0.01$) in the vaccinates than in the controls over the entire study period, even though a clinical ileitis break occurred between finishing days 57–70 in both groups [2]. Also, the level of ADG improvement over finishing (940 in vaccinates vs. 904 g/d in controls, $p < 0.01$) was found to be comparable to that in the present study (36 and 38 g/d). However, the Canadian herd had a high-health status, with higher growth performance levels than in our trial. In our study design, piglets of the two groups were not commingled in pens, but allocated to separate pens. This might hamper the distinction between the pen-effect and the group-effect. However, the farm in the study was built recently and all pens had an identical structure and equipment; the only difference being the symmetrical disposition around the alley. As the groups were alternately distributed on either side of the alley, it is highly likely that the pen-effect on the measured results is at most limited, if not negligible.

Risk of *M. hyopneumoniae* seropositivity increases with age and production system [11]. In our study, pigs from both groups had comparable serological profiles, with a continuous antibody level decline after week 12. This is suggestive of a vaccine-related seroconversion, rather than one triggered by field challenge.

PCV2 seroconversion took place between 12 and 16 weeks of age, as a result of exposure to the virus, with a marked increase later on. In the MycPCV group, vaccination was followed by a steady increase in PCV2 antibodies until week 12, followed by a drop in week 16. The subsequent seroconversion might be interpreted as the consequence of a delayed PCV2 circulation, due to 'herd immunity'. Differences in levels of PCV2 viremia between both groups confirm that non-PCV2-vaccinated pigs develop a significantly higher viremia and for a longer duration than vaccinated ones. The viremia levels observed in the Myc group (5.6 log10 genome copies/ml serum) were consistent with the 'high' viral load in pigs from a Spanish study of two 5000-sow farms that had a strongly decreased ADG between 3 to 21 weeks [12].

The shorter and lower viremia, the improved ADG, the tendency to an improved homogeneity and an absence of PCV2-like pathological lesions in the lymph nodes of the necropsied PCV2-vaccinated pigs support the protective efficacy of PCV2 vaccination in the face of a subclinical PCV2 infection in a conventional pig farm in Western France.

In terms of economic benefit, age at slaughter was significantly improved by 4.7 days ($p < 0.05$, Table 1). Also, a cost simulation was performed with the online tool designed by IFIP,[3] which calculated that, for a given 196-sow French farrow-to-finish farm under a 7-week management, the improvement of the fattening ADG by

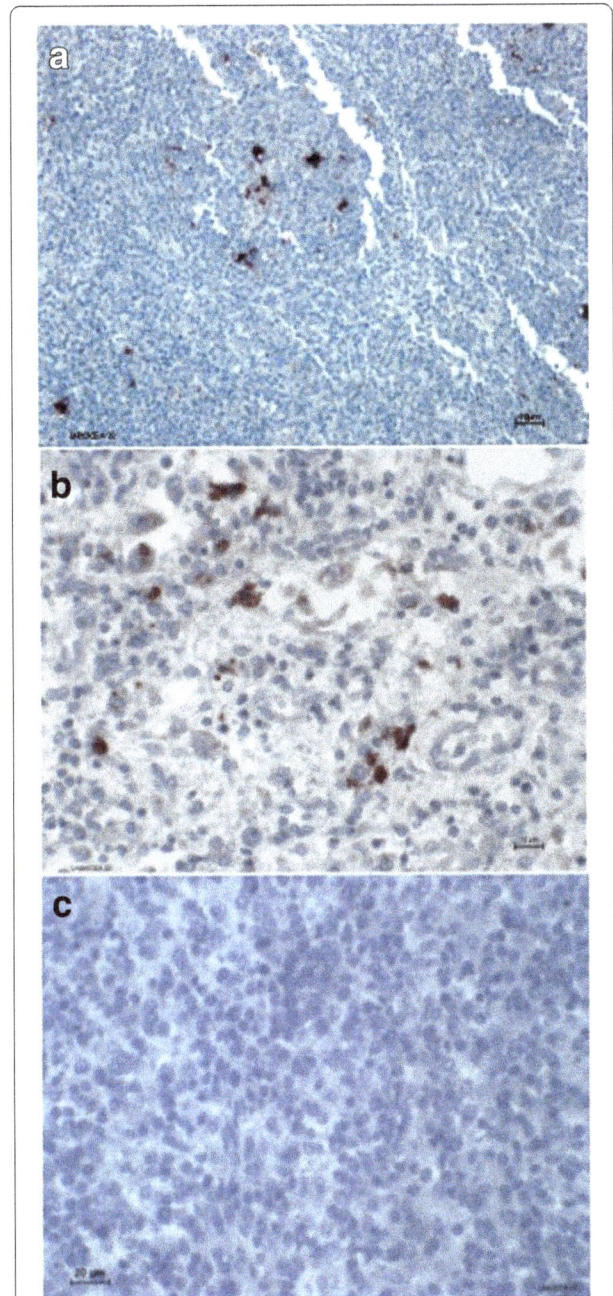

Fig. 5 Immunohistochemistry results on lymph nodes of pigs dead during the fattening period (scale bars: A, 40 μm; B, 15 μm; C, 20 μm). **a**. Weakly PCV2-positive immunohistochemistry of a lymph node from a dead pig of the Mhyo group, whose pathology presented a marked granulomatous lymphadenitis, highly suggestive of PCV2-associated lesions. **b**. PCV2-positive (+ and ++) immunohistochemistry stains of a lymph node from a dead pig of the Mhyo group, whose pathology presented a moderate lymphadenitis, suggestive of PCV2-associated lesions. **c**. No obvious PCV2-positive IHC in a lymph node from a pig dead of gastric ulceration in of the Mhyo group

34 g/d corresponded to €1.7 extra revenue per slaughtered pig (€39 additional revenue per sow per year). This calculation takes into account the higher price of the

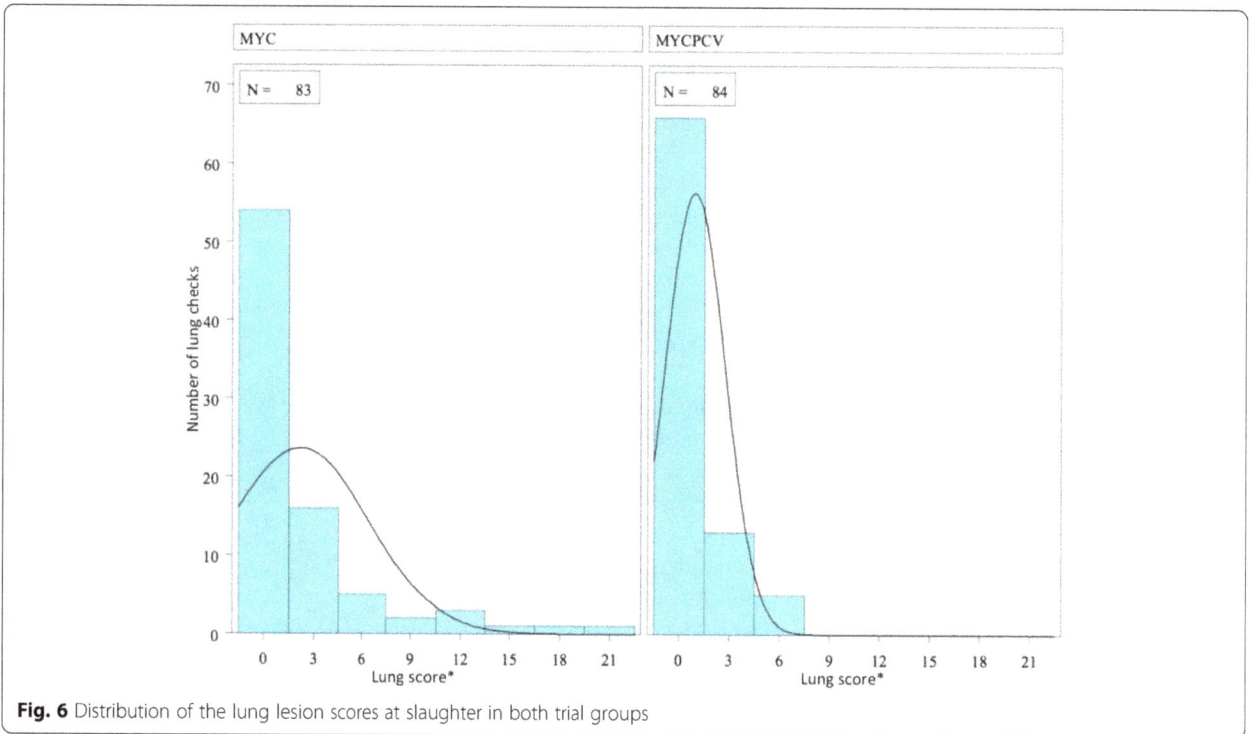

Fig. 6 Distribution of the lung lesion scores at slaughter in both trial groups

combination vaccine (as compared to the one-shot *M. hyopneumoniae* vaccine). This estimate seems conservative, even for the year of the trial. A British model estimated that each sub-clinically infected (unvaccinated) pig that reaches slaughter represents a mean loss of €9.52 (90% confidence interval: €2.56–17.75, Alarcon, 2013[4]), at a time when price for live swine was comparable between France and UK.

Conclusion

The trial was conducted in a farm with housing conditions and health status reflecting those of conventional facilities in Western France. The growth and reproductive performance levels of the farm are in the top-third of the French farrow-to-finish farms. Piglets were routinely vaccinated at weaning (4 weeks of age) with a one-shot *M. hyopneumoniae* bacterin vaccine. The study shows that, compared to that vaccine, the use of Porcilis® PCV M Hyo had no detrimental effect on growth performance post-weaning. It also significantly increased the growth performance during fattening (+34 g/d), while decreasing the age at slaughter by 5 days. These results led to an increase of the net profit by at least €1.7 per slaughtered pig (€39 per sow per year), including the extra-cost of the bivalent vaccine.

Improved FCR and homogeneity of pig batches were also observed, although the changes were not significant, possibly because of the limited number of pigs in the trial (*n* = 140), due to the automatic feeding system constraints.

The positive outcome observed in the MycPCV group suggests an improved control of PCV2 infection (lower viremia, of shorter duration, absence of PCV2-like lesions) through vaccination with Porcilis® PCV M. Hyo.

Endnotes

[1]These references are available online for 2015 and previous years, in French, at: http://www.ifip.asso.fr/fr/resultats-economiques-gttt-graphique.html

[2]Sixteen pigs died during the trial: 10 in the MycPCV group and 6 in the Myc group (no significant difference, exact Fischer test). This higher than usual mortality was associated with heat stress (gastric ulcers were the cause of 63% of deaths): a heat wave occurred during fattening.

[3]This tool is freely available at: http://pigsim.com/EN/Presentation/Pages/default.aspx

[4]This estimate was expressed in GBP in the original article, with 8.1 GBP mean loss per subclinically infected pig to reach slaughter.

Abbreviations

ADG: Average daily gain; AUC: Area under the curve; EU: European Union; FCR: Feed Conversion Rate; GBP: British Pound; LLS: Lung lesion score; PCR: Polymerase Chain Reaction; PCV2: Porcine Circovirus type 2; PRRS: Porcine Reproductive and Respiratory Syndrome; PRRSV: Porcine Reproductive and Respiratory Syndrome Virus; SIV: Swine Influenza Virus

Acknowledgements

The authors are grateful to Dr. Nadia Amenna (Labocea22, Ploufragan, France) for processing, reading and interpreting the organs submitted for pathological examination, and for providing the corresponding figures.

Field evaluation of piglet vaccination with a Mycoplasma hyopneumoniae bacterin as compared...

157

Funding
MSD Animal Health France and IFIP each funded half of the study costs.

Authors' contributions
CI was investigator and statistician of the study and main author of the manuscript. DD was monitor of the study, took part in animal manipulation and data collection and reviewed the manuscript. JR was in charge of sponsor management and reviewed the manuscript. HA, RM and RD took part in animal manipulation and data collection. All authors read and approved the final manuscript.

Competing interests
With the exception of the second and third authors, all other authors of this case report are employees of the sponsor company.

Author details
[1]MSD Santé Animale, 7, rue Olivier de Serres - Angers Technopole, C.S. 17144, 49071 Beaucouzé cedex, France. [2]IFIP, La Motte au Vicomte, 35650 Le Rheu, France. [3]MSD Animal Health, 2 Giralda Farms, Madison, NJ 07940, USA.

References
1. Segalés J. Porcine circovirus type 2 (PCV2) infections: clinical signs, pathology and laboratory diagnosis. Virus Res. 2012;164(1–2):10–9.
2. Young MG, Cunningham GL, Sanford SE. Circovirus vaccination in pigs with subclinical porcine circovirus type 2 infection complicated by ileitis. J Swine Health Prod. 2011;19(3):175–80. https://www.aasv.org/shap/issues/v19n3/v19n3p175.pdf
3. Alarcon P, Rushton J, Wieland B. Cost of post-weaning multi-systemic wasting syndrome and porcine circovirus type-2 subclinical infection in England - an economic disease model. Prev Vet Med. 2013;110(2):88–102. http://ac.els-cdn.com/S016758771300041X/1-s2.0-S016758771300041X-main.pdf?_tid=e48e5672-6940-11e6-a676-00000aab0f6c&acdnat=1471963991_ae5fbc7ceca31363d6858814eb0b9f26
4. Fraile L, Grau-Roma L, Sarasola P, Sinovas N, Nofrarías M, López-Jimenez R, López-Soria S, Sibila M, Segalés J. Inactivated PCV2 one shot vaccine applied in 3-week-old piglets: improvement of production parameters and interaction with maternally derived immunity. Vaccine. 2012;30(11):1986–92.
5. Heißenberger B, Weissenbacher-Lang C, Hennig-Pauka I, Ritzmann M, Ladinig A. Efficacy of vaccination of 3-week-old piglets with Circovac against porcine circovirus diseases (PCVD). Trials Vaccinology 2013;2(2):1-9. http://ac.els-cdn.com/S1879437813000028/1-s2.0-S1879437813000028-main.pdf?_tid=5b7a35ce-6a10-11e6-ba18-00000aacb362&acdnat=1472053096_62450311b083a2ad9ec4245db65cc952.
6. Kurmann J, Sydler T, Brugnera E, Buergi E, Haessig M, Suter M, Sidler X. Vaccination of dams increases antibody titer and improves growth parameters in finisher pigs subclinically infected with porcine Circovirus type 2. Clin Vaccine Immunol. 2011;18(10):1644–9. http://cvi.asm.org/content/18/10/1644.full.pdf+html
7. Fablet C, Marois-Créhan C, Simon G, Grasland B, Jestin A, Kobisch M, Madec F, Rose N. Infectious agents associated with respiratory diseases in 125 farrow-to-finish pig herds: a cross-sectional study. Vet Microbiol. 2012;157(1–2):152–63.
8. Raith J, Kuchling S, Schleicher C, Schobesberger H, Köfer J. Influence of porcine circovirus type 2 vaccination on the probability and severity of pneumonia detected postmortem. Vet Rec. 2015;176(5):124–30. http://veterinaryrecord.bmj.com/content/176/5/124.full.pdf+html
9. Madec F, Kobisch M. Lung lesion scoring of finisher pigs at the slaughterhouse [in French]. Journées de la Recherche Porcine. 1982;14:405–12.
10. Opriessnig T, Meng XJ, Halbur PG. Porcine circovirus type 2 associated disease: update on current terminology, clinical manifestations, pathogenesis, diagnosis, and intervention strategies. J Vet Diagn Investig. 2007;19(6):591–615. http://vdi.sagepub.com/content/19/6/591.full.pdf+html
11. Giacomini E, Ferrari N, Pitozzi A, Remistani M, Giardiello D, Maes D, Alborali GL. Dynamics of Mycoplasma hyopneumoniae seroconversion and infection in pigs in the three main production systems. Vet Res Commun. 2016;40(2):81–8.
12. López-Soria S, Sibila M, Nofrarías M, Calsamiglia M, Manzanilla EG, Ramírez-Mendoza H, Mínguez A, Serrano JM, Marín O, Joisel F, Charreyre C, Segalés J. Effect of porcine circovirus type 2 (PCV2) load in serum on average daily weight gain during the postweaning period. Vet Microbiol. 2014;174(3–4):296–301.

18

Detection of *Cystoisospora suis* in faeces of suckling piglets – when and how? A comparison of methods

Anja Joachim[1][*] [iD], Bärbel Ruttkowski[1] and Daniel Sperling[2]

Abstract

Background: *Cystoisospora suis* is the causative agent of porcine neonatal coccidiosis, a diarrheal disease which affects suckling piglets in the first weeks of life. Detection of oocysts in the faeces of infected animals is frequently hampered by the short individual excretion period and the high fat content of faecal samples. We analysed oocyst excretion patterns of infected piglets, evaluated different detection methods for their detection limit and reproducibility, and propose a sampling scheme to improve the diagnosis of *C. suis* in faecal samples from the field using a protocol for reliable parasite detection.

Results: Based on a hypothesized model of the course of infection on a farm, three samplings (days of life 7–14-21 or 10–15-20) should be conducted including individual samples of piglets from each sampled litter. Samples can be examined by a modified McMaster method (lower detection limit: 333 oocysts per gram of faeces, OpG), by examining faecal smears under autofluorescence (lower detection limit: 10 OpG) or after carbol-fuchsin staining (lower detection limit: 100 OpG). Reproducibility and inter-test correlations were high with ($R^2 > 0.8$). A correlation of oocyst excretion with diarrhoea could not be established so samples with different faecal consistencies should be taken. Pooled samples (by litter) should be comprised of several individual samples from different animals.

Conclusions: Since oocyst excretion by *C. suis*-infected piglets is usually short the right timing and a sufficiently sensitive detection method are important for correct diagnosis. Oocyst detection in faecal smears of samples taken repeatedly is the method of choice to determine extent and intensity of infection on a farm, and autofluorescence microscopy provides by far the lowest detection limit. Other methods for oocyst detection in faeces are less sensitive and/or more labour- and cost intensive and their usefulness is restricted to specific applications.

Keywords: Piglets, Coccidia, *Isospora suis*, Methods, McMaster, Faecal scoring, Carbol-fuchsin, Autofluorescence

Background

Detection of coccidial infections in domestic animals including pigs can be necessary in a variety of cases. In post mortem examinations of dead piglets, stages of *Cystoisospora suis*, the most important species of coccidia in pigs [1] can be found in histological sections and impression smears (e.g. [2]). This can be helpful in cases of prepatent infections and to determine the extent of pathological changes in relation to parasite infection. As for other enteropathogens, the detection of stages in faeces is a frequent routine to determine an infection in a litter or a herd (usually in relation to clinical signs - in case of coccidiosis, diarrhoea and poor weight gain – or to determine the status of animals as oocyst shedders to estimate the extent of environmental contamination by clinically healthy carriers. In some cases, the efficacy of control strategies is evaluated by determining oocyst excretion after intervention, usually in experimental studies (cf. [3]). Drug resistance has been described for anticoccidial drugs in chicken and recently also in pigs [4, 5] and evaluation of treatment efficacy by faecal examination in the field may also become important in mammalian host species including piglets.

In suckling animals, several issues need to be taken into consideration to accurately determine infection in a litter or a herd. We evaluated sampling schemes and

---

* Correspondence: Anja.Joachim@vetmeduni.ac.at
[1]Institute of Parasitology, Department of Pathobiology, University of Veterinary Medicine Vienna, Veterinaerplatz 1, A-1210 Vienna, Austria
Full list of author information is available at the end of the article

compared the different methods available for the detection and quantification of *C. suis* in piglet faeces and propose a methodology for reliable detection of the parasite in a herd and to evaluate treatment efficacy in cases where treatment failure is suspected.

Results

Course of excretion and diarrhoea and sampling time point

Typically, individual animals show a biphasic excretion pattern upon infection with a steep onset at the beginning of patency, usually five to 6 days after infection (Fig. 1). Excretion can be observed for one to 10 days (median: 5 days) but can be longer in single animals. Similarly, diarrhoea lasts for two to 5 days (median: 4 days) in most animals after experimental infection but can be prolonged in single piglets and is poorly correlated with excretion (Fig. 2). With such a short duration of acute illness and parasite shedding, it can be difficult to determine infections in individual piglets. In a model assuming that all piglets become infected and excrete oocysts for at least 1 day during the suckling period, the prevalence on any 1 day of sampling still never exceeded one third of the animals (Fig. 3). Since it is unknown when infection in the field takes place in individuals or litters, repeated sampling increases the detection rates (Fig. 4). As diarrhoea and excretion are only weakly correlated and do not occur simultaneously (Fig. 1; [6]) a preference for collection of semi-liquid or liquid (diarrhoeic) samples is not indicated.

Detection of oocysts

After flotation by centrifugation parasitic objects could not be removed from the surface as all centrifugation tubes showed large fatty plugs on top of the flotation medium (Fig. 4) which prevented access to the oocysts. The plugs were removed and treated like faecal smears but could not be stained as crystals of sugar and/or salt interfered with the staining (not shown).

Autofluorescence of oocysts could be observed as the emission of blue light form the oocyst (and in sporulated oocysts the sporocyst) wall (Fig. 5). Oocysts of *C. suis* are 18×20 μm in size and can easily be differentiated from Eimeria oocysts by their roundish appearance, their thin, smooth wall and, after sporulation, by the number of sporocysts [1].

In stained smears, oocysts (which usually remain unstained against a coloured background) were detectable only in thin smears (dilution 1:10 compared to those for autofluorescence) but not in thick ones. In unstained samples no oocysts could be visualised under the light microscope. The staining protocol with carbol-fuchsin was the most convenient and the fastest and clearly showed colourless oocysts against the red background (Fig. 6). Counterstaining, e.g. with methylene blue, which is often used to visualised oocysts of cryptosporidia (e.g. [7]), was not necessary for *C. suis* oocysts due to their larger size compared to cryptosporidia (details not shown).

When carbol-fuchsin staining was compared to autofluorescence, all samples were positive for autofluorescence but only 30% were positive after carbol-fuchsin staining, and 43% of the samples that were McMaster positive were also positive upon carbol-fuchsin staining. In firm faeces the detection rate in carbol-fuchsin strained samples was higher (39%) than in loose faeces (28%). The latter also contained fewer oocysts on average (1748 vs. 8288 mean OpG).

Quantification of oocysts

As outlined above, oocysts can be evaluated semi-quantitatively in faecal smears. Counting in a counting

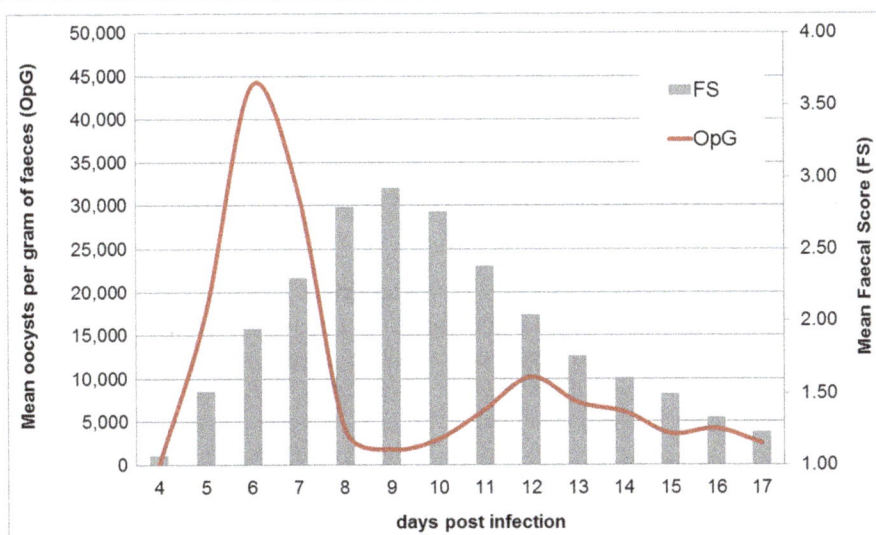

Fig. 1 Course of *C. suis* infections; $n = 117$ piglets from different infection trials, adapted from [8]

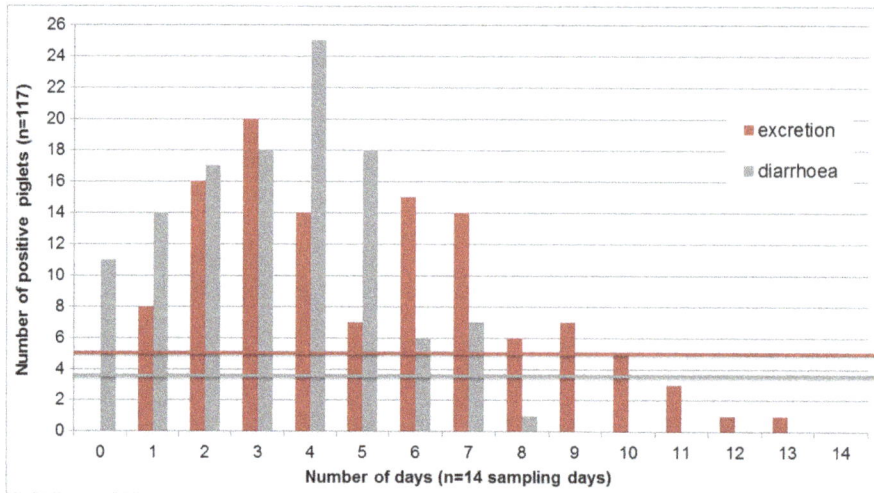

Fig. 2 Number of oocyst excretion days and diarrhoea days over a sampling period of 14 days (4–17 days post infection; n = 117 piglets); adapted from [8]. Horizontal bars: mean values (excretion: 5.1 days, diarrhoea: 3.6 days)

chamber is, however, more accurate since an exact amount of faecal matter can be used irrespective of the faecal consistency. Using the sugar-salt flotation solution in combination with filtration, oocysts could be suspended for floatation in the McMaster chambers. We have adapted this method to small amounts of faeces for the determination of OpGs in individual samples (standard amount of faeces 0.5 g; [6, 8]) or subsets of pooled samples from several individuals in a litter.

The correlations between OpG values and oocyst counts in smears were high with $R^2 = 0.90$ for autofluorescence and $R^2 = 0.98$ for carbol-fuchsin staining (and $R^2 = 0.97$ for autofluorescence v.s. carbol-fuchsin staining), but the mean oocyst counts were considerably higher in the samples examined by autofluorescence (mean: 28.1) than in the carbol-fuchsin-stained samples (mean: 8.5). The calculated lower cut-off for detection of oocysts is 10 OpG for autofluorescence, 100 OpG for the carbol-fuchsin staining (since it requires a 1:10 dilution in comparison to autofluorescence-based examination of faecal smears), and 333 OpG for McMaster. Consequently autofluorescence had the highest percentage of positive samples and the highest absolute oocyst counts (Fig. 7).

Comparison of oocyst counts in faecal smears (only positive samples) showed that 28.6% of these had a count > 50 by both examiners, and the inexperienced examiner evaluated two samples (4.1%) as above the cut-off of 50 oocysts (experienced examiner: counts: 46 and 49 oocysts). For the counted oocysts in samples < 50 oocysts (*n* = 35) the correlation (Pearson) was 0.993 (Fig. 8).

Examination of two separately prepared McMaster counts from 50 samples (2 preparations/sample) showed a correlation of 0.852 (Pearson's correlation coefficient)

between sample 1 and sample 2 (Fig. 9). Out of 50 samples, 18% were negative in both examinations, 20% were positive in 1 out of 2 examinations (with counts of 1 or 2 oocysts in the positive samples except one sample were seven oocysts were counted). Of the 31 samples that were positive in both examinations, 11 had OpG values between 333 and 3333 (low OpG), 13 and OpG of > 3333–10,000 in the first count (medium OpG) and 9 had an OpG > 10,000 (max 313,000; high OpG). Only two of the samples that were positive in both counts had identical OpGs (333 and 667, respectively). The deviations were highest in the low-OpG group with a mean of 3.2× (max: 9.0×) and similar in the medium- (mean 2.2-fold, max 5.0-fold) and high-OpG group (mean 2.1-fold, max 4.0-fold).

Comparison of count results of the same sample by two examiners (*n* = 175 McMaster samples) showed that 65.5% of the samples were evaluated as negative by both examiners and 33.3% were evaluated as positive by both. 1.5% were considered positive (single oocyst counts in each sample) by the unexperienced and negative by the experienced examiner. The correlation of OpGs was very high with 0.998 (Fig. 10).

Discussion

Lately, anecdotal reports of reduced efficacy of toltrazuril treatment and the first confirmed resistance case are pointing at *C. suis* as a "re-emerging" cause of diarrhoea in suckling piglets, and we aimed to encourage swine practitioners to include this parasite into the regular diagnostic panel irrespective of the treatment history, and we propose a sampling scheme to optimise detection in conjunction with evaluated methods of appropriate detection levels.

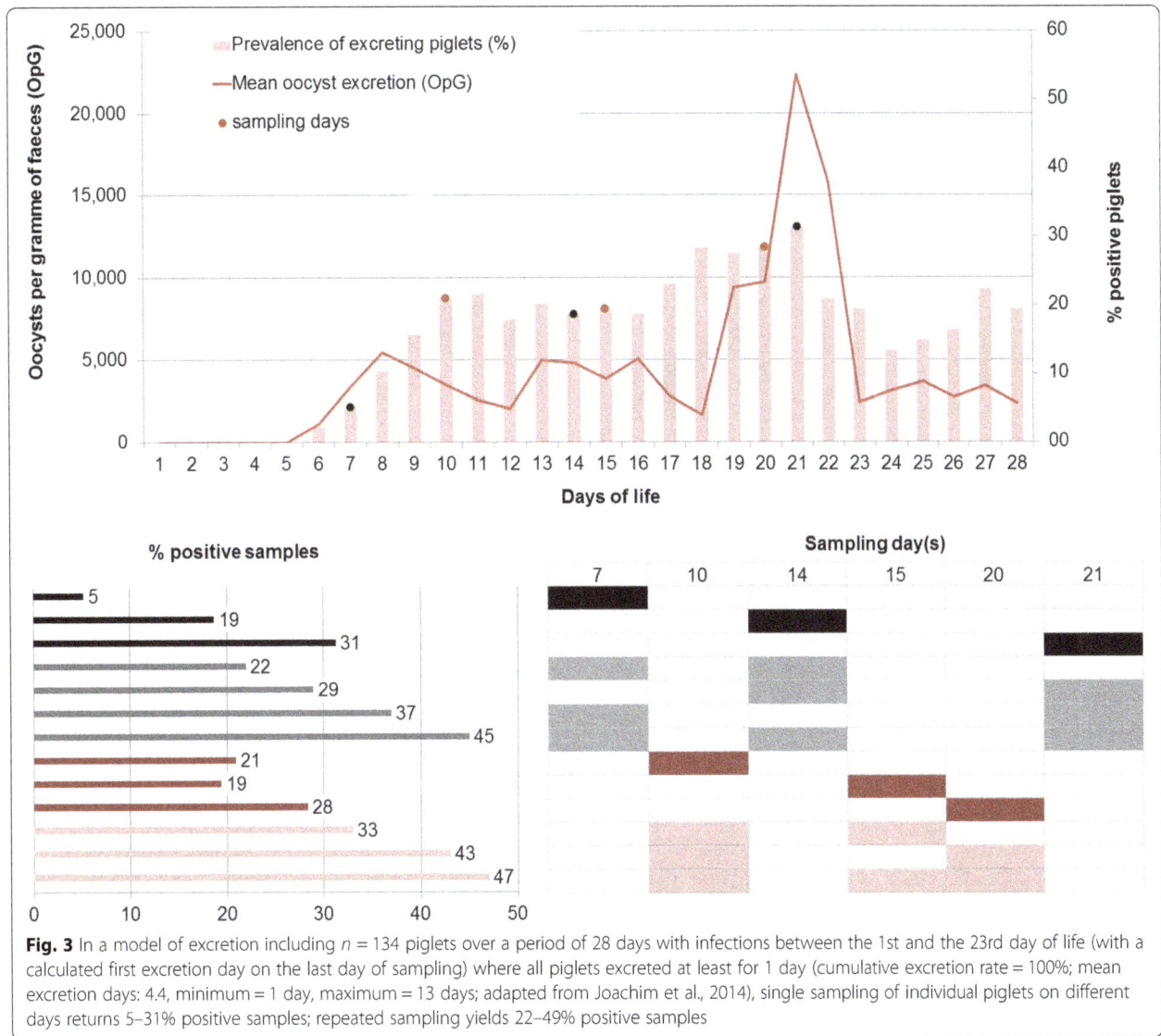

Fig. 3 In a model of excretion including *n* = 134 piglets over a period of 28 days with infections between the 1st and the 23rd day of life (with a calculated first excretion day on the last day of sampling) where all piglets excreted at least for 1 day (cumulative excretion rate = 100%; mean excretion days: 4.4, minimum = 1 day, maximum = 13 days; adapted from Joachim et al., 2014), single sampling of individual piglets on different days returns 5–31% positive samples; repeated sampling yields 22–49% positive samples

Patterns of excretion and diarrhoea – When to take samples

In most *primo* infections of piglets with *C. suis*, excretion shows a sudden onset, often accompanied by changes of faecal consistency. To determine the correlation between the onset of excretion with diarrhoea, field and experimental studies were evaluated [8–10] but no clear pattern could be determined. In experimental infections the correlation between quantitative oocyst excretion and faecal consistency was weak [6], probably due to the diluting effect of diarrhoea with larger amounts of faeces. It is therefore not advisable to take primarily samples from piglets wit diarrhoea, as such samples may contain few oocysts. Clinically, neonates are most severely affected while infections of older suckling piglets usually display few clinical signs and only low oocyst shedding [11–13]. Older pigs

are largely refractory to infection and excretion and diarrhoea are very unusual unless temporary immunosuppression occurs, e.g. in a case of acute viral infections, like in a herd of Swiss fatteners reported lately [14]. Sows usually show low shedding rates with few oocysts [15] which is in part supposedly due to acquired immunity, but also attributed to the pronounced age resistance in *C. suis* infections [12]. Therefore, sampling sows to determine infection on a farm is frequently unsuccessful and samples must be taken from suckling piglets. Prepatency of *C. suis* is four to 5 days so sampling piglets of younger age will not yield a positive result.

Since excretion is usually short (4–5 days on average in the evaluated experimental settings) it may be necessary to sample litters repeatedly to reliably detect oocysts on a farm to confirm the presence of the parasite, or to

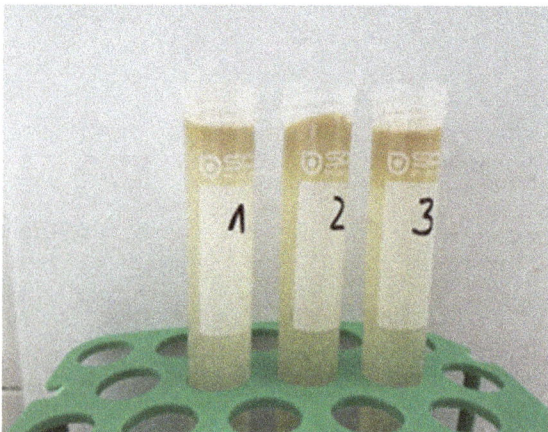

Fig. 4 Lipid plugs formed on top of the flotation solutions (1: Sheather's modified sugar solution, 2: sugar-salt solution, 3: sugar-salt solution + detergent; for details see Materials and Methods) preventing the removal of any parasite objects from the surface

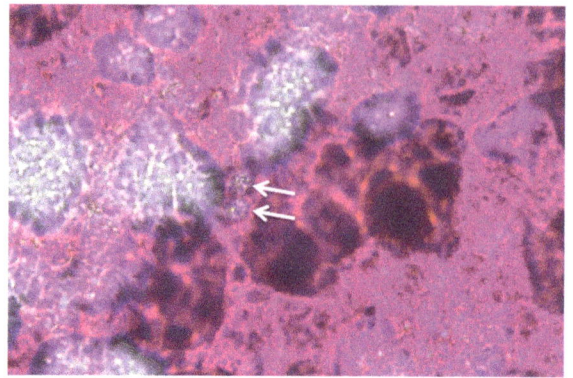

Fig. 6 Staining of thin faecal smears for detection of *C. suis* oocysts with carbol-fuchsin. Magnification: 200×. Arrows: unstained sporulated oocysts

sample a sufficient number of animals to evaluate treatment success. Even under the assumption that all piglets become infected and shed oocysts before weaning (which might not be the case when infection pressure is low) with a single sampling, the detection rate will not exceed one third of samples, while sampling three times (at 7, 14 or 21 days or 10, 15 and 20 days of age) detects almost half of the positive piglets. Assuming that in a litter all (or almost all) piglets become infected within 1 week, it is possible to reliably detect the parasite in a litter when it is sampled at least twice, and on farms when

samples are taken at three different time points. The number of samples to be taken varies with the size of the herd, but examining samples pooled by litter from a maximum of 30 litters (in herds with > 30 sows) will return sufficiently reliable results [15–17].

Detection and quantification of oocysts in faeces

Several methods of detection have been published that can be applied; however, many of them are not suitable for routine diagnostics. Molecular tools have been used to detect and differentiate stages in faeces with high sensitivity and specificity [18–21] but the processing of samples for DNA extraction from tough oocysts is time-consuming and the high costs of the assay are still prohibitive for routine examination.

Although oocysts are often present in high numbers in individual samples, detection by concentration before microscopic examination can be hampered by the high content of fat in suckling piglets' faeces (and especially in cases of steatorrhea as described for cystoisosporosis; [22, 23]), which can both prevent detection of oocysts by flotation and impede correct diagnosis in smears as lipid droplets may be taken for unsporulated oocysts. Concentration of oocysts from faecal material of suckling piglets can be problematic since the high fat content may lead to aggregation of a lipid layer with enclosed oocysts on top of the flotation solution after centrifugation. Several modifications of standard protocols are described in the literature. The most common flotation medium for *C. suis* oocysts is Sheather's sugar solution or modifications of it [24–30]. In our hands, however, none of the applied flotation solutions, even with the use of detergent, could prevent the formation of fat plugs. An alternative to remove most of the fat in piglet faeces is the use of Percoll® in an additional sedimentation step.

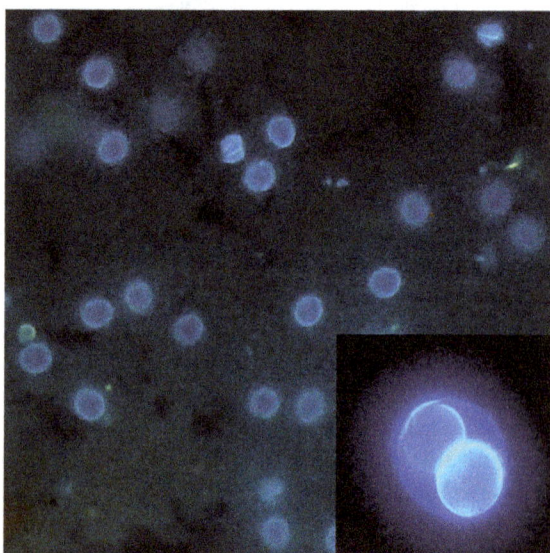

Fig. 5 Autofluorescence of unsporulated (large mage, 200× magnification) and sporulated (small image, 600× magnification) oocysts of *C. suis*

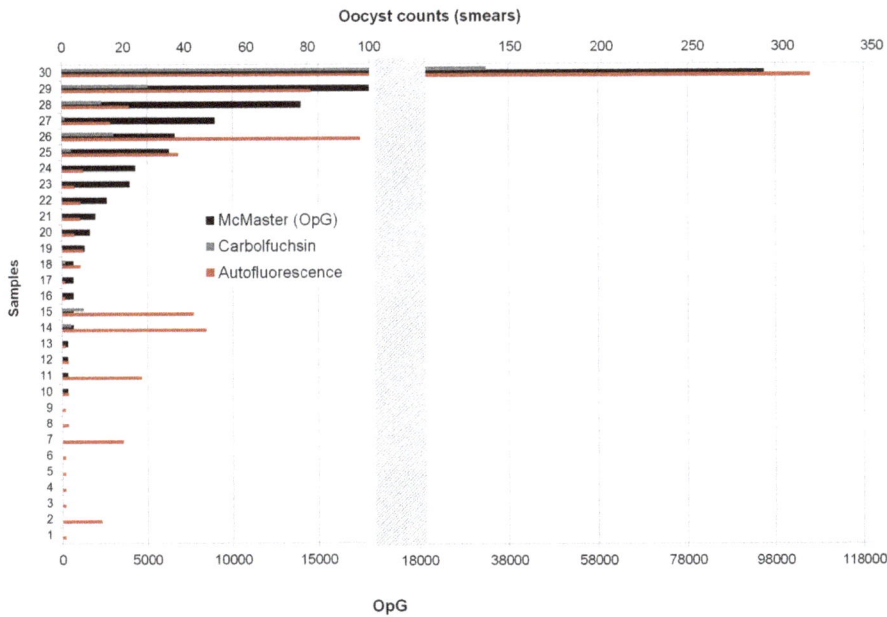

Fig. 7 Comparison of McMaster counting (given as OpG) and oocyst counts in smears examined by autofluorescence or light microscopy after carbol-fuchsin staining

Percoll® (GE Healthcare) is a density gradient separation medium of low viscosity, low osmolarity and low toxicity. It has been used as flotation solution for *C. suis* in piglet faeces with good success [31] but it is expensive and can be replaced by the cheaper sugar-salt flotation medium. It is, however, most suitable for concentration of oocysts from faeces by sedimentation for further processing of oocysts, e.g. for flotation (Joachim and Ruttkowski, unpublished data).

Some authors prefer the faecal smear with staining over the flotation concentration for reasons stated above [32, 33]. Detection in smears under light microscopy as suggested in earlier works [32, 34] is of poor sensitivity and specificity [35]. However, when autofluorescence is used both can be improved considerably [35]. Upon UV excitation, the walls of the oocysts (and in sporulated oocysts those of the sporocysts) emit a bright blue light that greatly facilitates detection. This phenomenon called autofluorescence has long been known to occur in oocysts of different coccidia [36–39] and is presumably due to tyrosine which is cross-linked in the oocyst wall [40].

Autofluorescence microscopy requires the use of a fluorescence microscope with suitable filters that are standard only in larger laboratories, but the running

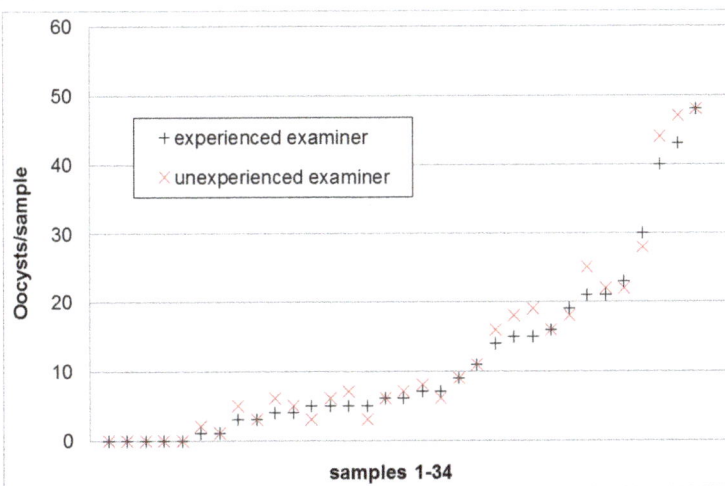

Fig. 8 Comparison of absolute oocyst counts by 2 different examiners, an experienced and an unexperienced one of the same faecal smear examined by the autofluorescence method

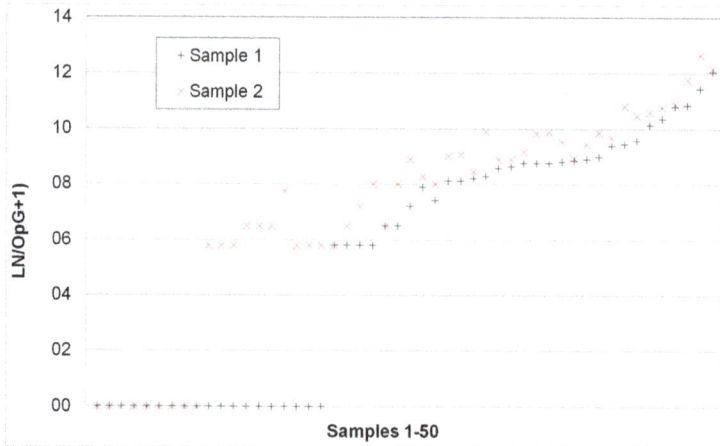

Fig. 9 Comparison of OpG counts from 2 independent preparations of the same faecal sample. For better visualisation the higher value was always defined as sample 1 and the lower value as sample 2

costs for material and manpower are lower than that of any concentration technique and it is superior to them in sensitivity [41].

If fluorescence equipment is not available faecal smears can be stained by various methods. Carbol-fuchsin staining is quick and easy and can aid the detection of oocysts in faecal smears [33]. Other staining protocols involving auramine O, Löffler's methylene blue, Lugol's solution, May-Grünwald or Gentiana violet have been proposed [33, 42] as useful and Ziehl-Neelsen and safranin staining were recently described for the detection of human *Cystoisospora belli* oocysts in faeces [43], carbol-fuchsin is easiest to apply and the contrast was sufficient to detect oocysts in smears, although autofluorescence is still far more sensitive.

For quantification of oocysts in faecal material, counting of oocysts in a McMaster chamber is standard [20, 23, 44, 45]. Since the confounding effect of lipid droplets can also occur in this method (albeit without centrifugation) Henriksen and Christensen suggested the use of saturated sugar solution instead of saturated sodium chloride [46]. A further modification was suggested by the same authors using gauze filtration of faeces in this sugar-salt solution before counting [47]. We have adapted the original method [6, 16] for the use on individual piglet samples (0.5 g/sample) but it can be used for larger amounts as well.

When counting of oocysts in smears by autofluorescence was compared to McMaster counting, there was a

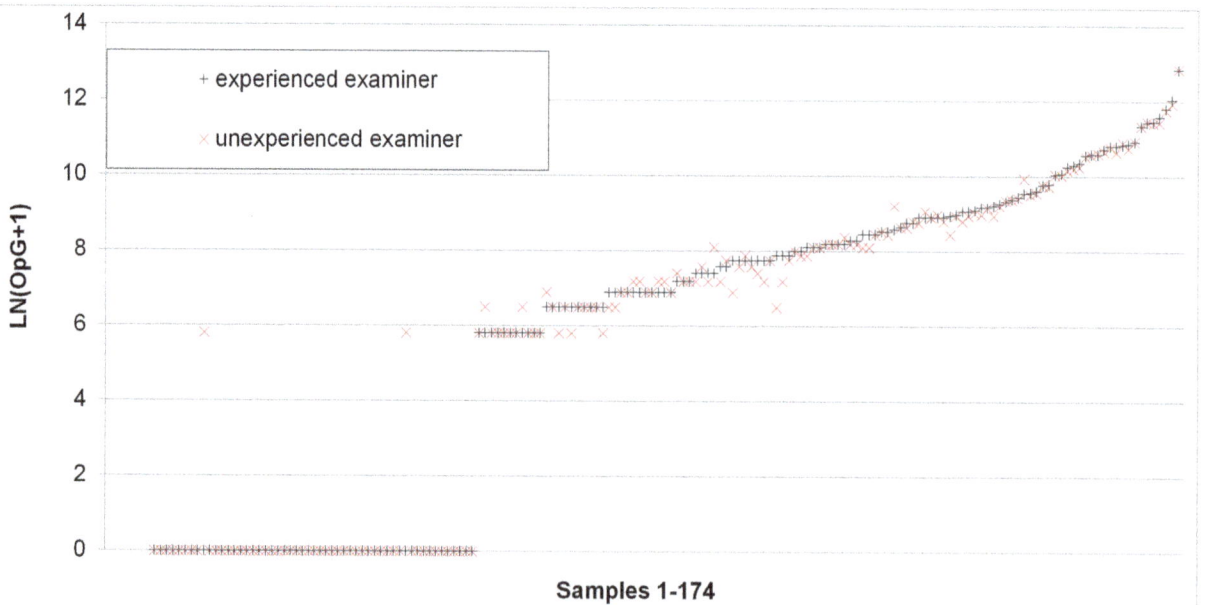

Fig. 10 Comparison of OpG counts by 2 examiners, an experienced and an unexperienced one of the same McMaster preparation

high correlation between the two methods; however, autofluorescence had a tendency for higher relative values so it must be assumed that with the McMaster method oocysts are lost during preparation or do not flotate. Also, McMaster counting has a cut-off value of 333.3 OpG while autofluorescence is much more sensitive with 10 OpG. Autofluorescence and McMaster counting both showed a high correlation between examinations by two different persons, with a slight tendency for higher values in case of the unexperienced examiner, especially in the autofluorescence microscopy, so false positive counts must be considered when staff is trained in this method. When McMaster counting was run on two independent preparations from the same sample, samples with a low OpG frequently gave back differing qualitative results and showed a high variation in the quantitation. When values for the area under curve of the OpG are statistically evaluated this has to be taken into account, especially when the results for this parameter are not supported by other parameters for oocyst excretion comparison between different groups in a treatment trial (ref. [46], for statistical evaluation of oocyst excretion in intervention studies).

For the sensitive qualitative and semiquantitative evaluation of oocysts in piglet faeces, autofluorescence appears the method of choice as previously shown [40]. It is easy and quick to do and can also be used to determine the extent of excretion when applied to samples from individual piglets, e.g. in prevalence studies [6]. If the equipment is not available, carbol-fuchsin staining according to Heine [48] can be applied. It is well correlated to autofluorescence, albeit less sensitive, but it could reliably detect oocysts in sample with an OpG of 6000 and more. Since during peak excretion average OpGs reach 45,000 this method can still be sued to determine the presence of oocysts on a farm when repeated sampling is applied (see above).

In summary, under field conditions oocyst of *C. suis* can be detected on a farm by repeated sampling of individual piglets and examination of pooled samples per litter. Oocyst detection can be accomplished by detection in faecal smears with autofluorescence or, with relatively lower sensitivity, after carbol-fuchsin staining, and can be judged semi-quantitatively. Determination of OpGs by adapted McMaster counting is usually applied under experimental conditions and for specific applications, such as an in vivo faecal oocyst reduction test to evaluate treatment efficacy [49]; however, this requires precise knowledge about the extent and intensity of infection and the course of infection on the farm in question.

In the light of recently reported reduced treatment efficacy for toltrazuril, *C. suis* should be re-considered as a diarrhoeal pathogen. We hereby suggest diagnostic procedures (repeated sampling and examination of faecal smears by autofluorescence or carbolfuchsin staining) that can be used to determine both the presence and the extent of infection on a farm to provide diagnostic tools for the evaluation of treatment efficacy and semi-quantitative determination of the infection rates in a herd.

Methods

Determination of prevalences of oocyst shedding at different time points

We used a subset of data obtained from experimental infections of neonatal piglets (*n* = 134 piglets) from previous studies with known infection days, onset and duration of excretion as determined by daily sampling and qualitative and quantitative oocyst excretion [8]. Over a period of 14 days (4th to 17th day after infection, i.e. during the patent period) the course of oocyst excretion and faecal consistency was determined for 117 piglets. Assuming that piglets can become infected for the first time from the first day of life until weaning we modelled 23 subgroups (*n* = 5–8 randomly allocated animals/group with a total of 134 modelled individuals) with *primo* infections on the 1st to 23rd day of life. This time span was chosen because the minimum pre-patent period for *C. suis* is 3 days (e.g. [24, 44, 50] but most piglets will not start excretion before the 5th day after infection [6, 8, 30, 51, 52]. The last day before weaning was assumed to be the 28th day of life so piglets older than 23 days could become infected but do not excrete oocysts before weaning. Different infection doses were not taken into consideration as these do not seem to have an appreciable influence on the onset and duration of excretion [8].

Detection methods for *C. suis* in faecal samples

We examined different methods of faecal concentration and faecal smears according to different protocols and compared their detection limit as well as the time needed to prepare and examine the samples. Faecal samples (firm or pasty consistency) of piglets with known status of excretion (from experimental studies) were pooled, mixed well and examined in parallel using different methods.

To concentrate oocysts from faecal samples by flotation different media were used: Sheather's sugar solution [25], sugar-saturated sodium chloride solution [44], or sugar-saturated sodium chloride solution with detergent (1/100 volume of household dishwasher detergent). For each sample 1.5 g of faeces were mixed with approx. 14 ml of flotation solution, filtered through sieve and funnel and centrifuged at 600 x *g* for 10 min.

Faecal smears were prepared from the same material (approximately 0.1 g/sample) and used natively for autofluorescence or stained with different methods prior to microscopic examination. For autofluorescence, the samples were covered with a glass cover slip and examined at 100× magnification under UV light (excitation wavelength: 340–380 nm; [35]).

Staining of faecal smears was carried out by mixing 0.1 g of faeces with 2–3 drops of the respective solution (1% carbol-fuchsin, 5% malachite green, 1/ nigrosine or 1% light green; ref. [48, 53]), and spreading the mix on a glass slide (a thick smear of 90% of the total amount and a thin smear with 10% of the volume further diluted 1:10 in tap water were prepared). Dried stained smears were examined by light microscopy as described above. In some cases the presence of oocysts had to be verified under 200× magnification.

To compare the detection limit of autofluorescence and carbol-fuchsin staining, 30 samples of piglets from experimental studies were examined as described above; 18 of them had a firm consistency, 12 were pasty to liquid. Nine had a low amount of oocysts (and were negative by McMaster counting, see below) and 21 had a countable oocyst per gram of faeces (OpG) value (median: 1665 OpG, maximum: 95571 OpG). Oocysts were counted in the smears to evaluate correlations with OpG values.

Quantification of oocysts

Oocyst numbers can be determined in faecal smears, but to obtain more accurate data on the number of oocysts per gram of faeces (OpG) modified McMaster methods are routinely used. Faecal matter (0.5 g) was mixed thoroughly with 4.5 g (3.55 ml) of a salt-sugar solution (50 g of sucrose added to 100 ml of saturated sodium chloride solution prepared from 400 g of sodium chloride ad 1 l of tap water); this suspension is then filtered by pressing a double-layered piece of gauze through the suspension to the bottom of a round-bottom tube (5 ml single-use plastic tube, 12 × 75 mm, round-bottom) using a metal loop (Fig. 11). This prevents the unsuspended lipid matter from floating in the suspension and trapping the oocysts. Immediately after filtering the suspension is further diluted 1:10 (200 µl + 1800 µl of solution) in the salt/sucrose solution, mixed well and filled into the McMaster chamber(s).

For the McMaster counting a cut-off of 666.6 for one field results from the dilution (1:100) and the size of the chamber (150 µl), and the oocysts per gram of faeces are calculated as follows:

$$OpG = \frac{X*100}{0.15\ ml} \text{ or } OpG = X*666.7$$

with X being the number of oocysts counted in one field. As a standard we calculate two fields/sample. This method was used to determine the OpG values for the first part of the evaluation (see above).

The reproducibility of oocyst counting in autofluorescence and McMaster was evaluated by examination of 49 autofluorescence-positive faecal smears analysed by autofluorescence by two different examiners, 174 McMaster preparations by two different examiners (an experienced and an unexperienced one) and by re-examining samples by one examiner in a second preparation (n = 50).

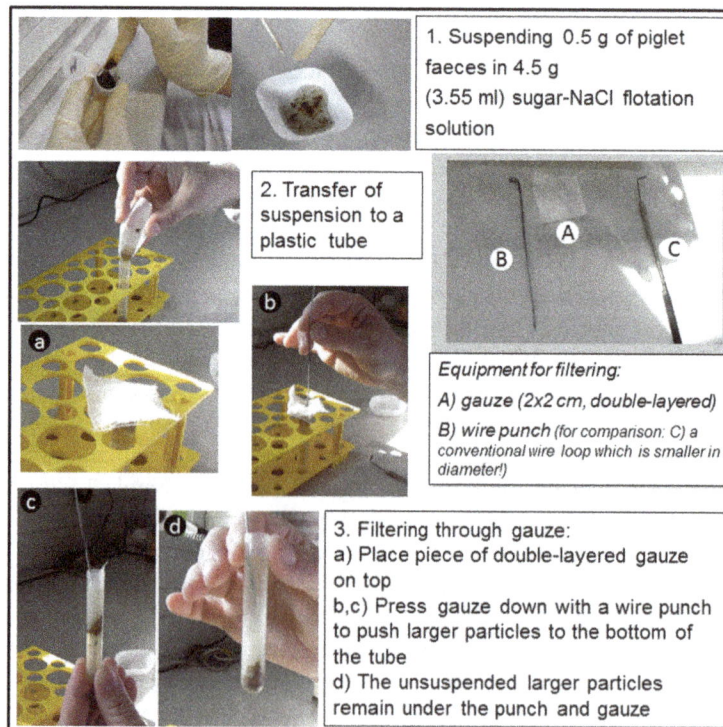

Fig. 11 Preparation of individual piglet samples for isolation of *C. suis* oocysts in flotation medium

Conclusion

C. suis-infected piglets usually excrete oocysts for short time periods, so the right timing and a sufficiently sensitive detection method are important to determine the presence and extent of the parasite in a herd. This should also be considered in cases of poor efficacy of toltrazuril treatment. Faecal samples should be taken repeatedly to improve sensitivity. Autofluorescence microscopy of faecal smears provides by far the highest sensitivity for oocyst detection. Other methods are less sensitive and/or more labour- and cost intensive and their usefulness is restricted to specific applications.

Abbreviations
C. suis: Cystoisospora suis; FS: Faecal score; OpG: Oocysts per gram of faeces

Acknowledgements
The authors gratefully acknowledge the technical support of Radinka Selista and Michaela Tischlinger.

Funding
This study was funded in part by CEVA Santé Animal, France.

Authors' contributions
AJ, BR and DS designed the study; AJ drafted the manuscript; BR evaluated the staining protocols and McMaster samples. All authors approved of the final version.

Competing interests
The authors declare that they have no competing interests. DS is employed by CEVA Santé Animale, France, who sponsored part of this study (staining evaluation).

Author details
[1]Institute of Parasitology, Department of Pathobiology, University of Veterinary Medicine Vienna, Veterinaerplatz 1, A-1210 Vienna, Austria. [2]CEVA Santé Animale, 10 avenue de la Ballastière, 33500 Libourne, France.

References
1. Joachim A, Schwarz L. Coccidia of swine: *Eimeria* species, *Cystoisospora* (syn. *Isospora*) *suis*. In: Mehlhorn H, editor. Encycloaedia of parasitology. Heidelberg: Springer; 2015. https://doi.org/10.1007/978-3-642-27769-6_3487-1.
2. Ruzicka CW, Andrews JJ. Porcine neonatal coccidiosis - a clinical review. Iowa State Univ Vet. 1984;45:90–5.
3. Joachim A, Altreuther G, Bangoura B, Charles S, Daugschies A, Hinney B, Lindsay DS, Mundt HC, Ocak M, Sotiraki S. W A A V P guidelines for evaluating the efficacy of anticoccidials in mammals (pigs, dogs, cattle, sheep). Vet Parasitol. 2018;53:102–19. https://doi.org/10.1016/j.vetpar.2018.02.029.
4. Blake DP, Tomley FM. Securing poultry production from the ever-present *Eimeria* challenge. Trends Parasitol. 2014;30(1):12–9. https://doi.org/10.1016/j.pt.2013.10.003.
5. Shrestha A, Freudenschuss B, Jansen R, Hinney B, Ruttkowski B, Joachim A. Experimentally confirmed toltrazuril resistance in a field isolate of *Cystoisospora suis*. Parasit Vectors. 2017;10(1):317. https://doi.org/10.1186/s13071-017-2257-7.
6. Mundt HC, Joachim A, Becka M, Daugschies A. *Isospora suis*: an experimental model for mammalian intestinal coccidiosis. Parasitol Res. 2006;98(2):167–75. https://doi.org/10.1007/s00436-005-0030-x.
7. Henriksen SA, Pohlenz JFL. Staining of cryptosporidia by a modified Ziehl-Neelsen technique. Acta Vet Scand. 1981;22:594–6.
8. Joachim A, Schwarz L, Hinney B, Ruttkowski B, Vogl C, Mundt HC. Which factors influence the outcome of experimental infection with *Cystoisospora suis*? Parasitol Res. 2014;113(5):1863–73. https://doi.org/10.1007/s00436-014-3834-8.
9. Niestrath M, Takla M, Joachim A, Daugschies A. The role of *Isospora suis* as a pathogen in conventional piglet production in Germany. J Vet Med B Infect Dis Vet Public Health. 2002;49(4):176–80. PMID: 12069269
10. Mundt HC, Mundt-Wüstenberg S, Daugschies A, Joachim A. Efficacy of various anticoccidials against experimental porcine neonatal isosporosis. Parasitol Res. 2007;100(2):401–11. https://doi.org/10.1007/s00436-006-0314-9.
11. Stuart BP, Gosser HS, Allen CB, Bedell DM. Coccidiosis in swine: dose and age response to Isospora suis. Can J Comp Med. 1982;46(3):317–20.
12. Koudela B, Kucerová S. Role of acquired immunity and natural age resistance on course of *Isospora suis* coccidiosis in nursing piglets. Vet Parasitol. 1999;82(2):93–9.
13. Worliczek HL, Mundt HC, Ruttkowski B, Joachim A. Age, not infection dose, determines the outcome of *Isospora suis* infections in suckling piglets. Parasitol Res. 2009;105:S157–62. https://doi.org/10.1007/s00436-009-1507-9.
14. Basso W, Marti H, Hilbe M, Sydler T, Stahel A, Bürgi E, Sidler X. Clinical cystoisosporosis associated to porcine cytomegalovirus (PCMV, Suid herpesvirus 2) infection in fattening pigs. Parasitol Int. 2017;66(6):806–9. https://doi.org/10.1016/j.parint.2017.09.007.
15. Meyer C, Joachim A, Daugschies A. Occurrence of *Isospora suis* in larger piglet production units and on specialized piglet rearing farms. Vet Parasitol. 1999;82(4):277–84.
16. Meyer CA. Vorkommen und Bedeutung von *Isospora suis* BIESTER und MURRAY 1934 in intensiv geführten Ferkelerzeugerbetrieben und in der spezialisierten Ferkelaufzucht. Germany: Thesis, University of Veterinary Medicine Hannover; 1998.
17. Noordhuizen JPTM, Frankena K, van der Hoofd C, Graat EAM. Application of quantitative methods in veterinary epidemiology. Wageningen: Wageningen Pers.; 1997. p. 445. ISBN: 9789074134897-429.
18. Ruttkowski B, Joachim A, Daugschies A. PCR-based differentiation of three porcine *Eimeria* species and *Isospora suis*. Vet Parasitol. 2001;95(1):17–23. PMID: 11163694
19. Johnson J, Samarasinghe B, Buddle R, Armson A, Ryan U. Molecular identification and prevalence of *Isospora* sp. in pigs in Western Australia using a PCR-RFLP assay. Exp Parasitol. 2008;120(2):191–3. https://doi.org/10.1016/j.exppara.2008.06.005.
20. Huang C, Wen F, Yue L, Chen R, Zhou W, Hu L, Chen M, Wang S. Exploration of fluorescence-based real-time loop-mediated isothermal amplification (LAMP) assay for detection of *Isospora suis* oocysts. Exp Parasitol. 2016;165:1–6. https://doi.org/10.1016/j.exppara.2016.03.001.
21. Lalonde LF, Gajadhar AA. Detection and differentiation of coccidian oocysts by real-time PCR and melting curve analysis. J Parasitol. 2011;97(4):725–30. https://doi.org/10.1645/GE-2706.1.
22. Nilsson O, Martinsson K, Persson E. Epidemiology of porcine neonatal steatorrhoea in Sweden. 1. Prevalence and clinical significance of coccidial and rotaviral infections. Nord Vet Med. 1984;36(3–4):103–10. PMID: 6330668
23. Lindsay DS, Dubey JP, Blagburn BL. Biology of *Isospora* spp. from humans, nonhuman primates, and domestic animals. Clin Microbiol Rev. 1997;10(1):19–34. PMCID: PMC172913
24. Vetterling JM. Prevalence of coccidia in swine from six localities in the United States, College Vet. Med. Urbana: University of Illinois; 1965. p. 155–66.
25. Stuart BP, Lindsay DS, Ernst JV, Gosser HS. *Isospora suis* enteritis in piglets. Vet Pathol. 1980;17(1):84–93.
26. Harleman JH, Meyer RC. Life cycle of *Isospora suis* in gnotobiotic and conventionalised piglets. Vet Parasitol. 1984;17:27–39.
27. Ernst JV, Lindsay DS, Current WL. Control of *Isospora suis*-induced coccidiosis on a swine farm. A J Vet Res. 1985;46:643–5.

28. Lindsay DS, Current WL, Taylor JR. Effects of experimentally induced *Isospora suis* infection on morbidity, mortality, and weight gains in nursing pigs. Am J Vet Res. 1985;46(7):1511–2.

29. Jarvinen JA, Zimmerman GL, Schons DJ, Guenther C. Serum proteins of neonatal pigs orally inoculated with *Isospora suis* oocysts. Am J Vet Res. 1988;49(3):380–5.

30. Vítovec J, Koudela B. Double alteration of the small intestine in conventional and gnotobiotic piglets experimentally infected with the coccidium *Isospora suis* (Apicomplexa, Eimeriidae). Folia Parasitol. 1990;37:21–33.

31. Karamon J, Ziomko I, Cencek T, Sroka J. Modified flotation method with the use of Percoll for the detection of *Isospora suis* oocysts in suckling piglet faeces. Vet Parasitol. 2008;156(3–4):324–8. https://doi.org/10.1016/j.vetpar.2008.05.020.

32. Lindsay DS. Diagnosing and controlling *Isospora suis* in nursing piglets. Vet Med. 1989;84:443–8.

33. Mathea J. Vorkommen von *Isospora suis* und *Cryptosporidium parvum* beim Ferkel in Schweinebeständen mit unterschiedlichen Haltungsbedingungen. Germany: Thesis, Veterinary Faculty, Free University of Berlin; 1993.

34. Tubbs RC. A review of porcine neonatal coccidiosis. Irish Vet News. 1987;2:24–7.

35. Daugschies A, Bialek R, Joachim A, Mundt HC. Autofluorescence microscopy for the detection of nematode eggs and protozoa, in particular *Isospora suis*, in swine faeces. Parasitol Res. 2001;87(5):409–12.

36. Vesey G, Deere D, Gauci MR, Griffiths KR, Williams KL, Veal DA. Evaluation of fluorochromes and excitation sources for immunofluorescence in water samples. Cytometry. 1997;29(2):147–54.

37. Berlin OG, Peter JB, Gagne C, Conteas CN, Ash LR. Autofluorescence and the detection of *Cyclospora* oocysts. Emerg Infect Dis. 1998;4(1):127.

38. Varea M, Clavel A, Doiz O, Castillo FJ, Rubio MC, Gómez-Lus R. Fuchsin fluorescence and autofluorescence in *Cryptosporidium*, *Isospora* and *Cyclospora* oocysts. Int J Parasitol. 1998;28(12):1881–3.

39. Lindquist HD, Bennett JW, Hester JD, Ware MW, Dubey JP, Everson WV. Autofluorescence of toxoplasma gondii and related coccidian oocysts. J Parasitol. 2003;89(4):865–7. https://doi.org/10.1645/GE-3147RN.

40. Belli SI, Wallach MG, Luxford C, Davies MJ, Smith NC. Roles of tyrosine-rich precursor glycoproteins and dityrosine- and 3,4-dihydroxyphenylalanine-mediated protein cross-linking in development of the oocyst wall in the coccidian parasite *Eimeria maxima*. Eukaryot Cell. 2003;2(3):456–64. PMCID: PMC161462

41. Kuhnert Y, Schmäschke R, Daugschies A. Vergleich verschiedener Verfahren zur Untersuchung von Saugferkelkot auf *Isospora suis*. Berl Münch tierärztl Wochenschr. 2006;119(7–8):282–6.

42. Hanscheid T, Cristino JM, Salgado MJ. Screening of auramine-stained smears of all fecal samples is a rapid and inexpensive way to increase the detection of coccidial infections. Int J Infect Dis. 2008;12(1):47–50. https://doi.org/10.1016/j.ijid.2007.04.008.

43. Pacheco FT, Silva RK, Martins AS, Oliveira RR, Alcântara-Neves NM, Silva MP, Soares NM, Teixeira MC. Differences in the detection of *Cryptosporidium* and *Isospora* (*Cystoisospora*) oocysts according to the fecal concentration or staining method used in a clinical laboratory. J Parasitol. 2013;99(6):1002–8. https://doi.org/10.1645/12-33.1.

44. Robinson Y, Morin M, Girard C, Higgins R. Experimental transmission of intestinal coccidiosis to piglets: clinical, parasitological and pathological findings. Ca J Com Med. 1983;47(4):401–7.

45. Girard C, Morin M. Amprolium and furazolidone as preventive treatment for intestinal coccidiosis of piglets. Can Vet J. 1987;28(10):667–9.

46. Henriksen SA, Christensen JPB. Demonstration of *Isospora suis* oocysts in faecal samples. Vet Rec. 1992;131:443–4.

47. Henriksen SA. *Isospora suis* of swine. In: Eckert J, Braun R, Shirley MW, Coudert P, editors. COST 89/20 biotechnology: guidelines on techniques in coccidiosis research. Brussels: European Coimmission, Directorate General XII, Science, Research and Development; Agrigulture Biotechnology, 2920 Luxembourg; 1995. p. 74–8.

48. Heine J. 1982. Eine einfache Nachweismethode für Kryptosporidien im Kot. Zbl Vetmed. 1982;29:324–7.

49. Joachim A, Shrestha A, Freudenschuss B, Palmieri N, Hinney B, Karembe H, Sperling D. Comparison of an injectable toltrazuril-gleptoferron (Forceris®) and an oral toltrazuril (Baycox®) + injectable iron dextran for the control of experimentally induced piglet cystoisosporosis. Parasit Vectors. 2018;11:206.

50. Lindsay DS, Stuart BP, Wheat BE, Ernst JV. Endogenous development of the swine coccidium, *Isospora suis* BIESTER 1934. J Parasitol. 1980;66(3):771–9.

51. Christensen JPB, Henriksen SA. Shedding of oocysts in piglets experimentally infected with *Isospora suis*. Act Vet Scand. 1994;35:165–72.

52. Matuschka FR, Heydorn AO. Die Entwicklung von *Isospora suis* Biester 1934 (Sporozoa: Coccidia: Eimeriidae) im Schwein. Zool Beiträge. 1980;26(3):405–76.

53. Rekha KMH, Puttalakshmamma GC, D'Souza PE. Comparison of different diagnostic techniques for the detection of cryptosporidiosis in bovines. VetWorld. 2016;9:211–5. https://doi.org/10.14202/vetworld.2016.211-215.

19

Long duration of immunity against a type 1 heterologous PRRS virus challenge in pigs immunised with a novel PRRS MLV vaccine

Jeremy Kroll[1*], Mike Piontkowski[2], Poul H. Rathkjen[3], Francois-Xavier Orveillon[3], Christian Kraft[4] and Oliver G. Duran[3]

Abstract

Background: Porcine reproductive and respiratory syndrome virus (PRRSV) is widespread in commercial pig farms worldwide, and has a significant cost to the swine industry. Herd owners need a vaccine that will confer long-lasting immunity to prevent PRRSV infection and transmission. The studies described here evaluated duration of immunity conferred by a European-derived PRRS (isolate 94,881) modified live virus (MLV) vaccine, Ingelvac PRRSFLEX® EU, at 20, 24, and 26 weeks post-vaccination. Primary endpoints were the assessment of gross and histological lung lesions and viral RNA load in lung tissue 10 days following heterologous PRRSV challenge. Secondary endpoints included clinical observations, average daily weight gain (ADWG) and viral RNA load in serum 10 days post-challenge. Three blinded, vaccination-challenge efficacy studies were performed using separate cohorts of pigs ($n = 56$ per study). Pigs received either Ingelvac PRRSFLEX® EU (Group 1) or placebo (Groups 2 and 3). Groups 1 and 2 were subsequently challenged with heterologous European PRRSV isolate 205,817 at 20, 24 or 26 weeks post-vaccination.

Results: Mean gross lung lesion scores were significantly lower in Group 1 than in Group 2 at 24 and 26 weeks ($p < 0.0001$), but not at 20 weeks ($p = 0.299$). Significantly lower mean histological lung lesion scores were observed in Group 1 versus Group 2 at 20 ($p = 0.0065$), 24 ($p < 0.0001$) and 26 weeks ($p < 0.0001$). Mean viral RNA load in lung tissue was significantly lower in Group 1 than in Group 2 ($p < 0.0001$) at 20 ($p < 0.0001$), 24 ($p < 0.0001$) and 26 weeks ($p < 0.0001$). Cumulative viral RNA loads in serum during days 1–10 post-challenge were significantly lower in Group 1 than in Group 2 ($p < 0.0001$) in all studies. A significant increase in ADWG was observed in Group 1 compared with Group 2 at 20 weeks ($p = 0.0027$) and 24 weeks ($p = 0.0004$), but not at 26 weeks ($p = 0.1041$). There were no significant differences in clinical signs post-challenge in any study.

Conclusion: These results suggest that Ingelvac PRRSFLEX® EU confers long-term immunity to European heterologous PRRSV, which is maintained up to 26 weeks after vaccination, corresponding to the expected lifespan of commercial pigs.

Keywords: Vaccine, Efficacy, PRRS, Immunity, Lung lesions, ADWG

* Correspondence: jeremy.kroll@boehringer-ingelheim.com
[1]Boehringer Ingelheim Animal Health, 2412 South Loop Dr, Ames, IA 50010, USA
Full list of author information is available at the end of the article

Background

Porcine reproductive and respiratory syndrome (PRRS) is a viral infection of pigs, causing pneumonia, reproductive failure, and increased mortality in young animals [1]. The disease was first identified in North America in the late 1980s [2] and soon after in Europe [3], and has since spread to other regions worldwide [4]. The disease has profound economic consequences, causing significant losses to the worldwide swine industry, and an estimated annual loss of 1 billion US dollars in North America alone [5]. The extent of animal suffering, along with these economic losses have led to a significant drive to develop effective prevention, control and elimination strategies.

PRRS is caused by the PRRS virus (PRRSV), which is a member of the *Arteriviridae* family of the order *Nidovirales*. Like all members of this family, PRRSV has a single-stranded, positive-sense RNA genome. There are two major genetic lineages: Type 1, which was originally isolated in Europe in 1990 [6], and Type 2, which was first isolated in North America [7]. These two genotypes emerged at approximately the same time, but their nucleotide sequences differ by approximately 40% [8, 9]. Indeed, there is also significant genetic variation within each genotype [5, 10]. This significant heterogeneity both between and within PRRSV genotypes has hindered attempts to develop an effective vaccine against PRRS.

At present, two types of vaccine are commercially available: killed-virus (KV) vaccines and modified-live virus (MLV) vaccines [11, 12]. KV vaccines are largely ineffective, or have only limited efficacy [13–15] while MLV vaccines are generally regarded as the most effective [5], reducing reproductive and respiratory symptoms of PRRS disease, and improving weight gain in growing pigs [16].

Despite their promising efficacy, PRRS MLV vaccines are still associated with multiple problems. Commercially available PRRS MLV vaccines are based on either PRRSV Type 1 or 2 viral strains, which effectively induce immunity against genetically similar PRRSV strains from within the same genotype [11, 12]. However, the level of efficacy conferred against heterologous PRRSV isolates is less clear. Vaccine efficacy can suffer from both the immune evasion strategies of the virus and the antigenic heterogeneity of the field strains. It is not possible to forecast precisely the level of protection afforded by a given PRRSV vaccine strain against a heterologous one, but it is clear that partial heterologous protection can be obtained [17–19].

Commercially-reared pigs are typically slaughtered between 18 and 26 weeks of age [20]; therefore, an optimal vaccine should quickly elicit an effective immune response, and maintain duration of immunity for at least 26 weeks. The absence of clear correlates of protection means that further in vivo studies are necessary [21]. Current PRRS MLV vaccines elicit humoral and cell-mediated immunity; both become detectable by 2–3 weeks post-vaccination [22, 25]. However, whilst levels of PRRS-specific antibodies rapidly reach their peak of detection 4 weeks after vaccination or infection, the cell-mediated response is profoundly delayed, remaining at low levels for over 3 months before reaching its highest levels after 32 weeks post-vaccination [22]. As well as their efficacy shortcomings, there also remain concerns over the safety of PRRS MLV vaccines due to their potential to revert to virulence [23, 24]. A vaccine conferring rapid, long-lasting as well as effective immunity against a broad range of heterologous viral strains is very much needed [11, 23].

An ideal vaccine would achieve a long duration of immunity to reduce the risk of re-infection with PRRS during an animal's lifetime. Simultaneously, it must effectively reduce clinical signs of PRRS disease, viraemia, viral RNA load in lung tissues and viral shedding, to help limit viral transmission. Such a vaccine would help limit both the acute economic losses caused by PRRS infection and animal suffering. Developing such a vaccine represents a significant challenge [23]. A new vaccine, PRRS 94881 (tradename: Ingelvac PRRSFLEX® EU), is derived from European PRRS isolate 94881, and has previously been shown to be clinically safe [25]. In order to determine whether PRRS 94881 MLV could provide long-term immunity to PRRSV challenge in 2-week old pigs, three vaccination-challenge studies following Good Clinical Practices (GCP) were carried out to evaluate the duration of immunity (DOI) at three different time points after vaccination. This paper details the results of these studies, which found that vaccinated pigs had reduced lung lesion scores, viraemia and viral RNA load in tissues at 20, 24 and 26 weeks.

Methods

Study designs

Three blinded, vaccination-challenge efficacy studies were performed using separate cohorts of pigs. Each study comprised three treatment arms. Group 1 (PRRS-vaccinated) received Ingelvac PRRSFLEX® EU (Boehringer Ingelheim Vetmedica, Inc., St. Joseph, MO, USA; Lot 390–005) followed by PRRSV challenge. Group 2 (challenge controls) received control product (CP; Boehringer Ingelheim Vetmedica, Inc.; Lot N240–191-062409) followed by PRRSV challenge. Group 3 (negative controls) received CP, but no PRRSV challenge. Ingelvac PRRSFLEX® EU vaccine and CP were administered to 14–17 day-old pigs on Day 0, and then Group 1 and Group 2 were challenged with heterologous European PRRSV isolate 205,817 (Boehringer Ingelheim Vetmedica, Inc.) at 20, 24 or 26 weeks after vaccination. This day was denoted day post-challenge (DPC) 0. All studies were carried out following Good Clinical Practice (GCP) guidelines.

Randomisation and blinding

Animals were randomised to one of three groups by the study investigator or a designee prior to study commencement. The randomisation sequence was created using Excel 2003 (Microsoft, Redmond, WA, US) with a 1:1 allocation using random block sizes of 0 and 1. Both the Ingelvac PRRSFLEX® EU and CP were administered by individuals not collecting study data in order to maintain study blinding. Both the study investigator and all laboratory personnel were blinded to treatment assignment.

Animals

These three studies were each conducted with 56 commercial crossbred female or castrated male pigs (Prairie View Farms, N5627 Hwy DD, Burlington, WI 53105, USA). The animals were healthy, aged between 14 and 17 days, weighed between 2.7–6.3 kg and were PRRSV-negative on Day 0. All pigs were housed at Veterinary Resources, Inc. (VRI) in Cambridge, IA, USA, for the duration of the study. Pigs were housed in multiple pens (each containing 11–12 pigs) per room. Vaccinated (Group 1) and control (Groups 2 and 3) animals were housed in uniform but separate rooms to prevent PRRSV cross-contamination between groups. Feeds provided were appropriate for the size, age and condition of pigs according to acceptable animal husbandry practices for the region. A minimum of 20 pigs were included in Groups 1 and 2, and 12 pigs were included in Group 3.

Vaccines and challenge material

Both Ingelvac PRRSFLEX® EU vaccine and CP were reconstituted with phosphate-buffered saline. Ingelvac PRRSFLEX® EU was reconstituted and administered to Group 1 animals per manufacturer's instructions [26]. Ingelvac PRRSFLEX® EU vaccine and CP were administered intramuscularly (IM) as a 1.0 mL dose to the right neck region of Group 1 and 2 pigs, respectively. Challenge material was PRRSV isolate 205,817, a heterologous Type 1 isolate with 88.3% homology to Ingelvac PRRSFLEX® EU (based on ORF5 sequence). The challenge strain was originally isolated from a herd with a severe outbreak of PRRS causing abortions in sows and respiratory disease in fattening pigs. Challenge material had a mean viral titre of $1 \times 10^{6.27}$ $TCID_{50}$/3 mL dose administered 1 mL per each nostril (2 mL in total) and 1 mL intramuscularly. The CP was a lyophilised placebo product that contained an inert material comprising the vaccine vehicle without Ingelvac PRRSFLEX® EU.

Variables for efficacy and safety assessments

The primary efficacy outcome variable for the three studies was lung pathology (gross and histological lesions) at 20, 24 or 26 weeks after PRRS 94881 MLV vaccination. The DOI at 20, 24 and 26 weeks post-vaccination was achieved if Group 1 had statistically significant decreased lung pathology (gross or histological) post-challenge compared with Group 2 at the same time point. Secondary efficacy outcomes included post-challenge viraemia (in both lung and serum), average daily weight gain (ADWG), post-vaccination safety assessments and post-challenge clinical assessments of disease.

Sample analysis and outcome measurements

Gross and histological lung lesions

Gross pathology was determined following examination of lung tissue following necropsy on DPC 10. A percentage of affected lung tissue was recorded for each lung lobe and the total percentage was subsequently calculated based on the weighing formula recommended in the draft monograph 'Porcine enzootic Pneumonia Vaccine (inactivated)' (PA/PH, Exp 15 V/T[07]2 ANP). To determine histological pathology, a single slide containing seven sections (one each for all seven lung lobes) was created for each pig. Slides were examined for pneumocytic hypertrophy and hyperplasia, septal infiltration with mononuclear cells, necrotic debris, intra-alveolar accumulation of inflammatory cells, and perivascular accumulation of inflammatory cells. For each histological parameter (except necrotic debris), samples were scored either 0 (not present: no detectable lesions present within an area of view), 1 (mild lesions: few positive cells [1–5 cells/area] present within an area of view), 2 (moderate lesions: multiple positive cells [> 5 cells/area] within an area of view) or 3 (severe lesions: multiple positive cells [> 5 cells/area] at multiple locations within an area of view). Necrotic debris was scored either 0 (not present) or 1 (yes present).

Serum PRRSV quantitative polymerase chain reaction

Two to 5 mL venous whole blood samples were collected from all pigs on Day 0 to confirm the PRRSV-negative status. Blood samples were also taken on DPC 0, 3, 7, 9 and 10 in all three studies. Reverse transcription and quantitative PCR (qPCR) were performed [27] on serum samples to determine serum PRRSV RNA levels; results were reported as genome equivalent/mL ($\log_{10}$ GE/mL).

Lung PRRSV qPCR

Tissue samples from left and right lung lobes were homogenised, and qPCR following reverse transcription was performed (BioScreen GmbH, Hannover, Germany) to determine lung PRRSV RNA levels [27]; results were reported as Log_{10} GE/mL.

Average daily weight gain

Body weights were recorded on Day 0, DPC 0 and DPC 9 in all studies, and individual daily weight gains were calculated between DPC 0–9.

Post-vaccination and post-challenge clinical safety observations

Post-vaccination clinical safety assessments were performed daily on Days – 1 to 21, then three times per week thereafter until DPC – 2 in all studies. These clinical assessments were recorded as either 'normal' or 'abnormal'. Pigs were observed for clinical signs of disease from DPC – 1 to 10 in all three studies. Clinical parameters included respiratory symptoms, behaviour and cough, and were scored 0–3 based on severity of symptoms (Respiration: 0 = normal respiration; 1 = panting/rapid respiration; 2 = dyspnoea; 3 = dead. Behaviour: 0 = normal; 1 = mild to moderate lethargy; 2 = severely lethargic or recumbent; 3 = dead. Cough: 0 = no coughing; 1 = soft or intermittent cough; 2 = harsh or severe, repetitive cough; 3 = dead).

Statistical methods

For each study, pigs were randomly assigned to one of three groups. Data were summarised using descriptive statistics with a 95% confidence interval (CI), and analysed assuming a completely random design structure. All tests on differences between Groups 1 and 2 were designed as two-sided tests using an alpha value of 5% (p-value < 0.05 for indicating statistical significance). Differences between treatment groups in each study were tested using analysis of variance in case of quantitative variables with normally distributed data (ADWG) and Wilcoxon Mann-Whitney tests for scores and other variables with not normally distributed data. Statistical analyses were performed using SAS software release 8.2 (SAS 2001, SAS Institute Inc., Cary, North Carolina, USA). No statistical analyses were performed on Group 3 pigs.

Results

Animals

In total, 56 animals were included per study, and assigned to one of three groups. For each study, Groups 1 and 2 comprised 22 animals each, and Group 3 comprised 12 animals. In the 20-week study, two pigs assigned to Group 2 died. In the 24-week study, one Group 1 pig and three Group 2 pigs died, and in the 26-week study, one Group 1 pig and two Group 2 pigs died. All of these animals died pre-challenge, and were not included in the analyses presented here.

Lung lesion scores

The mean gross lung lesion scores for Group 1 pigs following challenges at 20, 24 and 26 weeks were 0.156%, 0.084% and 1.099%, respectively, whilst those for Group 2 pigs were 0.26%, 3.38% and 15.84%, respectively (Table 1). The differences between the two groups were significant after challenges at 24 and 26 weeks, but not after 20 weeks (Table 1).

Table 1 Gross lung lesion scores at necropsy

| Study | | Gross lung lesion score (%) | | | | |
	Group	n	Mean	95% CI	Median (IQR)	p-value*
20-week	1	22	0.156	0.00–0.16	0.000 (0.160)	0.2989
	2	20	0.261	0.00–0.16	0.060 (0.185)	
24-week	1	20	0.084	0.00–0.10	0.000 (0.130)	< 0.0001
	2	19	3.378	0.61–4.74	2.050 (4.59)	
26-week	1	21	1.099	0.05–0.55	0.060 (0.400)	< 0.0001
	2	19	15.842	2.69–22.65	13.80 (20.85)	

CI distribution free confidence interval of the median, *IQR* interquartile range, *MLV* modified live virus, *n* number of pigs included in analysis, *PRRS* porcine reproductive and respiratory syndrome
Group 1 = PRRS 94881 MLV vaccinated; Group 2 = challenge controls
*p-values were calculated using the Wilcoxon-Mann-Whitney test

Group 1 pigs exhibited significantly lower mean histological lung lesion scores than Group 2 pigs after challenges at 20, 24 and 26 weeks (Table 2).

Viral RNA load in serum

PRRSV RNA was not detected in the serum of any pigs on Day 0, meeting the inclusion criteria for the study. Also, no PRRSV RNA was detected in any group on the day of challenge (DPC0), meaning that the vaccine virus was cleared at this point in time.

Group 1 pigs in all three studies exhibited significantly lower serum PRRSV RNA levels than Group 2 pigs at both DPC 7 and DPC 10 (Table 3). During DPC 1–10, the mean area under the curve (AUC) values for Group 1 pigs were 14.3, 12.9 and 17.6 $\log_{10}$ GE/mL, and 37.4, 35.3 and 44.8 $\log_{10}$ GE/mL for Group 2 pigs in the 20, 24 and 26-week studies, respectively (Table 4).

AUC values during DPC 3–10 were also significantly lower for Group 1 than Group 2 pigs in all three studies. Group 1 pigs exhibited mean AUC values of 8.57, 7.83 and 11.0 $\log_{10}$ GE/mL compared with 29.4, 27.7 and 36.1 $\log_{10}$ GE/mL for Group 2 pigs in the 20, 24 and 26-week studies, respectively (Table 4).

Table 2 Mean histological lung lesion scores at necropsy

| Study | | Histological lung lesion score (mean) | | | | |
	Group	n	Mean	95% CI	Median (IQR)	p-value*
20-week	1	22	13.0	4.0–18.0	9.5 (14.0)	0.0065
	2	20	24.7	16.0–35.0	23.0 (20.5)	
24-week	1	20	7.3	2.0–10.0	7.0 (8.5)	< 0.0001
	2	19	20.6	12.0–28.0	19.0 (16.0)	
26-week	1	21	6.6	3.0–8.0	6.0 (5.0)	< 0.0001
	2	20	20.2	15.0–23.0	19.5 (10.0)	

CI distribution free confidence interval of the median, *IQR* interquartile range, *MLV* modified live virus, *n* number of pigs included in analysis, *PRRS* porcine reproductive and respiratory syndrome
Group 1 = PRRS 94881 MLV vaccinated; Group 2 = challenge controls
*p-values were calculated using the Wilcoxon-Mann-Whitney test

Table 3 PRRSV-viral RNA load in serum

Study	DPC	Group	n	Mean	95% CI	Median (IQR)	p-value*
				PRSSV-viral RNA load in serum (log$_{10}$ GE/mL)			
20-week	0	1	22	0.00	0.00–0.00	0.00 (0.00)	1.0000
		2	20	0.00	0.00–0.00	0.00 (0.00)	
	3	1	22	3.84	3.00–4.29	3.79 (1.29)	< 0.0001
		2	20	5.30	5.06–5.52	5.34 (0.54)	
	7	1	22	0.14	0.00–0.00	0.00 (0.00)	< 0.0001
		2	20	4.00	3.44–4.59	3.95 (1.26)	
	10	1	22	0.27	0.00–0.00	0.00 (0.00)	< 0.0001
		2	20	3.23	3.00–3.37	3.00 (0.51)	
24-week	0	1	20	0.00	0.00–0.00	0.00 (0.00)	1.0000
		2	19	0.00	0.00–0.00	0.00 (0.00)	
	3	1	20	3.39	3.00–4.04	3.78 (1.13)	< 0.0001
		2	19	5.06	4.85–5.36	5.13 (0.56)	
	7	1	19	0.32	0.00–0.00	0.00 (0.00)	< 0.0001
		2	19	3.85	3.00–4.53	3.87 (1.53)	
	10	1	20	0.00	0.00–0.00	0.00 (0.00)	< 0.0001
		2	19	2.75	3.00–3.37	3.00 (0.37)	
26-week	0	1	21	0.00	0.00–0.00	0.00 (0.00)	1.0000
		2	20	0.00	0.00–0.00	0.00 (0.00)	
	3	1	21	4.42	3.93–5.28	4.44 (1.51)	< 0.0001
		2	20	5.81	5.75–6.00	5.88 (0.32)	
	7	1	21	0.61	0.00–0.00	0.00 (0.00)	< 0.0001
		2	20	5.30	4.86–5.69	5.30 (1.08)	
	10	1	21	0.00	0.00–0.00	0.00 (0.00)	< 0.0001
		2	20	3.97	3.71–4.42	4.24 (1.18)	

CI distribution free confidence interval of the median, *DPC* day post-challenge, *GE* genome equivalent, *IQR* interquartile range, *MLV* modified live virus, *n* number of pigs included in analysis, *PRRS* porcine reproductive and respiratory syndrome, *PRRSV* PRRS virus
Group 1 = PRRS 94881 MLV vaccinated; Group 2 = challenge controls
*p-values were calculated using the Wilcoxon-Mann-Whitney test

Viral RNA load in lung tissues at necropsy

Lung PRRSV RNA levels at necropsy for Group 1 pigs were significantly lower than for Group 2 pigs in all three studies ($p < 0.0001$; Table 5).

Average daily weight gain

At the time of challenge, the mean weight difference between respective groups was insignificant. A significant increase in ADWG was observed in Group 1 pigs compared with Group 2 pigs in the 9 days following challenge at 20 ($p = 0.0027$) and 24 ($p = 0.0004$) weeks, but not at 26 weeks ($p = 0.1041$) (Table 6). Mean ADWG in Group 3 pigs was 1.016, 0.771 and 0.5 kg/day in the 9 days following challenge at 20, 24 and 26 weeks, respectively. This was greater than the ADWG of both Group 1 and 2 pigs in all three studies.

Clinical signs post-challenge

For all three studies, no difference was observed between Group 1 and Group 2 for each of the clinical signs considered: abnormal respiration, abnormal behaviour and coughing. No pigs in either Group 1 or Group 2 exhibited any coughing following challenge at 20, 24 or 26 weeks. No abnormal respiration, behaviour or coughing was observed in any pigs challenged at 20 weeks.

Adverse events

No adverse events attributed to the test product (Ingelvac PRRSFLEX® EU) was noted in any of the three studies. Also, no deaths were attributed to either control product or Ingelvac PRRSFLEX® EU.

Table 4 PRRSV-viral RNA cumulative loads in serum

Study	DPC	Group	n	Mean	95% CI	Median (IQR)	p-value*
				AUC values (log$_{10}$ GE/mL)			
20-week	0–10	1	22	14.33	10.50–17.80	13.32 (7.3)	< 0.0001
		2	20	37.40	35.02–39.37	37.44 (4.54)	
	3–10	1	22	8.57	6.00–10.46	7.61 (4.46)	< 0.0001
		2	20	29.44	27.71–31.08	29.74 (3.76)	
24-week	0–10	1	19	12.87	10.50–15.16	13.23 (4.66)	< 0.0001
		2	19	35.31	32.78–38.22	36.07 (5.68)	
	3–10	1	19	7.83	6.00–8.86	7.56 (2.86)	< 0.0001
		2	19	27.72	25.16–30.72	28.29 (5.70)	
26-week	0–10	1	21	17.61	13.76–19.53	15.54 (5.95)	< 0.0001
		2	20	44.84	43.23–48.03	44.77 (6.24)	
	3–10	1	21	10.97	7.86–11.16	8.88 (3.40)	< 0.0001
		2	20	36.12	34.60–38.53	36.43 (5.23)	

AUC area under the concentration-time curve, *CI* distribution free confidence interval of the median, *DPC* day post-challenge, *GE* genome equivalent, *IQR* interquartile range, *MLV* modified live virus, *n* number of pigs included in analysis, *PRRS* porcine reproductive and respiratory syndrome, *PRRSV* PRRS virus
Group 1 = PRRS 94881 MLV vaccinated; Group 2 = challenge controls
*p-values were calculated using the Wilcoxon-Mann-Whitney test

Table 5 PRRSV-viral RNA load for lung tissues at necropsy

Study	Group	n	Mean	95% CI	Median (IQR)	p-value[*]
			PRRSV-viral RNA load in lung tissues at necropsy (mean $\log_{10}$ GE/mL)			
20-week	1	22	4.26	3.70–5.18	4.20 (1.51)	< 0.0001
	2	20	6.31	5.94–6.73	6.51 (0.86)	
24-week	1	20	2.36	1.50–4.17	1.50 (3.42)	< 0.0001
	2	19	5.33	4.85–5.97	5.34 (1.23)	
26-week	1	21	3.36	1.50–5.21	3.69 (3.18)	< 0.0001
	2	20	6.22	5.62–6.68	6.25 (1.26)	

CI distribution free confidence interval of the median, *GE* genome equivalent, *IQR* interquartile range, *MLV* modified live virus, *n* number of pigs included in analysis, *PRRS* porcine reproductive and respiratory syndrome, *PRRSV* PRRS virus
Group 1 = PRRS 94881 MLV vaccinated; Group 2 = challenge controls
[*]p-values were calculated using the Wilcoxon-Mann-Whitney test

Discussion

These three GCP laboratory efficacy studies were performed in seronegative 2–week old pigs. Each study contained three groups; Group 1 was vaccinated on Day 0 with Ingelvac PRRSFLEX® EU, and Groups 2 and 3 were vaccinated with a placebo vaccine. This study aimed to evaluate DOI at 20, 24 and 26 weeks following vaccination. After 20, 24 or 26 weeks, Groups 1 and 2 were challenged with a heterologous European PRRS viral isolate 205,817, which shared 88.3% sequence homology at the GP5 gene with Ingelvac PRRSFLEX® EU. The GP5 gene encodes the major envelope protein of PRRSV, and carries the major neutralising epitope of PRRSV [28]. Groups 1 and 2 were subsequently evaluated for lung pathology, serum and lung viremia, and observed for clinical signs of disease. No infections were observed in Group 3 pigs in any study, and there were no signs of co-infection. Therefore, the results presented here were attributed to the effects of PRRS 94881 MLV vaccine.

PRRS respiratory infection models using EU type 1 PRRSV are rare due to them being difficult to develop. In the current study, we have modelled a novel PRRSV type I isolate 205,817 that can consistently infect and cause severe PRRS respiratory lesions at different ages of a growing and fattening pig; however, the amount of

Table 6 Mean group ADWG during DPC 0–9

Mean ADWG (kg/day)					
Study	Group	n	Mean (SD)	Median	p-value[*]
20-week	1	22	0.740 (0.333)	0.739	0.0027
	2	20	0.155 (0.783)	0.339	
24-week	1	20	0.737 (0.295)	0.683	0.0004
	2	19	0.068 (0.705)	0.189	
26-week	1	21	0.412 (0.317)	0.411	0.1041
	2	20	0.235 (0.365)	0.289	

ADWG average daily weight gain, *MLV* modified live virus, *n* number of pigs included in analysis, *PRRS* porcine reproductive and respiratory syndrome, *SD* standard deviation
Group 1 = PRRS 94881 MLV vaccinated; Group 2 = challenge controls
[*]p-values were calculated using the analysis of variance (t-test)

expected clinical signs and respiratory disease is reduced the older the pig gets.

Reduction in gross and histological lung lesion scores was the primary efficacy endpoint of three studies. Lung lesion development is one of the hallmarks of PRRSV in growing pigs [29], and can be considered the source for all subsequent manifestations of secondary PRRS disease characteristics, including clinical signs, pyrexia, decreased ADWG and secondary infection with other pathogens. Therefore, these are the most clinically relevant and convincing parameters for measurement of PRRS vaccine efficacy. Macroscopic gross lung lesions are usually mild in adult animals, so slides were examined for multiple microscopic lung lesions typically observed following PRRSV infection [30]. The results of these three studies showed significant improvements in both gross and histological lung lesion scores among Group 1 compared with Group 2 pigs at 24 and 26 weeks after vaccination. Additionally, a significant reduction in histological lung lesions was seen at 20 weeks in Group 1 pigs. In the 20-week study, the lung lesion score of Group 1 animals was in a similar range to that of Group 1 animals in the two adjacent studies; however, significance could not be reached due to the fact that lung lesions in Group 2 pigs were low as well. These findings suggest that Ingelvac PRRSFLEX® EU vaccine is highly effective in providing long-term (up to 26 weeks) immunity against a virulent challenge with PRRS. Some histological lung lesions were observed in negative control pigs, despite their confirmed absence of PRRSV RNA in serum at all time points throughout the study. Pigs housed under normal swine husbandry conditions for extended periods of time can develop minor lung lesions that are inconsequential, and not related to specific pathogens [31].

Post-challenge viremia was selected as the most important secondary efficacy parameter because it represents the level of viral replication occurring within the host animal upon exposure. Furthermore, pathogenic and humoral immune responses to PRRSV are related to viral loads in acute infection [32]. Therefore, a significant reduction in PRRS viral load following vaccination would indicate that the vaccine could efficiently limit PRRSV pathogenesis in the host. Significant reductions in post-challenge viremia were observed in Group 1 pigs compared with Group 2 pigs 7 and 10 days post-challenge at 20–26 weeks. Cumulative exposure (AUC) from Days 3–10 post-challenge was also decreased in these pigs. Both findings indicate that Ingelvac PRRSFLEX® EU is efficient in limiting PRRSV viremia following virulent challenge, and confers a duration of immunity up to 26 weeks. Furthermore, a significant reduction in PRRSV-viral RNA load in lung tissue was observed in Group 1 pigs compared with Group 2 pigs at 20, 24 and 26 weeks. Viral RNA load in lung tissue is associated with viral replication and persistence in the host [33]. The results of these studies showed that Ingelvac PRRSFLEX® EU can effectively reduce PRRS-viral RNA load in lung tissue.

PRRSV infection contributes to a reduction in daily weight gain in young pigs [34]. In the 9 days following PRRSV challenge at 20 and 24 weeks, the ADWG of the Group 1 pigs was significantly higher than that of Group 2 pigs, whose ADWG was lower than that of Group 3 pigs. Following challenge at 26 weeks, ADWG in Group 1 pigs was increased compared with Group 2, but this increase did not reach statistical significance. These results indicate that Ingelvac PRRSFLEX® EU is effective at diminishing weight gain reduction caused by PRRS, possibly representing substantial economic importance. A recently published field study also supports this conclusion. This study found that vaccinating 4-week old piglets with Ingelvac PRRSFLEX® EU improved weight gain and reduced clinical signs during the growing period, even when the piglets are infected shortly after vaccination [35]. However, the current study is limited by the lack of statistical power due to the small sample size and findings need to be confirmed in larger studies. Also, this study used young pigs that were negative for PRRSV RNA; further studies are therefore required to determine whether these results apply to pigs of different ages and immune status.

PRRS MLV vaccines are considered the most effective PRRS vaccines available [5, 12]. The results of the previous studies provide evidence that Ingelvac PRRSFLEX® EU effectively confers immunity to PRRSV, which is maintained for up to 26 weeks. Since commercially-reared animals are typically slaughtered between 18 and 26 weeks of age [20], this long DOI conferred by Ingelvac PRRSFLEX® EU may help reduce the chance of PRRSV-related disease for the whole lifespan of vaccinated animals.

Conclusions

The three studies described here show that Ingelvac PRRSFLEX® EU was highly effective at conferring long-term immunity (up to 26 weeks) against virulent challenge with a heterologous European isolate of PRRSV in young pigs. After challenge at 24 and 26 weeks, gross and histological lung lesion scores, post-challenge viremia and viral RNA load in lung tissue, and ADWG were improved in PRRS-vaccinated pigs compared with challenge controls, with most measures reaching statistical significance. These results show that protection against heterologous PRRSV is achieved with the Ingelvac PRRSFLEX® EU, and can be maintained for the expected lifespan of young pigs, with beneficial effects on animal health and production.

Abbreviations
ADWG: average daily weight gain; AUC: area under the concentration-time curve; CI: confidence interval; CP: control product; DOI: duration of immunity; DPC: day post-challenge; GCP: good clinical practices; GE: genome equivalent; IM: intramuscular; IQR: interquartile range; KV: killed virus; MLV: modified live virus; PRRS: porcine reproductive and respiratory syndrome; PRRSV: porcine reproductive and respiratory syndrome virus; qPCR: quantitative polymerase chain reaction; TCID: tissue culture infective dose; VRI: Veterinary Resources, Inc.

Acknowledgements
The authors thank Dr. Ryan Saltzman, Dr. Lyle Keel, Dr. Stephan Perch, Mr. Rex Smiley, Dr. Alicia Zimmerman and Ms. Sarah Layton for technical assistance. The authors would also like to thank Dr. Zoe Kelly of InterComm International Ltd., Cambridge, UK, for providing medical writing support in accordance with Good Publication Practice (GPP3) guidelines (http://www.ismpp.org/gpp3).

Funding
The three studies were funded by Boehringer Ingelheim Vetmedica, Inc. Medical writing support with this manuscript was provided by InterComm International, Cambridge, UK, and this service was funded by Boehringer Ingelheim Vetmedica, Inc.

Authors' contributions
JK, F-XO, CK and MP designed the study outlines, monitored the studies, reviewed, analysed and reported the data. PR and OD reviewed the manuscript. All authors read and approved the final manuscript.

Competing interests
Jeremy Kroll is an employee of Boehringer Ingelheim Vetmedica, Inc. Poul H Rathkjen, Francois-Xavier Orveillon, and Oliver G. Duran are employees of Boehringer Ingelheim Vetmedica GmbH, Christian Kraft is an employee of Boehringer Ingelheim Veterinary Research Center GmbH & Co. KG. Michael Piontkowski is a retired employee of Boehringer Ingelheim Vetmedica, Inc.

Author details
[1]Boehringer Ingelheim Animal Health, 2412 South Loop Dr, Ames, IA 50010, USA. [2]Boehringer Ingelheim Animal Health, 2621 North Belt Highway, St. Joseph, MO 64506, USA. [3]Boehringer Ingelheim Vetmedica GmbH, Binger Straße 173, 55216 Ingelheim, Germany. [4]Boehringer Ingelheim Veterinary Research Center GmbH & Co. KG, Bemeroder Str. 31, 30559 Hannover, Germany.

References

1. Lunney JK, Benfield DA, Rowland RR. Porcine reproductive and respiratory syndrome virus: an update on an emerging and re-emerging viral disease of swine. Virus Res. 2010;154(1–2):1–6. Epub 19 Oct 2010
2. Keffaber KK. Reproductive failure of unknown etiology. Am Assoc Swine Pract Newsl. 1989;1:1–9.
3. Office International des Epizooties: World Animal Health 1991. Animal health status and disease control methods (part one: reports). 1992. http://www.oie.int/doc/ged/D7827.PDF Accessed 10 Sept 2017.
4. Wills RW, Zimmerman JJ, Yoon KJ, Swenson SL, McGinley MJ, Hill HT, et al. Porcine reproductive and respiratory syndrome virus: a persistent infection. Vet Microbiol. 1997;55(1–4):231–40. Epub 01 Apr 1997
5. Renukaradhya GJ, Meng XJ, Calvert JG, Roof M, Lager KM. Live porcine reproductive and respiratory syndrome virus vaccines: current status and future direction. Vaccine. 2015;33(33):4069–80. Epub 08 July 2015
6. Terpstra C, Wensvoort G, Pol JM. Experimental reproduction of porcine epidemic abortion and respiratory syndrome (mystery swine disease) by infection with Lelystad virus: Koch's postulates fulfilled. Vet Q. 1991;13(3):131–6. Epub 01 July 1991
7. Benfield DA, Nelson E, Collins JE, Harris L, Goyal SM, Robison D, et al. Characterization of swine infertility and respiratory syndrome (SIRS) virus (isolate ATCC VR-2332). J Vet Diagn Invest. 1992;4(2):127–33. Epub 01 Apr 1992
8. Nelsen CJ, Murtaugh MP, Faaberg KS. Porcine reproductive and respiratory syndrome virus comparison: divergent evolution on two continents. J Virol. 1999;73(1):270–80.
9. PGW P. Porcine reproductive and respiratory syndrome virus: origin hypothesis. Emerg Infect Dis. 2003;9(8):903–8.
10. Kim WI, Lee DS, Johnson W, Roof M, Cha SH, Yoon KJ. Effect of genotypic and biotypic differences among PRRS viruses on the serologic assessment of pigs for virus infection. Vet Microbiol. 2007;123(1–3):1–14. Epub 01 May 2007
11. Charerntantanakul W. Porcine reproductive and respiratory syndrome virus vaccines: immunogenicity, efficacy and safety aspects. World J Virol. 2012;1(1):23–30. Epub 12 Feb 2012
12. Rowland RR, Lunney J, Dekkers J. Control of porcine reproductive and respiratory syndrome (PRRS) through genetic improvements in disease resistance and tolerance. Front Genet. 2012;3:260. Epub 14 Feb 2013
13. Nielsen TL, Nielsen J, Have P, Baekbo P, Hoff-Jorgensen R, Botner A. Examination of virus shedding in semen from vaccinated and from previously infected boars after experimental challenge with porcine reproductive and respiratory syndrome virus. Vet Microbiol. 1997;54(2):101–12. Epub 01 Feb 1997
14. Nilubol D, Platt KB, Halbur PG, Torremorell M, Harris DL. The effect of a killed porcine reproductive and respiratory syndrome virus (PRRSV) vaccine treatment on virus shedding in previously PRRSV infected pigs. Vet Microbiol. 2004;102(1–2):11–8. Epub 04 Aug 2004
15. Scortti M, Prieto C, Alvarez E, Simarro I, Castro JM. Failure of an inactivated vaccine against porcine reproductive and respiratory syndrome to protect gilts against a heterologous challenge with PRRSV. Vet Rec. 2007;161(24):809–13. Epub 18 Dec 2007
16. Cano JP, Dee SA, Murtaugh MP, Pijoan C. Impact of a modified-live porcine reproductive and respiratory syndrome virus vaccine intervention on a population of pigs infected with a heterologous isolate. Vaccine. 2007;25(22):4382–91. Epub 25 Apr 2007
17. Park C, Choi K, Jeong J, Chae C. Cross-protection of a new type 2 porcine reproductive and respiratory syndrome virus (PRRSV) modified live vaccine (Fostera PRRS) against heterologous type 1 PRRSV challenge in growing pigs. Vet Microbiol. 2015;177(1–2):87–94. Epub 15 Mar 2015
18. Prieto C, Alvarez E, Martinez-Lobo FJ, Simarro I, Castro JM. Similarity of European porcine reproductive and respiratory syndrome virus strains to vaccine strain is not necessarily predictive of the degree of protective immunity conferred. Vet J. 2008;175(3):356–63. Epub 15 June 2007
19. Roca M, Gimeno M, Bruguera S, Segales J, Diaz I, Galindo-Cardiel IJ, et al. Effects of challenge with a virulent genotype II strain of porcine reproductive and respiratory syndrome virus on piglets vaccinated with an attenuated genotype I strain vaccine. Vet J. 2012;193(1):92–6. Epub 24 Oct 2012
20. Marchant-Forde JN. Introduction to the welfare of pigs. In: Marchant-Forde JN, editor. The welfare of pigs. Dordrecht: Springer Netherlands; 2009. p. 1–12.
21. Murtaugh MP, Genzow M. Immunological solutions for treatment and prevention of porcine reproductive and respiratory syndrome (PRRS). Vaccine. 2011;29(46):8192–204. Epub 20 Sept 2011
22. Meier WA, Galeota J, Osorio FA, Husmann RJ, Schnitzlein WM, Zuckermann FA. Gradual development of the interferon-gamma response of swine to porcine reproductive and respiratory syndrome virus infection or vaccination. Virology. 2003;309(1):18–31. Epub 03 May 2003
23. Hu J, Zhang C. Porcine reproductive and respiratory syndrome virus vaccines: current status and strategies to a universal vaccine. Transbound Emerg Dis. 2014;61(2):109–20.
24. Madsen KG, Hansen CM, Madsen ES, Strandbygaard B, Botner A, Sorensen KJ. Sequence analysis of porcine reproductive and respiratory syndrome virus of the American type collected from Danish swine herds. Arch Virol. 1998;143(9):1683–700. Epub 27 Oct 1998
25. Piontkowski M, Kroll J, Kraft C, Coll T. Safety and early onset of immunity with a novel European porcine reproductive and respiratory syndrome virus vaccine in young piglets. Can J Vet Res. 2016;80(2):124–33.
26. Summary of product characteristics. Ingelvac PRRSFLEX EU lyophilisate and solvent for suspension for injection for pigs. 2015: Health Products Regulatory Authority; 2017. http://www.hpra.ie/img/uploaded/swedocuments/LicenseSPC_10007-052-001_02042015120937.pdf Accessed 10 Sept 2017
27. Revilla-Fernandez S, Wallner B, Truschner K, Benczak A, Brem G, Schmoll F, et al. The use of endogenous and exogenous reference RNAs for qualitative and quantitative detection of PRRSV in porcine semen. J Virol Methods. 2005;126(1–2):21–30. Epub 26 Apr 2005
28. Roques E, Girard A, St-Louis M-C, Massie B, Gagnon CA, Lessard M, et al. Immunogenic and protective properties of GP5 and M structural proteins of porcine reproductive and respiratory syndrome virus expressed from replicating but nondisseminating adenovectors. Vet Res. 2013;44(1):17.
29. Christianson WT, Joo HS. Porcine reproductive and respiratory syndrome: a review. J Swine Health Prod. 1994;2(2):10-28.
30. Rossow KD. Porcine reproductive and respiratory syndrome. Vet Pathol. 1998;35(1):1–20. Epub 17 Apr 1998
31. Grest P, Keller H, Sydler T, Pospischil A. The prevalence of lung lesions in pigs at slaughter in Switzerland. Schweizer Archiv fur Tierheilkunde. 1997;139(11):500–6. Epub 01 Jan 1997
32. Johnson W, Roof M, Vaughn E, Christopher-Hennings J, Johnson CR, Murtaugh MP. Pathogenic and humoral immune responses to porcine reproductive and respiratory syndrome virus (PRRSV) are related to viral load in acute infection. Vet Immunol Immunopathol. 2004;102(3):233–47. Epub 28 Oct 2004
33. Rossow KD, Collins JE, Goyal SM, Nelson EA, Christopher-Hennings J, Benfield DA. Pathogenesis of porcine reproductive and respiratory syndrome virus infection in gnotobiotic pigs. Vet Pathol. 1995;32(4):361–73. Epub 1995/07/01
34. Li MM, Seelenbinder KM, Ponder MA, Deng L, Rhoads RP, Pelzer KD, et al. Effects of porcine reproductive and respiratory syndrome virus on pig growth, diet utilization efficiency, and gas release from stored manure. J Anim Sci. 2015;93(9):4424–35. Epub 07 Oct 2015
35. Cano G, Cavalcanti MO, Orveillon F-X, Kroll J, Gomez-Duran O, Morillo A, et al. Production results from piglets vaccinated in a field study in Spain with a type 1 porcine respiratory and reproductive virus modified live vaccine. Porcine Health Management. 2016;2(1):22.

20

Clinical efficacy of two vaccination strategies against *Mycoplasma hyopneumoniae* in a pig herd suffering from respiratory disease

Vojislav Cvjetković[1], Sabine Sipos[2], Imre Szabó[3] and Wolfgang Sipos[4*] [iD]

Abstract

Background: A randomised field trial was conducted on an Austrian farrow-to-finish farm for one year to compare the efficacy of two commercial *Mycoplasma hyopneumoniae* vaccines. 585 piglets either received the one-shot formulation in group 1 (Hyogen®, 23.9 days of age) or a two-shot vaccine (Stellamune® Mycoplasma, 4.3 and 24.0 days of age) in group 2. Assessment of vaccine efficacy was evaluated by regression analyses through cough monitoring from nursery to slaughter, average daily weight gain from inclusion to slaughter, antibiotic treatment rate (ATR), mortality rate, and lung lesion scoring at slaughter.

Results: In general, coughing was more frequent during late nursery and finishing. No significant differences were found in the coughing index (0.02 vs 0.03) and mean average daily weight gain (560 vs 550 g) between the two groups. ATR was higher in group 2 (3.8 vs 9.6%). At the slaughterhouse check, significant differences in the prevalence of bronchopneumonia (62.9 vs 71.2%) could be found. Extension of lung lesions was also significantly lower in group 1 in terms of enzootic pneumonia (EP) values ($p = 0.000$, $z = -4.269$). There were no significant differences in the rate of scarred lungs (20.0 vs 24.0%) or those affected by dorsocaudal pleurisy (36.8 vs 34.3%).

Conclusions: This trial demonstrated that Hyogen® was superior to Stellamune® Mycoplasma in reducing (I) the prevalence of bronchopneumonic lungs and those affected by cranioventral pleurisy, (II) the extension and severity of EP-like lung lesions, and (III) the rate of antibiotically treated animals against respiratory disease.

Keywords: Mycoplasma hyopneumoniae, One-shot vaccine, Two-shot-vaccine, Randomised field trial, Lung health

Background

Mycoplasma hyopneumoniae (*M. hyopneumoniae*) is considered a primary pathogen of the porcine respiratory system, playing an important role in the porcine respiratory disease complex. The first stage of pathogenesis is the adhesion of *M. hyopneumoniae* to the ciliated epithelial cells of the respiratory mucosa by means of the adhesins P97, P102, and P159 [1–3]. In addition, *M. hyopneumoniae* is able to produce hydrogen peroxide, thus leading to inflammatory lesions at the respective sites [4]. Thus ciliostasis, clumping and loss of the cilia, and direct toxic harm to the respiratory epithelium are induced, which eventually leads to a decreased clearance of bacteria and opens the gate to secondary respiratory infections [5]. Genetic analyses showed that there is a strong heterogeneity in *M. hyopneumoniae* isolates originating from different herds [6]. A recent study reported that different *M. hyopneumoniae* strains can also be isolated from different batches of slaughter pigs of the same herd, with the severity of pneumonia at slaughter being significantly higher in those batches where multiple strains co-existed [7].

Possible methods to prevent and control *M. hyopneumoniae* are optimization of management practices such

---
* Correspondence: wolfgang.sipos@vetmeduni.ac.at
[4]Clinic for Swine, University of Veterinary Medicine Vienna, Veterinärplatz 1, 1210 Vienna, Austria
Full list of author information is available at the end of the article

as all-in/all-out production and multisite-operations, the use of antimicrobials, and vaccination. Although national eradication programs have been carried out in some countries, reinfection of herds frequently occurs, as documented in Switzerland [8, 9]. The *M. hyopneumoniae*-free state of herds is difficult to maintain especially in pig-dense areas, since airborne spread of the pathogen may occur over several kilometers [10]. Tetracyclines and macrolides are used most frequently to control and treat respiratory disease induced by *M. hyopneumoniae* [8]. Other potentially active antimicrobials include lincosamides, pleuromutilins, fluoroquinolones, florfenicol, aminoglycosides, and aminocyclitols [11]. Nevertheless, antibiotics are neither able to eliminate *M. hyopneumoniae* from the respiratory tract nor restore already developed lung lesions [5]. Additionally, the massive and often not justified use of antibiotics has led to a rise in antibiotic resistances, which has important drawbacks for animal and human health.

Commercial vaccines are extensively used in controlling *M. hyopneumoniae*. Several vaccination schemes exist: traditional two-shot formulations, which are still favoured in some European countries like Austria, one-shot formulations, and bivalent one-shot formulations containing both *M. hyopneumoniae* and porcine circovirus type 2 (PCV2) antigens. In general, vaccination reduces the occurrence of clinical signs and lung lesions and improves performance, but on the other hand does not prevent colonization of the respiratory tract epithelia by mycoplasma organisms [12, 13]; yet variable results can be observed under field conditions. Vaccine storage, administration and compliance play an important role in the efficacy of the products [14]. Furthermore, according to a field study comparing two different one-shot and a two-shot vaccine, vaccine efficacy is more likely to be dependent on the composition of vaccines used and to a lesser degree on the number of vaccinations [15]. Aim of this study was to compare the efficacy of a single-shot vaccine against *M. hyopneumoniae* based on a novel bacterin using the 2940 strain and Imuvant™ (combination of light liquid paraffin O/W and *Escherichia coli* J5 lipopolysaccharide (ECJ5L)) as adjuvant with a two-shot product based on the strain P-5722-3 (NL 1042) adjuvated by a mixture of Amphigen base and Drakeol 5, by assessment of clinical signs, performance, and macroscopic lung lesions at slaughter.

Methods
Animals and trial setting
The study was performed on a closed combined family-owned single-site farm in Lower Austria, housing 84 Large White sows working in a 3-weeks rhythm. 600 fattening places were assigned to 10 pens in one stable and therefore also one air space. Every four months, all

sows were vaccinated with a modified-live porcine reproductive and respiratory syndrome virus (PRRSV) vaccine as well as with a combined vaccine against Erysipelas and Parvovirosis. The PRRS-MLV vaccine was administered also to the piglets at their fourth week of life immediately after weaning. Other piglet vaccinations included a live, attenuated vaccine against *Lawsonia intracellularis* (week 3) and an inactivated PCV2 vaccine (week 4).

After anamnestic reporting of dry recurrent coughing beginning in the nursery, PCR testing for *M. hyopneumoniae* out of lung samples at a local Animal Health Service Lab in May 2015 gave positive results and therefore a two-shot vaccination program using a commercial vaccine (Stellamune® Mycoplasma, Elanco Animal Health) was introduced. However, coughing persisted and the pathogen was isolated again in 2016 before the start of the study. At that time, an additional PCR for *M. hyorhinis*, *Haemophilus parasuis* (HPS), and *Actinobacillus pleuropneumoniae* (APP), as well as serological analyses for APP- and HPS-antibodies gave no positive results. Additional serological survey for PRRSV-antibodies showed homogeneous titers with higher levels in sows due to vaccination and negative results in fatteners. Two slaughter lung checks in March and April 2016 revealed high rate bronchopneumonia (BP) lesions with prevalences of 84 and 92%, respectively, and extended cranioventral consolidations. The combined occurrence of clinical signs, enzootic pneumonia (EP)-like lesions at slaughter, and detection of *M. hyopneumoniae* by PCR were indicative of a still ongoing infection with this pathogen. The veterinary practitioner and the farm owner then decided to perform a comparative study between the actual two-shot vaccine and Hyogen® (Ceva Santé Animale), a novel single-shot bacterin. When doing random microbiological analyses from lungs of four euthanized animals in the course of the study, one animal was found to be completely free of lung pathogens in PCR and bacteriology, another animal exhibited infection with only *M. hyopneumoniae*, but was negative in bacteriology, the third animal was positive for *M. hyopneumoniae*, *M. hyorhinis*, HPS, and APP, and the fourth animal was positive for *M. hyopneumoniae*, *M. hyorhinis*, and *Pasteurella spp.*.

The field trial began in May 2016 and ended a year later in May 2017. In summary, 585 healthy, on average 4-day-old piglets of six consecutive farrowings were individually weighed and sexed. Then, starting with the heaviest piglet and ending with the smallest one, piglets were alternately assigned to the two groups and ear-tagged at the same time within each farrowing group, so that in the end we had an approximately 50:50 proportion of both vaccination groups within each litter. On average sow parity was 3.3 in group 1 with 62 sows included and 3.1 in group 2 with 63 sows included. Both vaccines were administered intramuscularly according to manufacturers' instructions: group 1 piglets were injected in the neck once with 2 ml of the one-shot vaccine at 23.9 days of age in the mean. Group 2 piglets were injected in the neck twice on average at days 4.3 and 24.0 with the two-shot product. Male piglets were castrated in their first week of life. Animals of each group were raised in different pens in the nursery and fattening unit but shared the same air space. Cough monitoring was performed by only one veterinarian once weekly in each group starting from weaning until the end of the fattening period. Pigs in each pen were solicited to get up and the number of coughs was counted during a period of two minutes. The coughing index (CI) was obtained by dividing the number of coughs by the number of observed animals and examination days. Weights were measured at the end of nursery and before slaughter beside the time point of inclusion, when piglets had an age of 4 days. Average daily weight gain (ADG) from inclusion to slaughter, overall mortality rate, as well as the antibiotic treatment rate (ATR) against respiratory disease with amoxicillin, fluoroquinolones, and florfenicol were also documented. Animals were only treated by injectables by the farmer, who was blinded. No oral-route antibiotics were used.

Assessment of lung lesions

Lungs were blindly scored at the slaughterhouse according to a methodology combining the detection of four different types of lesions [16]. Due to the high speed of the line process, the two investigators, who were always the same, shared the work. One person did the lung check and the second one was responsible for the documentation by using the software tool Ceva Lung Program®, meaning, they stood side by side at the site of the line, where lung and heart were prepared from the carcass. First, each lung lobe was individually evaluated according to a scoring system for EP-like lesions based on the Madec and Kobisch score [17, 18]. Scores 0–4 are attributed to lesions according to the percentage of surface affected per lobe with score 0 representing 0% affected surface, score 1 representing 1–25%, score 2 representing 26–50%, score 3 representing 51–75%, and score 4 representing 76–100%. Consequently, each lung can achieve an EP value between 0 and 28, with values > 0 being considered a bronchopneumonic lung.

Second, for each lung, pleuritic lesions exclusively affecting the dorsocaudal lobes were evaluated according to a modified Slaughterhouse Pleurisy Evaluation System (SPES), with no lesion being score 0, score 2 resembling a dorsocaudal monolateral focal lesion, score 3 resembling a dorsocaudal bilateral focal lesion or extended monolateral lesion (at least 1/3 of one diaphragmatic lobe), and score 4 resembling a severely extended

bilateral lesion (at least 1/3 of both diaphragmatic lobes) [19].

Third, each lung was inspected for the presence of cranioventral pleurisy (CP) without describing the extension of the lesion. Finally, each lung was also visually inspected for the presence scars or fissures.

Statistical analysis

During the analyses the following three regression models were used.

Mixed effect ANOVA:

$$y_{jkl} = \mu + \sum_{i}^{n} \beta_i x_{ijkl} + \gamma_l + \delta_{kl} + \varepsilon_{jkl}$$

Mixed effect logistic regression:

$$\ln\left(\frac{p_{jkl}}{1-p_{jkl}}\right) = \mu + \sum_{i}^{n} \beta_i x_{ijkl} + \gamma_l + \delta_{kl} + \varepsilon_{jkl}$$

Mixed effect Poisson regression:

$$\ln\left(y_{jkl}\right) = \mu + \sum_{i}^{n} \beta_i x_{ijkl} + \gamma_l + \delta_{kl} + \varepsilon_{jkl}$$

In these models y represents the observed result, p represents the probability of occurrence of the observed event, μ represents the constant term, β represents the fixed factor effects (treatment group, sex, sow parity and in case of ADG time between first and last weighing), n represents the number of fix factors used in the model, x represents the factor configurations, γ represents random intercept of the farrowing group factor, δ represents the random intercept of the mother sow number factor, and ε represents the residual error.

ADG was compared with mixed-effect analysis of variance (ANOVA) models with vaccination group, gender, time between first and last weighing as well as sow parity as fixed factors and farrowing group and sow number as random factors. Indicator variable data (0 and 1) were compared with mixed-effect logistic regression models with vaccination group, gender, and sow parity as fixed factors and farrowing group and sow number were used as random factors. Ordinal data were compared with generalized Wilcoxon-Mann-Whitney ranksum test (van Elteren's test) using farrowing groups as strata. Here the z score is the measure of the deviation of central tendency from the hypothetical perfect equivalence of the two groups. A negative z score means that the examined population is stochastically smaller than the other population. The results of the ordinal data evaluations were supplemented with mixed-effect logistic regression models using the indicator value categorization of the ordinal data where vaccination group, gender, and sow parity were used as fixed factors and farrowing group and sow number were used as random factors. Score zero was coded as 0; score values higher than zero were coded as 1. Mortality data were compared with mixed-effect logistic regression models, where the vaccination group was used as fixed factor and farrowing groups and sow numbers were used as random factors. As the time of the events (deaths) was not available, Kaplan-Meier estimation was not possible. ATR was compared with mixed-effect logistic regression models where the vaccination group was used as fixed factor and the farrowing group was used as random factor. Cough monitoring data were compared with mixed-effect Poisson regression models. Here, again the vaccination group was used as the fixed factor and the farrowing group as the random factor. If an estimate of a random effect was negligible (less than 10^{-4}), the effect was omitted with the exception of cough monitoring and the regression model was refitted to the data. Model outcomes were described using the 95% confidence interval, effect sizes (ES) and odds ratios (OR) are representing the one-shot vs two-shot vaccination comparison in that order. All statistical computations were performed using Stata 15 software (StataCorp. 2017. Stata Statistical Software: Release 15. College Station, TX: StataCorp LLC). The type I error for all statistical tests was set to 5% ($p < 0.05$).

Results
Performance
Animals tolerated vaccinations very well. Neither local nor systemic reactions could be observed. No significant difference in ADG ($p = 0.96$, ES = 0.000 (−0.006, 0.006)) between the two vaccination groups was found. Overall mortality was 13/293 in group 1 (2 suckling piglets, 5 animals in nursery, and 6 fatteners) and 21/292 in group 2 (7 piglets, 9 growers, and 5 fatteners) ($p = 0.16$, ES = 0.51 (−0.2, 1.22), OR = 1.67 (0.82, 3.40)). CI did not differ significantly between the two groups ($p = 0.65$, ES = 0.36 (−1.17, 1.90)), however, coughing was generally more prominent in late nursery and finishing. In terms of ATR, the groups differed significantly ($p = 0.005$, ES = 1.036 (0.310, 1.762), OR = 2.817 (1.363, 5.822)). It can be estimated from the regression model that in the one-shot group 3.2% (0.6, 5.8%) of the animals and in the two-shot group 8.6% (3.2, 14.0%) of the animals will need antibiotic treatment.

Lung health
In terms of bronchopneumonia prevalence at slaughter, the supplementary logistic regression model exhibited a significant difference between the treatment groups ($p = 0.028$, ES = 0.439 (0.048, 0.829), OR = 1.550 (1.049, 2.292)). It can be estimated from the regression model that 59.6% (42.5, 76.6%) of the animals in the one-shot group will show a bronchopneumonic lung at any

severity level, whereas in in the two-shot group 69.6% (54.6, 84.5%) of the animals will be affected. However, no significance could be demonstrated concerning the influence of gender ($p = 0.07$, ES = 0.37 (−0.03, 0.77), OR = 1.45 (0.97, 2.15)) or sow parity ($p = 0.94$, ES = −0.01 (−0.15, 0.14), OR = 0.99 (0.86, 1.15)). EP values were significantly lower in group 1 ($p = 0.000$, z = −4.269) (Fig. 1).

Furthermore, a significant difference in the presence of cranioventral pleurisy between the vaccination groups was found ($p = 0.038$, ES = 0.368 (0.020, 0.715), OR = 1.444 (1.020, 2.045)). It can be estimated from the regression model that 50.1% (38.7, 61.5%) of the animals in the one-shot group will suffer from CP, whereas in the two-shot group 59.2% (48.3, 70.1%) of the animals will be affected. Both gender ($p = 0.47$, ES = −0.13 (−0.47, 0.22), OR = 0.88 (0.62, 1.24)) and sow parity ($p = 0.30$, ES = 0.06 (−0.05, 0.16) OR = 1.06 (0.95, 1.18)) showed no significant effect on CP. No significant differences were found in modified SPES values ($p = 0.58$, z = 0.55) or numbers of scarred lungs ($p = 0.26$, ES = 0.25 (−0.18, 0.68), OR = 1.28 (0.84, 1.98)) between the two vaccination groups. Dorsocaudal pleurisy was not affected by gender ($p = 0.41$, ES = 0.15 (−0.20, 0.50), OR = 1.16 (0.82, 1.65)) or sow parity ($p = 0.09$, ES = 0.09 (−0.01, 0.19), OR = 1.09 (0.99, 1.21)), in similarity to scarring and gender ($p = 0.45$, ES = 0.17 (−0.27, 0.60), OR = 1.18 (0.76, 1.83)) and scarring and sow parity ($p = 0.46$, ES = 0.06 (−0.09, 0.21), OR = 1.06 (0.91, 1.23)).

Prevalences and descriptive statistics of all data sets are presented in Tables 1 and 2.

Discussion
Although vaccination against *M. hyopneumoniae* is applied worldwide, variable results are observed [14]. Most current vaccines are still based on the J-strain, isolated in 1963 from a pig herd in the United Kingdom [20]. The one-shot formulation used in this study is based on the *M. hyopneumoniae* strain 2940, isolated in 1999 from a farm facing a severe outbreak of enzootic pneumonia, which might be beneficial for vaccine efficacy as low virulent strains might not be the best choice [21]. Furthermore, adjuvants also play a key role in the efficacy of vaccines [22]. Apart from light liquid paraffin O/W-formulation, the vaccine tested in this study is also adjuvated by inactivated *Escherichia coli* J5 non-toxic LPS (ECJ5L), which was shown to exert a significantly stronger cell-mediated immune response in terms of specific interferon-γ producing T cells when compared to solely paraffin-adjuvated or non-adjuvated test vaccines [23]. Furthermore, Hyogen® has been shown to be efficacious against experimental challenge with both low and highly virulent *M. hyopneumoniae* strains [24].

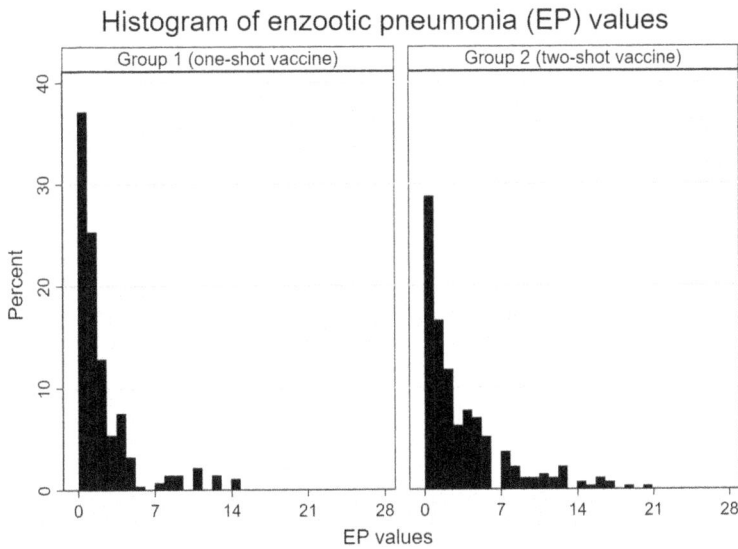

Fig. 1 Comparison of EP-value distributions between vaccination group 1 (*n* = 280) and vaccination group 2 (*n* = 271)

Although EP-like lesions are generally not considered pathognomonic of *M. hyopneumoniae*, they are considered suggestive for previous EP due to mixed infections with *M. hyopneumoniae* and other pathogens [25]. *M. hyopneumoniae* was demonstrated to be a key factor for respiratory disease and EP-like lung lesions at slaughter in the herd under investigation, although besides *M. hyopneumoniae* also other respiratory pathogens had been isolated in the herd under investigation, and therefore the decision was made to introduce a new vaccination program against *M. hyopneumoniae*, as the two-shot vaccination regimen against *M. hyopneumoniae* and additional management optimizations had not yielded any improvement. The present study was therefore conducted in order to compare the efficacy of a novel one-shot vaccine against the two-shot vaccine, which was already in use. To the authors' knowledge, this is the first randomised field trial comparing 6 consecutive batches of differently *M. hyopneumoniae*-vaccinated groups for an entire year. Also,

we also had the opportunity to verify if gender had a significant impact on the development of gross lung lesions as previously described in literature [26, 27].

In terms of clinical observations, coughing generally became more prominent in late nursery and finishing but CI did not differ between the two groups, which contrasts with the results of the slaughter lung lesions. This is in accordance with a study suggesting that weekly assessment of coughing is not a predictive indicator of lung lesions at slaughter [28]. ADG did not differ between the groups, which is also in accordance with other field studies [29, 30]. However, a recent study investigating the impact of lung lesions on production performance showed that each categorial increase in EP-like lesion severity, according to a 5-step scoring system different from the one used in this study, resulted in a reduction of 0.37 kg in post-trimming carcass weight [31]. Mortality accounted for 13/293 of the animals in group 1 and 21/292 in group 2 without showing any

Table 1 Descriptive statistics of evaluated data

Parameter	Treatment group	N	Mean	SD	Min	Median	Max
Weight at inclusion with 4 days (grams)	Group 1	280	1890.6	442.4	927.0	1839.5	3099.0
	Group 2	271	1918.6	494.2	670.0	1858.0	3235.0
Average daily weight gain (grams)	Group 1	280	560	60	350	560	710
	Group 2	271	550	60	390	560	700
EP-like lesion values	Group 1	280	2.02	2.98	0.00	1.00	14.00
	Group 2	271	3.39	4.12	0.00	2.00	20.00
SPES values	Group 1	280	0.98	1.33	0.00	0.00	4.00
	Group 2	271	0.92	1.31	0.00	0.00	4.00
Coughing index	Group 1	118	0.02	0.04	0.00	0.00	0.19
	Group 2	118	0.03	0.08	0.00	0.02	0.83

Table 2 Prevalences of observed data sets

Parameter	Treatment group	N	Lack of parameter	Lack of parameter (%)	Presence of parameter	Presence of parameter (%)
Pneumonia	Group 1	280	104	37.1	176	62.9
	Group 2	271	78	28.8	193	71.2
Cranial pleurisy	Group 1	280	131	46.8	149	53.2
	Group 2	271	104	38.4	167	61.6
Dorsocaudal pleurisy	Group 1	280	177	63.2	103	36.8
	Group 2	271	178	65.7	93	34.3
Lung tissue scars	Group 1	280	224	80.0	54	20.0
	Group 2	271	206	76.0	65	24.0
Mortality	Group 1	293	280	95.6	13	4.4
	Group 2	292	271	92.8	21	7.2
Antibiotic treatments	Group 1	293	282	96.2	11	3.8
	Group 2	292	264	90.4	28	9.6

significance, which is in accordance with most field studies comparing *M. hyopneumoniae* vaccines [29, 30]. Mortality rates in our study can be explained to some extent by crushing of piglets to death by the sows. Remaining animals died due to fibrinous bronchopneumonia or septicemic heart disease, thus reflecting the additional problems caused by HPS and APP in that herd.

Individual treatment against respiratory disease was recorded by the farmer and later evaluated. The Hyogen®-group had a significantly lower ATR than the two-shot group for the whole observation period and in some way the ATR refined what was previously missing for the CI. This finding is of importance, as a low ATR against respiratory disease can be used as indicator of lung health on the one hand and support the rationale of using effective vaccines to avoid otherwise indicated antibiotic treatment regimens on the other hand. However, our results are in contrast to the results of another field study, where no reduction in antibiotic treatment between differently vaccinated groups and the control group could be found [29].

Over the study period the proportion of lungs affected by bronchopneumonia was significantly lower in the Hyogen®-group. Also, severity of lung lesions in terms of EP-values was significantly lower in this group. However, gender and sow parity had no influence on lung lesion prevalences. The same applied to CP values. In a comparable field-study, three *M. hyopneumoniae* vaccines (two one-shot vaccines and a two-shot vaccine) were compared in terms of lung lesions, lung histopathology, and *M. hyopneumoniae* load [15]. One one-shot vaccine showed significantly higher median Madec and Kobisch lung lesion scores (3) than the other one-shot vaccine and the two-shot product (both 0). Although mean lesions between the latter two vaccines did not differ significantly, the two-shot vaccine had a higher prevalence of lungs with score 0 (64.2% vs. 55.6%) and a lower

prevalence of lungs with score 5–9 (5.3% vs. 14.9%) and 10–20 (1.6% vs. 2.3%). Thus, in this study the two-shot formulation proved to be higher protective in terms of lung health than the two one-shot formulations. This is in contrast to our study and demonstrates that continuous development of vaccines can lead to even unexpected results.

The study presented has two major limitations. First, only one farm has been included. This farm represents a typical Austrian farm, although production units in other countries house much higher numbers of sows. Second, no continuous monitoring of the *M. hyopneumoniae* load was performed. However, our primary aim was to demonstrate clinical non-inferiority of Hyogen® in comparison to an established two-shot regimen, which could be clearly shown.

Conclusions

Under the conditions of the present study, pigs vaccinated with the one-shot vaccine Hyogen® did not differ from the two-shot group in terms if coughing index, ADG, or mortality rate, but exhibited a significantly better lung health status at slaughter in terms of a lower proportion of bronchopneumonic lungs and lower Madec and Kobisch score values as well as lower incidences of cranioventral pleurisies. Furthermore, a significantly higher proportion of pigs needed antibiotic treatment against respiratory infections in the two-shot group.

Abbreviations
ADG: Average daily weight gain; ANOVA: analysis of variance; ATR: antibiotic treatment rate; BP: bronchopneumonia; CP: cranioventral pleurisy; EP: enzootic pneumonia; ES: effect size; OR: odds ratio; SPES: Slaughterhouse Pleurisy Evaluation System

Acknowledgements
The authors would like to thank the farmer and his family for their support. The authors also want to thank the Izsler Institute for their support in designing the lung scoring online tool.

Funding
This study was funded by Ceva Tiergesundheit GmbH.

Authors' contributions
WS conducted the study design, supervised the study, participated in data collection and corrected the manuscript. IS performed the statistics. SS chose the farm for the study and participated in data collection. VC participated in data collection and wrote the manuscript. All authors read and approved the final manuscript.

Competing interests
First and third author of this research article are employees from the company sponsor.

Author details
¹Ceva Tiergesundheit GmbH, Kanzlerstraße 4, 40472 Düsseldorf, Germany. ²Veterinary Practice Schwertfegen, Schwertfegen 2, 3040, Neulengbach, Austria. ³Ceva-Phylaxia, Co., Szállás u.5, Budapest 1107, Hungary. ⁴Clinic for Swine, University of Veterinary Medicine Vienna, Veterinärplatz 1, 1210 Vienna, Austria.

References
1. Hsu T, Minion FC. Identification of the cilium binding epitope of the mycoplasma hyopneumoniae P97 Adhesin. Infect Immun. 1998;66:4762–6.
2. Adams C, Pitzer J, Minion FC. In vivo expression analysis of the P97 and P102 paralog families of Mycoplasma hyopneumoniae. Infect Immun. 2005;73:7784–7.
3. Burnett TA, Dinkla K, Rohde M, Chhatwal GS, Uphoff C, Srivastava M, Cordwell SJ, Geary S, Liao X, Minion FC, Walker MJ, Djordjevic SP. P159 is a proteolytically processed, surface adhesin of Mycoplasma hyopneumoniae: defined domains of P159 bind heparin and promote adherence to eukaryote cells. Mol Microbiol. 2006;60(3):669–86.
4. Ferrarini MG, Siquiera FM, Mucha SG, Palama TL, Jobard E, Elena-Hermann B, Vasconcelos ATR, Tardy F, Schrank IS, Zaha A, Sagot MF. Insights on the virulence of swine respiratory tract mycoplasmas through genome-scale metabolic modeling. BMC Genomics. 2016;17:353.
5. Thacker EL, Minion FC. Mycoplasmosis. In: Zimmerman JJ, Karriker LA, Ramirez A, Schwartz KJ, Stevenson GW, editors. Diseases of Swine. 10th ed. Chichester: John Wiley & Sons Ltd; 2012. p. 779–86.
6. Charlebois A, Marois-Créhan C, Hélie P, Gagnon CA, Gottschalk M, Archambault M. Genetic diversity of Mycoplasma hyopneumoniae isolates of abattoir pigs. Vet Microbiol. 2014;168:348–56.
7. Michiels A, Vranckx K, Piepers S, Del Pozo Sacristán R, Arsenakis I, Boyen F, Haesebrouck F, Maes D. Impact of diversity of Mycoplasma hyopneumoniae strains on lung lesions in slaughter pigs. Vet Res. 2017;48:2.
8. Maes D, Segales J, Meyns T, Sibila M, Pieters M, Haesebrouck F. Control of Mycoplasma hyopneumoniae in pigs. Vet Microbiol. 2008;126:297–309.
9. Hege R, Zimmermann W, Scheidegger R, Stärk KDC. Incidence of reinfections with Mycoplasma hyopneumoniae and Actinobacillus pleuropneumoniae in pig farms located in respiratory-disease-free regions of Switzerland – identification and quantification of risk factors. Acta Vet Scand. 2002;43:145–6.
10. Otake S, Dee S, Corzo C, Oliveira S, Deen J. Long-distance airborne transport of infectious PRRSV and Mycoplasma hyopneumoniae from a swine population infected with multiple viral variants. Vet Microbiol. 2010;145:198–208.
11. Vicca J. Virulence and antimicrobial susceptibility of Mycoplasma hyopneumoniae isolates from pigs. http://www.rohh.ugent.be/v3/research/phd/2005/Vicca_J.pdf (2005). Accessed 16 Feb 2018.
12. Thacker EL, Thacker BJ, Young TF, Halbur PG. Effect of vaccination on the potentiation of porcine reproductive and respiratory syndrome virus (PRRSV)-induced pneumonia by mycoplasma hyopneumoniae. Vaccine. 2000;18:1244–52.
13. Meyns T, Dewulf J, de Kruif A, Calus D, Haesebrouck F, Maes D. Comparison of transmission of mycoplasma hyopneumoniae in vaccinated and non-vaccinated populations. Vaccine. 2006;24:7081–6.
14. Maes D, Sibila M, Kuhnert P, Segales J, Haesebrouck F, Pieters M. Update on Mycoplasma hyopneumoniae infections in pigs: knowledge gaps for improved disease control. Transbound Emerg Dis. 2017; https://doi.org/10.1111/tbed.12677.
15. Hillen S, Von Berg S, Köhler K, Reinacher M, Willems H, Reiner G. Occurrence and severity of lung lesions in slaughter pigs vaccinated against Mycoplasma hyopneumoniae with different strategies. Prev Vet Med. 2014;113:580–8.
16. Krejci R, Munoz R. Lung scoring program as a monitoring tool in Asia. In: Proceedings of the 23 rd International Pig Veterinary Society Congress, Cancun, Mexico, vol. 397; 2014.
17. Madec F, Kobisch M. Bilan lésionnel des poumons de porcs charcutiers à l'abattoir. Journees. Rech porcine en France. 1982;14:405–12.
18. Ostanello F, Dottori M, Gusmara C, Leotti G, Sala V. Pneumonia disease assessment using a slaughterhouse lung-scoring method. J Vet Med A. 2007;54:70–5.
19. Dottori M, Nigrelli AD, Bonilauri P, Merialdi G, Gozio S, Cominotti F. Proposal for a new grading system for pleuritis at slaughterhouse. The S.P.E.S. (slaughterhouse Pleuritis evaluation system) grid [in Italian]. Large Anim Rev. 2007;13:161–5.
20. Villareal I, Vranckx K, Calus D, Pasmans HF, Maes D. Effect of challenge of pigs previously immunised with inactivated vaccines containing homologous and heterologous Mycoplasma hyopneumoniae strains. BMC Vet Res. 2012;8:2.
21. Villareal I, Maes D, Meyns T, Gebruers F, Calus D, Pasmans F, Haesebrouck F. Infection with a low virulent mycoplasma hyopneumoniae isolate does not protect piglets against subsequent infection with a highly virulent M. Hyopneumoniae isolate. Vaccine. 2009;27(12):1875–9.
22. Elicker S, Sipos W. The tissue compatibility of different Mycoplasma hyopneumoniae vaccines is mainly dependent upon their adjuvants. Berl Münch Tierärztl Wochenschr. 2009;122:348–53.
23. Tenk M, Rozsnyay Z, Pálmai N, Szórádi MA, Tóth I, Márton Z, Baranyai B, Kollár A, Halas M, Vetró P, Imre A, Nagy Z, Krejči R, Pénzes Z. Potentiation of the Mycoplasma hyopneumoniae vaccine efficacy with a novel adjuvant. In: Proceedings of the 9th European Symposium of Porcine Health Management, Prague, Czech Republic; 2017.
24. Michiels A, Arsenakis I, Boyen F, Krejci R, Haesebrouck F, Maes D. Efficacy of one dose vaccination against experimental infection with two Mycoplasma hyopneumoniae strains. BMC Vet Res. 2017;13:274.
25. Sibila M, Pieters M, Molitor T, Maes D, Haesebrouck SJ. Current perspectives on the diagnosis and epidemiology of Mycoplasma hyopneumoniae infection. Vet J. 2009;181:221–31.
26. Andreasen M, Mousing J, Thomsen LK. No simple association between time elapsed from seroconversion until slaughter and the extent of lung lesions in Danish swine. Prev Vet Med. 2001;52:147–61.
27. De Kruijf JM, Welling AA. Incidence of chronic inflammations in gilts and castrated boars [in Dutch]. Tijdschr Diergeneeskd. 1988;113(8):415–7.
28. Morris CR, Gardner IA, Hietala SK, Enzootic Pneumonia CTE. Comparison of cough and lung lesions as predictors of weight gain in swine. Can J Vet Res. 1995;59:197–204.
29. Kristensen CS, Vinther J, Svensmark B, Bækbo P. A field evaluation of two vaccines against Mycoplasma hyopneumoniae infection in pigs. Acta Vet Scand. 2014;56:24.
30. Baccaro MR, Hirose F, Umehara O, Gonçalves LCB, Doto DS, Paixão R, Shinya LT, Moreno AM. Comparative efficacy of two single-dose bacterins in the control of Mycoplasma hyopneumoniae in swine raised under commercial conditions in Brazil. Vet J. 2006;172(3):526–31.
31. Brewster VR, Maiti HC, Tucker AW, Nevel A. Associations between EP-like lesions and pleuritis and post trimming carcass weights of finishing pigs in England. Livest Sci. 2017;201:1–4.

21

An efficiency comparison of different in vitro fertilization methods: IVF, ICSI, and PICSI for embryo development to the blastocyst stage from vitrified porcine immature oocytes

Fahiel Casillas[1,2]*, Miguel Betancourt[3], Cristina Cuello[4], Yvonne Ducolomb[3], Alma López[3], Lizbeth Juárez-Rojas[1] and Socorro Retana-Márquez[1]

Abstract

Background: Most studies carried out to evaluate recovery and development after porcine oocyte vitrification, reported better rates when cryopreserved in embryonic development stages or zygotes, but not in immature oocytes. For this reason, many studies are performed to improve immature oocyte vitrification protocols testing the use of different cryoprotectant concentrations, cooling devices, incubation times; but only a few of them have evaluated which fertilization procedure enhances blastocyst rates in vitrified oocytes. Therefore, this study was aimed to evaluate: 1) if the sperm selection with hyaluronic acid (HA) or polyvinylpyrrolidone (PVP) before injection could play a key role in increasing fertilization and blastocyst formation and 2) the embryo developmental ability and blastocyst production of porcine immature oocytes retrieved after vitrification-warming and co-cultured with granulosa cells during IVM, using different fertilization techniques: in vitro fertilization (IVF), intracytoplasmic sperm injection (ICSI) and conventional ICSI with hyaluronic acid (HA) sperm selection, known as physiological intracytoplasmic sperm injection (PICSI) and.

Results: Sperm selected with HA-PICSI displayed a higher percentage of live/acrosome reacted status compared to those in control and exposed to PVP. Higher dead/acrosome reacted rates were obtained after PVP exposure compared to control and HA. In oocytes, viability significantly decreased after IVM in vitrified oocytes. Besides, IVM rates were not different between control denuded oocytes cultured with granulosa cells (DO-GC) and vitrified oocytes. Regarding fertilization parameters, IVF showed higher percentages of total fertilization rate than those obtained by ICSI and PICSI. However, results demonstrate that PICSI fertilization increased the blastocysts formation rate in control DO-GC and vitrified oocytes compared to IVF and ICSI.

Conclusions: To achieve high blastocyst formation rates from vitrified GV oocytes, it is recommended that sperm should be selected with HA instead of PVP before injection since high viability and acrosome reaction rates were obtained. Also, PICSI fertilization was the best method to produce higher blastocyst rates compared to the IVF and ICSI procedures.

Keywords: Porcine, Immature oocytes, Embryo development, Blastocyst, Vitrification, IVF ICSI, PICSI

* Correspondence: fahiel@xanum.uam.mx
[1]Departamento de Biología de la Reproducción, División de Ciencias Biológicas y de la Salud, Universidad Autónoma Metropolitana-Iztapalapa, 09340 CDMX, Mexico
[2]Doctorado en Ciencias Biológicas y de la Salud. Universidad Autónoma Metropolitana-Iztapalapa, 09340 CDMX, Mexico
Full list of author information is available at the end of the article

Background

The improvement of oocyte cryopreservation techniques allows the creation of valuable genetic banks. The development of different oocyte cryopreservation and in vitro fertilization (IVF) methods in swine have significant applications in biomedical research and livestock production [1]. Pigs are considered an important experimental model due to their biological similarities to humans, but also as potential organ donors for xenotransplants [2]. Different cryopreservation methods such as vitrification and slow freezing are applied for organ and tissue preservation; however, gametes represent a major challenge [3]. At present, vitrification is proposed as the best method for oocyte cryopreservation [4], and several studies are performed to improve vitrification protocols testing cryoprotectant agents (CPAs) concentrations [5–7], cooling devices [8–11], co-culture systems [12, 13], incubation times and temperatures [14], but few of them are focused on establishing the best fertilization procedure for vitrified-warmed oocytes [15]. Compared to other meiotic stages and species, porcine oocytes at the germinal vesicle stage (GV) are reported to be more difficult to recover after vitrification due to their high intracytoplasmic lipid content [16, 17]. Low viability, maturation, fertilization and blastocyst rates are obtained after GV oocyte vitrification [10, 18–20], mainly due to different morphological and physiological damage caused by the exposure to high CPAs concentrations, ice crystal formation, abnormal mitochondrial distribution and plasma membrane disruption [21, 22]. Despite this, it has been previously demonstrated that vitrified porcine GV oocytes can complete their nuclear and cytoplasmic maturation, and sustain the subsequent embryo development (ED) until the blastocysts stage. Therefore, the generation of live piglets from vitrified GV oocytes, fertilized with in vitro fertilization (IVF) has already been achieved [10]; however, blastocyst rates were reported to be low (5.2%). In a previous study [15] we used intracytoplasmic sperm injection (ICSI) to fertilize vitrified oocytes because it has the advantage of avoiding polyspermy and zona pellucida (ZP) hardening issues compared to IVF. However, we observed that vitrified oocytes fertilized by conventional IVF displayed higher blastocyst formation rates than those subjected to ICSI. Another study showed that it is possible to obtain blastocysts after ICSI from porcine oocytes vitrified at the GV stage [19]. However, when performing ICSI in control and vitrified oocytes, cleavage and blastocyst rates remain significantly low [19]. This fact could be due to the physiological lacks of ICSI, where some of the sperm checkpoints of natural fertilization are bypassed, such as the sperm-oocyte recognition and acrosome reaction [23–26]. Also, the sperm selection during ICSI is carried out by a visual approach based on motility and sperm morphology, which does not reflect sperm quality. The use of polyvinylpyrrolidone (PVP) is required during ICSI for sperm immobilization; however, this molecule is known to be toxic when injected into the oocyte cytoplasm, possibly affecting fertilization and sperm head decondensation [27]. In this regard, other studies reported low ED rates after ICSI using fresh oocytes [28–30], which are mainly ascribed to an inadequate sperm selection, resulting in sperm chromatin decondensation failures and sex chromosome abnormalities [23, 25]. Therefore, some efforts to increase the efficiency of ICSI are based on the establishment of new sperm selection criteria. For this purpose, some studies performed in fresh oocytes have previously reported the use of ZP [31] or hyaluronic acid (HA) for sperm selection prior to ICSI [32]. The improvement of ICSI using HA is also known as physiological intracytoplasmic sperm injection (PICSI) [33, 34]. One study reported that the use of HA is superior to the use of conventional ICSI in producing chromosomally normal embryos with low aneuploidy rates, suggesting that the ED and quality rates can be significantly improved [35]. However, this study was only performed in fresh oocytes, and to our knowledge, the present study is the first one to evaluate the effect of sperm selection with HA before injection in vitrified porcine immature oocytes. During HA selection, the adhesion of sperm to an HA gel stimulates the natural sperm-granulosa cells recognition and acrosome reaction which improves fertilization [36]. This is highly important because sperm quality is also crucial for the subsequent ED and implantation. Also, other studies reported that sperm bound to HA exhibit increased viability, maturity, acrosome integrity, reduced aneuploidy and DNA fragmentation [37, 38]. For this reason, sperm selection using HA could play a key role by increasing fertilization and ED rates, not only in fresh but also in vitrified immature oocytes. Therefore, the aims of the present study were 1) to evaluate the sperm viability and acrosome status after PVP and HA exposure and 2) to evaluate if the PICSI procedure is a useful tool for improving the fertilization and ED to the blastocyst stage of vitrified porcine GV oocytes compared to IVF and ICSI.

Methods
Chemicals culture media and culture conditions

Unless otherwise stated, all reagents were purchased from Sigma Chemical Co. (St. Louis, MO, USA) and different culture media were prepared. For cumulus-oocytes complexes (COCs) collection and washing, Tyrode's medium containing 10 mM HEPES, 10 mM sodium lactate and 1 mg/mL polyvinyl alcohol (TL-HEPES-PVA) was used [39]. For vitrification and warming, TCM-199-HEPES (product number TCM-199: 170929 ME-044, HEPES: H4034) medium was supplemented with 0.5 mM L-glutamine and 0.1% PVA (V-W medium). To perform in vitro maturation (IVM), the maturation medium (MM) was comprised of TCM-199-Earle's salts supplemented with 26.2 mM sodium bicarbonate, 0.1% PVA, 3.05 mM D-glucose, 0.91 mM sodium pyruvate, 0.57 mM cysteine and 10 ng/mL EGF (In Vitro, Mexico City). In control denuded oocytes cultured with granulosa cells (control DO-GC) and vitrified oocytes, IVM was performed using an oocyte-granulosa cells co-culture. Granulosa cells were collected from immature oocyte mechanical denudation in MM containing 0.1% hyaluronidase and from the follicular fluid. A total of 1×10^6 granulosa cells were added to each maturation well [40]. Briefly, 500 µL of follicular fluid containing granulosa cells were vortexed in 0.1% hyaluronidase for 5 min, then washed twice in phosphate buffered saline (PBS) and centrifuged at 200 X g for 5 min. The pellet was resuspended in MM and cells were counted on a Neubauer chamber. Finally, 50 µL of the suspension were added to 4-well culture dishes. The medium used for fertilization was modified Tris-buffered (mTBM) containing 3 mM KCl, 13.1 mM NaCl, 7.5 mM CaCl$_2$·2H$_2$O, 20 mM Tris, 11 mM glucose and 5 mM sodium pyruvate, 0.4% fraction V bovine serum albumin (BSA) and 2.5 mM caffeine [41]. For embryo culture, North Carolina State University-23 (NCSU-23) medium supplemented with 0.4% BSA was used [42]. All culture media and samples were incubated under mineral oil at 38.5 °C with 5% CO$_2$ in air and humidity at saturation.

Oocyte collection

Porcine ovaries were obtained from pre-pubertal Landrace gilts at "Los Arcos", Edo. de México slaughterhouse and transported to the laboratory in 0.9% NaCl solution at 25 °C. The aforementioned facility has the animal health federal law authorization under the number 6265375. For COCs collection, ovarian follicles between 3 and 6 mm in diameter were aspirated using an 18-gauge needle set to a 10 mL syringe. Oocytes with intact cytoplasm and surrounded by two to four layers of cumulus cells (CC) were selected to perform all experiments.

Vitrification and warming

For vitrification, immature COCs were denuded mechanically in MM, then washed twice in V-W medium and equilibrated in the first vitrification solution containing 7.5% dimethylsulphoxide (Me$_2$SO) and 7.5% ethylene glycol (EG) for 3 min. Later, oocytes were exposed to the second vitrification solution containing 16% Me$_2$SO, 16% EG and 0.4 M sucrose for 1 min. Later, at least nine oocytes were immersed in a 2 µL drop and loaded into the Cryolock device (Importadora Mexicana de Materiales para Reproducción Asistida S. A. de C.V.

México). Finally, in less than 1 min, the Cryolock was plunged horizontally into liquid nitrogen and the vitrified oocytes were stored for 30 min before warming [12].

For warming, the one-step method was performed [43]. Briefly, the Cryolock was immersed vertically in a four-well dish containing 800 µL of V-W medium with 0.13 M sucrose. Later, warmed oocytes were incubated in the same medium for 5 min and then recovered for IVM [44].

In vitro maturation (IVM)

Control DO-GC and vitrified-warmed denuded immature oocytes were washed in 500 µL of MM three times. Afterwards, 30 to 40 oocytes were randomly distributed in a four-well dish (Thermo-Scientific Nunc, Rochester NY) containing 500 µL of MM with 0.5 µg/mL LH and 0.5 µg/mL FSH for 44 h and incubated under mineral oil at 38.5 °C with 5% CO$_2$ in air and humidity at saturation [42]. Control DO-GC and vitrified oocytes were matured in MM adding a granulosa cell co-culture system as described above.

Oocyte selection before IVF, ICSI or PICSI

After 44 h of IVM, to perform fertilization, co-cultured granulosa cells were removed in the control DO-GC and vitrification group. Before fertilization, oocytes were evaluated by stereomicroscopy, and only matured oocytes with uniform cytoplasm and intact ZP intended to each experimental group were subjected to IVF, ICSI or PICSI. Oocytes with lysed cytoplasm membranes were considered degenerated and were discarded.

In vitro fertilization (IVF)

After IVM, mature oocytes were rinsed twice in 500 µL of MM and later in 500 µL of mTBM. Groups of 30 to 40 denuded oocytes from control and vitrified groups were placed into a four-well dish with 50 µL drops of mTBM covered with mineral oil and incubated for 45 min.

To perform insemination, the semen sample was obtained from one Landrace boar, using the gloved hand method at a commercial insemination center, diluted in Duragen (Magapor, México) 1:2 (v:v), then transported to the laboratory at 16 °C within 2 h after collection. Sperm evaluation was performed and motility was determined; only if the semen sample had greater than 80% motile spermatozoa was used. Then, 5 mL of the semen sample were diluted with 5 mL of Dulbecco's phosphate buffered saline (DPBS; In Vitro, S.A., México) medium supplemented with 0.1% BSA fraction V, 75 µg/mL potassium penicillin G and 50 µg/mL streptomycin sulfate. Then, this suspension was centrifuged (61 X g for 5 min). The pellet was discarded and 5 mL of the supernatant were diluted 1:1 (v:v) with DPBS and centrifuged (1900 X g for 5 min). The supernatant was discarded, and the pellet was diluted with 10 mL of DPBS and centrifuged twice under the same conditions. Later, the pellet was diluted in 100 μL of mTBM to assess the final sperm concentration (5 X 10^5 spermatozoa/mL) and after dilution, 50 μL of the suspension were added to the medium containing oocytes. Finally, gametes were co-incubated in mTBM for 6 h.

Intracytoplasmic sperm injection (ICSI)

Microinjection was carried out using an inverted optical differential interference contrast microscope (Nikon eclipse, TE300, Japan). Holding pipettes (COOK medical, USA) exhibit an external 130 μm and internal 23 μm diameter and injection pipettes (COOK medical, USA) had an outer diameter of 7 μm and an inner diameter of 5.5 μm, both pipettes with an angle of 30°.

For oocyte preparation, an oil covered 35 mm diameter Petri dish (Thermo-Scientific Nunc, Rochester NY) previously incubated at 38.5 °C for 2 h with eight drops of 10 μL mTBM medium for oocytes (3 oocytes/drop) and a drop of 4 μL of mTBM containing 10% PVP (mTBM-PVP) for spermatozoa was used. A 1 μL drop of mTBM medium with the sperm sample was added in the extreme of the 4 μL drop of 10% PVP. To carry out microinjection, progressive motile and normal sperm were immobilized by hitting its tail with the injection needle. Sperm capture was performed by the introduction of the tail into the injection pipette. Then, mature oocytes were aspirated carefully by the holding pipette to prevent polar body damage. The sperm was carefully expelled from inside the injection needle and reloaded for washing to remove the PVP surrounding the sperm before injection. Subsequently, in the position of the three o'clock, the injection pipette was inserted into the oocyte so that the sperm head could be in touch with the cytoplasm to facilitate oocyte activation. To ensure that the injection took place correctly, a small volume of cytoplasm was aspirated and immediately after, the sperm was introduced. Micropipettes were removed and the oocyte was released. Finally, microinjected oocytes were washed twice and IVC [15].

Physiological intracytoplasmic sperm injection (PICSI)

A 1 μL sperm droplet from the diluted sample described formerly (when performing IVF) was added to the PICSI dish (ORIGIO, Denmark) containing a previously hydrated HA gel drop. To hydrate the gel drop, 1 μL of MM was added in each drop and incubated at 38.5 °C for 3 min. Before injection, the Petri dish containing the sperm sample was incubated at 38.5 °C for 15 min. After that, only spermatozoa bound to the HA drop were selected and subsequently injected into the oocytes as described above by the ICSI method.

Evaluation of the sperm viability and acrosomal status

Sperm samples used for ICSI or PICSI were stained with propidium iodide (PI) and fluorescein isothiocyanate lectin from the peanut plant, *Arachis hypogaea* (FITC-PNA) for simultaneous evaluation of sperm viability and acrosomal status, respectively. For evaluation, 5 μL of the sperm sample were diluted in 100 μL of mTBM containing 5 μL of PI: 1000 μg/mL solution in distilled water and 5 μL of FITC-PNA: 1000 μg/mL solution in PBS. The sample was homogenized and then incubated for 5 min. Later, 10 μL of the suspension were fixed with 10 μL of 1.6% glutaraldehyde on a slide and evaluated under an epifluorescence microscope (Zeiss Axiostar) with a FITC-TRITC filter set. Sperm observations were classified as follows: live/non-acrosome reacted (A/NAR): positive FITC-PNA at the acrosome and negative PI at the post-acrosomal region. Live/acrosome reacted (A/AR): both FITC-PNA and PI negative. Dead/ non-acrosome reacted (D/NAR): both FITC-PNA and PI positive. Dead/acrosome reacted (D/AR): negative FITC-PNA and positive PI [44].

Evaluation of oocyte viability

Viability was measured at T 0 h = immediately after collection or vitrification and at T 44 h = after IVM. Oocytes were added in 100 μL drop of 0.5 mg/mL Thiazolyl blue (MTT) diluted in PBS. After 1 h, oocytes were analyzed under a light microscope (Zeiss Axiostar) and classified as viable cells (with purple coloration) and non-viable (colorless).

Evaluation of maturation and fertilization parameters

For IVM and IVF parameters, oocytes were stained using 10 μg/mL bisbenzimide (Hoechst 33,342) diluted in PBS for 40 min and washed in PBS. The oocytes were fixed with 2% glutaraldehyde and mounted in a PBS-glycerol solution (1:9). Oocytes and putative zygotes were analyzed under an epifluorescence microscope (Zeiss Axiostar) at 400 X magnification. For maturation parameters evaluation, a random subset of oocytes was fixed after 44 h of IVM and classified as: immature, those oocytes in GV or in metaphase I (MI) and matured, those in metaphase II (MII) [45]. Fertilization parameters were assessed 16 h after IVF or injection in a subset of putative zygotes. Fertilization was evaluated by visualizing pronucleus (PN) formation by the Hoechst staining method. Oocytes were considered activated showing: one pronucleus (PN), monospermic: 2 PN + 2 PBs (Fig. 1, a and b), and polyspermic: > 2PN [46]. Total fertilization rate was calculated as % 2PN + > 2PN oocytes/total oocytes and non-fertilized as % non-pronuclear formation/total oocytes.

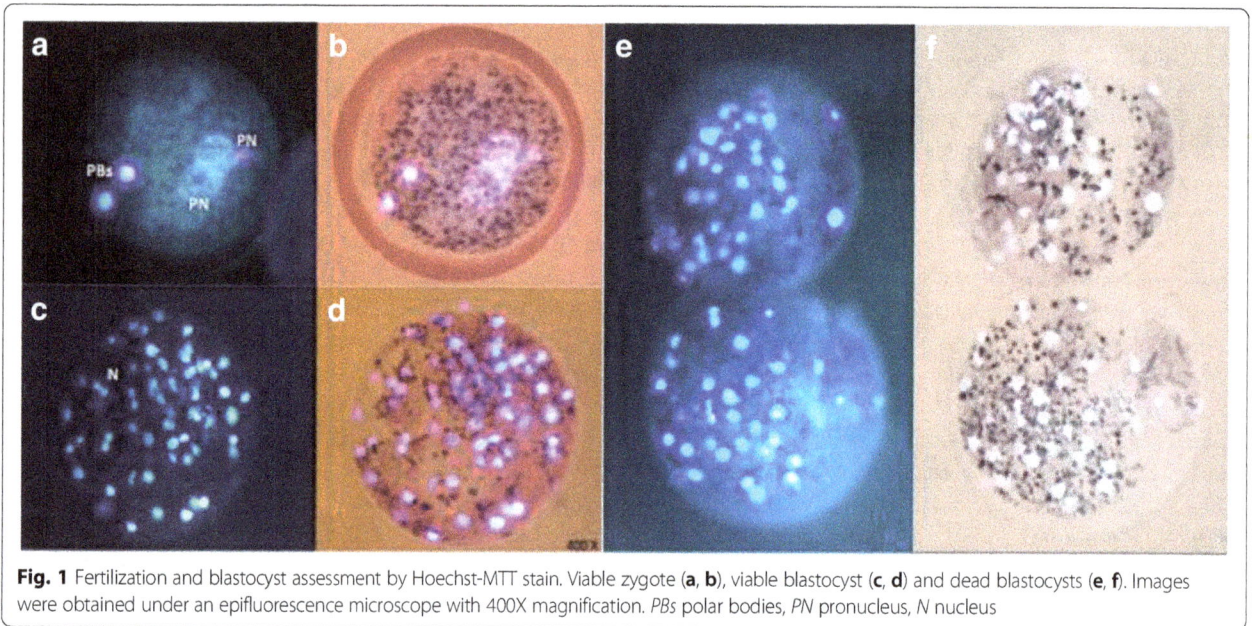

Fig. 1 Fertilization and blastocyst assessment by Hoechst-MTT stain. Viable zygote (**a, b**), viable blastocyst (**c, d**) and dead blastocysts (**e, f**). Images were obtained under an epifluorescence microscope with 400X magnification. *PBs* polar bodies, *PN* pronucleus, *N* nucleus

Embryo culture and evaluation of the embryo development, blastocyst quality and viability

After 6 h of gametes co-incubation during IVF or immediately after injection (ICSI and PICSI), 30 to 40 putative zygotes were transferred to four-well dishes containing 500 µL drops of NCSU-23. The embryo cleavage (number of zygotes cleaved per total cultivated) and blastocyst (number of blastocysts per total cultivated) rates were determined at 48 and 168 h after IVC, respectively, by morphological evaluation under an inverted microscope (Olympus Optical) (Fig. 2). At day 7 (d0 = day of IVF or injection) to count the total number of nuclei, blastocysts were stained with 10 µg/mL bisbenzimide (Hoechst 33,342) in MM for 40 min and evaluated (Zeiss Axiostar) at 400 X magnification (Fig. 1, c and e). For cell viability assessment, day 7 blastocysts

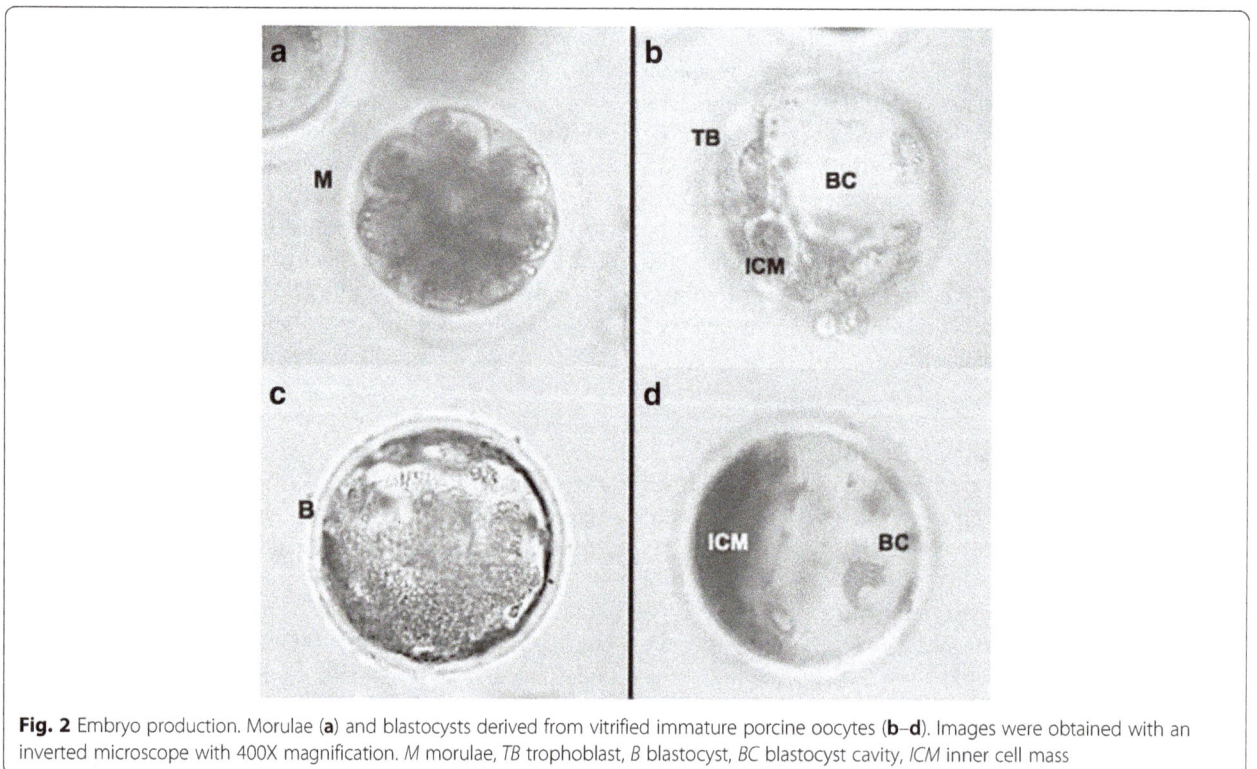

Fig. 2 Embryo production. Morulae (**a**) and blastocysts derived from vitrified immature porcine oocytes (**b–d**). Images were obtained with an inverted microscope with 400X magnification. *M* morulae, *TB* trophoblast, *B* blastocyst, *BC* blastocyst cavity, *ICM* inner cell mass

were added in 100 μL drop of 0.5 mg/mL MTT diluted in PBS. After 1 h, embryos were analyzed under a light microscope (Zeiss Axiostar) and classified as viable (with purple coloration) (Fig. 1, d) and non-viable (colorless) (Fig. 1, f). Results are presented as percentages of viable cells in blastocysts.

Experimental design

Experiment 1: Viability and acrosomal status of PVP exposed spermatozoa and HA-bound sperm

Three replicates were performed to compare the viability and acrosomal status of spermatozoa diluted for ICSI in mTBM and exposed to PVP or HA. The number of sperm evaluated in each replicate was $n = 200$ per treatment. Sperm sample was divided into three groups: 1) non-treated spermatozoa (Control group, $n = 600$), 2) spermatozoa treated with PVP (PVP-ICSI, n = 600) and 3) spermatozoa treated with HA (HA-PICSI, n = 600). Sperm viability and acrosome status were evaluated 15 min after treatment in all groups using the FITC-PNA-PI stain.

Experiment 2: Oocyte viability, IVM and IVF parameters obtained after GV oocyte vitrification

Oocytes used to evaluate each parameter correspond to independent samples. At least five experiments were performed to evaluate oocyte viability and maturation in fresh and vitrified oocytes. Viability was assessed immediately after selection (T 0 h) (Control DO-GC, $n = 80$ and Vitrification, $n = 67$) and at the end of IVM (T 44 h) (Control DO-GC, n = 60 and Vitrification, n = 67). After IVM, oocytes were fixed to assess the maturation rate (Control DO-GC, $n = 100$ and Vitrification, $n = 121$). To evaluate IVF parameters, three replicates were performed and the oocytes were distributed in the following groups: 1) non-vitrified oocytes subjected to IVF (Control DO-GC, $n = 41$), ICSI (Control DO-GC, $n = 30$), and PICSI (Control DO-GC, $n = 45$); 2) vitrified GV oocytes matured and subjected to IVF (Vitrification, $n = 62$), ICSI (Vitrification, $n = 43$) and PICSI (Vitrification, $n = 40$). After fertilization, oocytes were cultured for 16 h and fixed to evaluate IVF parameters.

Experiment 3: ED and blastocyst quality obtained with vitrified GV oocytes after IVF, ICSI or PICSI

Ten replicates were performed to evaluate ED and three for blastocyst quality. Fresh and vitrified immature oocytes were matured and then randomly allocated in the following groups: 1) non-vitrified oocytes subjected to IVF (Control DO-GC, $n = 100$), ICSI (Control DO-GC, $n = 74$), and PICSI (Control DO-GC, $n = 60$), 2) vitrified GV oocytes subjected to IVF (Vitrification, $n = 210$), ICSI (Vitrification, $n = 113$) and PICSI (Vitrification, $n = 158$). Selected oocytes from each experimental group were subjected to IVF, ICSI or PICSI and cultured as described above to evaluate ED.

Statistical analysis

To evaluate sperm viability and acrosomal status, oocyte viability, maturation, fertilization parameters, ED and blastocyst quality, data were analysed using ANOVA followed by a non-parametric Duncan test using number cruncher statistical software (NCSS[11]). Percentage data are presented as mean ± standard deviation (SD) values. Differences were considered significant when $P < 0.05$.

Results

Spermatozoa viability and acrosomal status

In experiment 1, it was observed that both groups of treated spermatozoa differed ($P < 0.05$) from the control group in terms of the percentage of A/AR spermatozoa (Table 1). Higher A/AR sperm rate was obtained in the HA-PICSI group ($P < 0.05$) when compared to control and PVP. No significant difference was observed between the control and HA-PICSI group in D/AR rates. However, results demonstrate that PVP exposure significantly affects viability and AR (D/AR). The HA-PICSI group displayed lower A/NRA rates than control and PVP ($P < 0.05$) and no differences were obtained in all D/NAR sperm ($P > 0.05$) groups.

Oocyte viability, IVM and IVF parameters obtained after GV oocyte vitrification

In experiment 2, oocyte viability after vitrification (T 0 h) was not affected compared to control DO-GC; however, it decreased significantly after IVM (T 44 h) up

Table 1 Viability and acrosomal status in spermatozoa selected for ICSI or PICSI

Treatment	Total Spermatozoa n	A/AR (%)	D/AR (%)	A/NAR (%)	D/NAR (%)
Control	600	432 (72 ± 1.4)[a]	29 (5 ± 1.4)[a]	108 (18 ± 1.8)[a]	31 (5 ± 0.4)[a]
PVP-ICSI	600	319 (53 ± 0.9)[b]	180 (30 ± 1.1)[b]	82 (14 ± 2.3)[a]	19 (3 ± 0.2)[a]
HA-PICSI	600	504 (84 ± 2.3)[c]	50 (8 ± 1.9)[a]	42 (7 ± 1.8)[b]	4 (1 ± 0.3)[a]

Percentage data are presented as mean ± SD values
PVP Polyvinilpyrrolidone, *HA* Hyaluronic acid, *A/AR* live/acrosome reacted, *D/AR* dead/acrosome reacted, *A/NAR* live/non-acrosome reacted, *D/NAR* dead/non-acrosome reacted, *n* number of sperm examined
[a,b,c]Values in the same column with different letters are significantly different ($P < 0.05$)

to 66% in the vitrification group (Table 2). Regarding maturation, the percentage of MII oocytes in control DO-GC and vitrified oocytes were not statistically different. However, the percentage of oocytes in GV was higher in control DO-GC compared to vitrified oocytes. Also, GVB (MI + MII) rates were higher (P < 0.05) in vitrified oocytes compared to control DO-GC (Table 3). Regarding fertilization parameters, pronuclear formation was evaluated and 2PN rates were higher in control DO-GC, and vitrified IVF oocytes than ICSI and vitrified PICSI groups. Also, percentages up to 20% of >2PN were obtained after IVF. The total fertilization rate was significantly higher after IVF in control and vitrified oocytes compared to ICSI and PICSI. Lower fertilization rates were obtained after ICSI than IVF and PICSI. Consequently, higher non-fertilized rates (non pronuclear formation) were obtained after ICSI compared to IVF and PICSI procedures (Table 4).

Blastocyst formation obtained with vitrified GV oocytes
In experiment 3, vitrification did not impair the embryo cleavage rates obtained after IVF, ICSI and PICSI (Table 5). Cleavage rates were not statistically different between IVF and PICSI procedures. However, cleavage decreased (P < 0.05) after ICSI. Blastocyst formation was significantly higher after PICSI compared to IVF and ICSI. Also, higher (P < 0.05) percentages of viable cells in blastocysts were obtained after PICSI and ICSI control DO-GC group compared to IVF. In terms of total number of nuclei, IVF and PICSI were not statistically different; however, it decreased significantly after ICSI.

Discussion
Experiment 1 results indicated that HA-PICSI sperm displayed higher A/AR rates than control and PVP exposed sperm. For fertilization, high A/AR rates are needed to promote sperm head decondensation. Also, reduced D/AR, A/NAR and D/NAR sperm were obtained after HA exposure. Compared to IVF and PICSI, during ICSI, PVP is often used for sperm manipulation decreasing motility and facilitating capture. However, it was reported that PVP could be toxic for the spermatozoa [47], reducing fertilization [27], male PN formation and blastocyst development [48]. These observations agree with our results, where the PVP exposed

spermatozoa displayed a higher proportion of D/AR sperm than those exposed to HA and control, suggesting that the HA does not affect sperm viability. Also, the HA-binding mechanism is related to sperm maturity [49]. Only mature sperm have HA specific ligand-receptors, which are implicated in the fertilization potential. Thus, conventional sperm preparation techniques prior to fertilization [50] such as removal of seminal plasma (sperm washing), filtration, centrifugation, swim up, PVP, and observational selection based on motility, have important limitations. These procedures do not select functional, mature and competent spermatozoa, and are possibly involved in reducing sperm viability, fertilization and ED [38, 51]. Important aspects of sperm functions such as motility; maturation and capacitation appear to be partially mediated through HA [52]. In human and porcine oviduct fluid, HA is also found [36], suggesting that great amounts of HA are in contact with the sperm through the oviduct, possibly maintaining their viability until fertilization. Interactions between the oviduct fluid and sperm are required for fertilization. Only mature sperm have hyaluronic specific ligand-receptor that facilitates HA-binding, hyaluronidase activity, ZP recognition and acrosome reaction [53, 54]. Therefore, our results demonstrate that sperm viability is less affected when sperm are exposed to HA (P < 0.05).

Experiment 2 results demonstrate that oocyte viability is not affected immediately after vitrification (T 0 h). However, it was significantly reduced after IVM (T 44 h) in the vitrification group compared to control DO-GC. In agreement, other studies reported that viability decreases after IVM in vitrified porcine [55] and goat oocytes and embryos [56]. This fact could be due to the high sensitivity of the GV oocytes during vitrification compared to other meiotic or developmental stages [22], mainly because of their high lipid content [16], reducing CPAs permeation, causing cell damage and lowering viability [19]. Other studies support that the oocyte viability after vitrification decreases after IVC [12, 15, 57, 58]. This fact could be since, during IVC, O_2 and reactive oxygen species levels increase, affecting oocyte viability [59]. Also, buffalo [60] and porcine oocytes [61] exhibit an increased intracytoplasmic lipid content [16], affecting in vitrified oocytes the glutathione levels and increased production of H_2O_2, decreasing viability rates [61]. Concerning maturation, in the present study, it was possible to obtain maturation rates up to 46% in control DO-GC and 54% after vitrification. In agreement, several studies reported rates from 3 to 61% MII oocytes after GV oocyte vitrification [10, 18, 19, 58]. Also, our results indicate that maturation was not affected in vitrified GV oocytes compared to control DO-GC. Other studies indicate that porcine GV oocytes are less cryotolerant. Other factors responsible for decreasing IVM rates after

Table 2 Viability of porcine oocytes after vitrification and IVM

Treatment	Viability T 0 h (%)	Viability after IVM T 44 h (%)
Control (DO-GC)	75/80 (94 ± 0.8)[a]	52/60 (87 ± 2.3)[a]
Vitrification	65/67 (97 ± 0.2)[a]	44/67 (66 ± 2.1)[b]

Percentage data are presented as mean ± SD values
DO-GC Denuded oocytes cultured with granulosa cells
[a,b]Values in the same column with different letters are significantly different (P < 0.05)

Table 3 IVM of porcine oocytes after vitrification

Treatment	Total Oocyte n	Maturation MII (%)	Meiotic stages (%)		
			GV	MI	GVB
Control (DO-GC)	100	46 (46 ± 4)[a]	49 (49 ± 1.8)[a]	5 (5 ± 0.3)[a]	51 (51 ± 1.2)[a]
Vitrification	121	65 (54 ± 1.2)[a]	44 (36 ± 4.3)[b]	12 (10 ± 0.6)[a]	77 (64 ± 3.2)[b]

Percentage data are presented as mean ± SD values

DO-GC Denuded oocytes cultured with granulosa cells, *GV* Germinal vesicle, *MI* Metaphase I, *MII* Metaphase II, *GVB* Germinal vesicle breakdown (MI + MII), *n* number of oocytes examined

[a,b]Values in the same column with different letters are significantly different (P < 0.05)

vitrification include ZP damage, reduced mitochondrial matrix density and irreversible cytoskeleton damage [22, 62]. In the present study, the DO co-cultured with isolated CC can partially recover meiotic and developmental competence. These cells have a pH regulatory mechanism during culture and paracrine factors display antioxidant properties allowing maturation [63, 64]. However, co-culture of DO with granulosa cells does not reestablish gap junctions and IVM rates remain low. Premature nuclear maturation, oocyte aging and GAP junction damage occurs after vitrification [18, 22, 65]. Regarding fertilization, several attempts were made to increase IVF and ED rates of vitrified porcine GV oocytes [10, 12, 15]. However, embryo production rates remain low due to a high incidence of vitrification-warming injuries [22]. In the present study, higher 1PN + 2PBs rates were obtained after IVF, control ICSI and PICSI than the vitrified ICSI group, suggesting that low oocyte activation and insufficient sperm head decondensation is obtained after ICSI. When evaluating pronuclear formation, higher 2PN rates were obtained after IVF and PICSI than the ICSI procedure. Other studies performed in control and vitrified GV oocytes reported 2PN rates up to 43 and 33%, respectively [58], 23 and 13%, respectively [66] and fresh oocytes [67, 68].

Nevertheless, significantly reduced male PN formation was obtained after ICSI. Also, results indicate that the IVF procedure increases total fertilization rates compared to ICSI and PICSI. However, with the IVF procedure, polyspermy (>2PN) rates up to 13–20% are obtained and polyspermic fertilization is one of the leading causes in producing low quality embryos. Therefore, the IVF method selection, sperm and oocyte factors could have detrimental effects on the fertilization and ED potential. In agreement to our results, another study reported that reduced oocyte activation and male PN formation are the main causes of low ICSI efficiency [69]. Results obtained in the present study demonstrate that less PN formation (non-fertilized oocytes) is obtained after ICSI compared to IVF and PICSI. Therefore, sperm selection with PVP may lead to a reduced PN formation. The ICSI efficiency was previously tested; results obtained in other studies showed 55% of 2PN fertilization in control oocytes that can be improved using roscovitine up to 72% [2]. Also, oocyte activation with ionomycin in parthenogenetic oocytes or calcium ionophore and sperm selection before injection with ZP binding were performed in porcine [70, 71] and ovine oocytes [44]. However, significantly low fertilization and cleavage rates were obtained. In the present study, the

Table 4 In vitro fertilization parameters of fresh and vitrified oocytes

Treatment	Total Oocyte n	Pronuclear formation (%)			Total Fertilization	Non-fertilized
		1PN	2PN + 2 PBs	>2PN		
IVF						
Control (DO-GC)	41	10 (24 ± 1.2)[a]	21 (51 ± 3.4)[a]	8 (20 ± 5)[a]	29 (71 ± 2)[a]	2 (5 ± 1.3)[a]
Vitrification	62	16 (26 ± 3.2)[a]	38 (61 ± 4.3)[a]	8 (13 ± 2.8)[a]	46 (75 ± 3.2)[a]	–
ICSI						
Control (DO-GC)	30	5 (17 ± 8)[a]	10 (33 ± 4.2)[b]	.	10 (33 ± 4.3)[b]	15 (50 ± 1.1)[b]
Vitrification	43	3 (7 ± 1.9)[b]	15 (35 ± 8)[b]	–	15 (35 ± 8)[b]	25 (58 ± 1.2)[b]
PICSI						
Control (DO-GC)	45	10 (22 ± 4)[a]	22 (49 ± 9.9)[a]	–	22 (49 ± 9.9)[c]	13 (29 ± 6.2)[c]
Vitrification	40	8 (20 ± 3)[a]	18 (45 ± 5.6)[c]	–	18 (45 ± 5.6)[c]	14 (35 ± 1.4)[c]

DO-GC Denuded oocytes cultured with granulosa cells, *PBs* polar bodies, *PN* pronucleus,

Total Fertilization = counted as 2PN + >2PN/total oocytes

Non-fertilized = non pronuclear formation/total oocytes

Percentage data are presented as mean ± SD values

[a,b,c]Values in the same column with different letters are significantly different (P < 0.05)

Table 5 In vitro embryo development and blastocyst quality of fresh and vitrified oocytes

Treatment	Total n	Cleavage (%)	Blastocyst (%)	Viable cells in blastocysts %	Total no. of nuclei (means ± S.D.)
IVF					
Control (DO-GC)	100	73 (73 ± 3.4)[a]	15 (15 ± 1.2)[a]	82 ± 3[a]	50 ± 0.6[a]
Vitrification	210	142 (68 ± 2)[a]	30 (14 ± 1.8)[a]	70 ± 5[b]	46 ± 3[a]
ICSI					
Control (DO-GC)	74	33 (45 ± 2)[b]	9 (12 ± 0.3)[a]	100[c]	44 ± 0.9[b]
Vitrification	113	45 (40 ± 9)[b]	10 (9 ± 0.2)[b]	42 ± 5[d]	41 ± 2[b]
PICSI					
Control (DO-GC)	60	38 (63 ± 2)[a]	18 (30 ± 1.5)[c]	100[c]	50 ± 2.5[a]
Vitrification	158	99 (63 ± 3.5)[a]	39 (25 ± 3)[c]	100[c]	54 ± 5[a]

DO-GC Denuded oocytes cultured with granulosa cells, *n* number of embryos examined
Cell viability was considered as the percentage of viable cells in blastocysts
Percentage data are presented as mean ± SD values
Cleavage = number of zygotes cleaved per total cultivated
Blastocyst = number of blastocysts per total cultivated
[a,b,c,d]Values in the same column with different letters are significantly different (P < 0.05)

use of HA increased 2PN formation up to 45%. Recently, it was reported that the use of lipase to select and inject oocytes, resulted in 29% of 2PN formation [48]. In addition, this study also evaluated the efficiency of PVP, reporting 24% of 2PN formation [48], similar to those obtained in the present study (35%). Fertilization and ED success depends on the quality of the spermatozoa selected for injection, but this is not possible to achieve by ICSI.

In experiment 3, regarding cleavage results, IVF and PICSI were not statistically different. However, significantly reduced cleavage rates were obtained after ICSI. Therefore, results demonstrate that sperm selection is crucial for improving ED. PVP sperm selection reduces viability, and could increase DNA fragmentation rates resulting in less oocyte activation, PN formation and ED. In agreement, other studies reported low blastocyst production after ICSI, in fresh oocytes (4–14%) [2, 19]. Our results demonstrate that cleavage and blastocyst rates are significantly affected after ICSI compared to IVF and PICSI. In contrast, another study reported blastocyst rates up to 40% in pigs after ICSI; however, different culture media and BSA supplementation were used [72]. When performing PICSI, blastocyst formation was improved in control DO-GC (30%) and in vitrified oocytes (25%). To increase ED rates, other studies add 10% of fetal bovine serum (FBS) or porcine follicular fluid (pFF) during IVM or IVF culture [35, 58, 73]; however, we avoided its use. In the present study, we obtained similar results in terms of cleavage rate with fresh oocytes in all treatments without using FBS or pFF. Supplementation with FBS or pFF has important limitations since pathogens such as viruses are present. Regarding blastocyst viability and quality, results indicate that viable day 7 blastocysts can be obtained by PICSI of matured oocytes

derived from vitrified GV oocytes. Higher percentages of viable cells in blastocysts and a total number of nuclei were obtained by PICSI than when using IVF and ICSI. Our results demonstrate that sperm selection with HA, ensures the injection of a sperm that has completed its maturation and that is able to recognize and attach to the HA, improving blastocysts formation. However, sperm selection with PVP during ICSI can significantly reduce the oocyte developmental potential to the blastocyst stage. Therefore, superior quality blastocysts can be obtained after HA sperm selection during PICSI. It has been stated that the contribution of sperm towards embryogenesis can be divided into two periods: the early period (fertilization to < 8-cell stage) and the late period (8-cell stage to birth) [74]. In the early period, an inadequate sperm selection can affect fertilization, syngamy and the mitotic division [75, 76]. In the late period, sperm can influence embryogenesis by a genome way. If the genome is altered by DNA fragmentation, it may result in a poor blastocyst development, lower implantation, early pregnancy loss or abortion [74]. According to this, other studies with PICSI fertilization have reported that HA-bound injected sperm increased embryo production in human [34]. But also, low pregnancy loss, high pregnancy rates [77, 78], and high DNA integrity [79] are obtained by PICSI. Therefore, our results demonstrate that sperm selection with HA improves blastocysts rates not only in control but also in vitrified oocytes. Compared to PVP-ICSI, sperm selection with HA improved blastocyst formation. The PICSI mechanism by which ED is improved is that only mature and competent sperm hold hyaluronan specific ligand receptors, facilitating fertilization. HA-selected sperm exhibit normal head morphology, reduced DNA fragmentation, reduced chromosomal aneuploidy rates and better fertilization potential [37]. In contrast, PVP has no selective function and its use can cause DNA fragmentation rates up to 11% [34] compared to 5.3% with HA. Also, higher percentages of spermatozoa with normal nucleus are selected with HA compared to PVP (14.5% vs. 11%, respectively) [34]. Consequently, oocyte fertilization with arrested sperm maturity and DNA damage may lead to a reduced blastocyst development. Also, lower oocyte activation and PN formation rates were obtained after ICSI compared to PICSI, reducing the ED potential. Therefore, the present study suggests that the PICSI procedure is the best method to fertilize and produce blastocysts from vitrified GV oocytes. This procedure compared to the conventional IVF in porcine oocytes has several advantages: 1) during PICSI, polyspermy is avoided, 2) only one selected sperm is used per oocyte and 3) sperm selection allows the injection of a high-quality sperm. The IVP of porcine blastocysts has been difficult to achieve mainly in vitrified GV oocytes. However, if nuclear maturation is performed with a granulosa cell co-culture system and sperm are selected with HA before injection, blastocyst production can be improved. The advantages of cryopreserving GV oocytes compared to other meiotic or developmental stages are that they can be collected in a greater quantity than MII oocytes, allowing the production of a high number of blastocysts for embryo transfer. Also, to obtain GV oocytes, no ovarian stimulation is required. They can be obtained from prepubescent females; however, IVM is required.

Conclusions

To achieve high blastocyst formation rates from vitrified GV oocytes, it is recommended that sperm should be selected with HA instead of PVP before injection since high viability and acrosome reaction rates were obtained. Also, PICSI fertilization was the best method to produce higher blastocyst rates compared to the IVF and ICSI procedures.

Abbreviations

A/AR: Live/acrosome reacted; A/NAR: Live/non-acrosome reacted; ART: Assisted reproduction technologies; BC: Blastocyst cavity; BSA: Bovine serum albumin; CC: Cumulus cells; COCs: Cumulus-oocyte complexes; CPAs: Cryoprotectant agents; D/AR: Dead/acrosome reacted; D/NAR: Dead/non-acrosome reacted; DO: Denuded oocytes; DO-GC: Denuded oocytes cultured with granulosa cells; DPBS: Dulbecco's phosphate buffered saline; ED: Embryo development; EG: Ethylene glycol; EGF: Epidermal growth factor; FBS: Fetal bovine serum; FITC-PNA: Fluorescein isothiocyanate-peanut agglutinin; FSH: Follicle stimulating hormone; GAGs: Glycosaminoglycan's; GV: Germinal vesicle; GVB: Germinal vesicle breakdown; HA: Hyaluronic acid; ICM: Inner cell mass; ICSI: Intracytoplasmic sperm injection; IVC: In vitro culture; IVF: In vitro fertilization; IVM: In vitro maturation; LH: Luteinizing hormone; M: Morulae; Me$_2$SO: Dimethylsulphoxide; MI: Metaphase I; MII: Metaphase II; MM: Maturation medium; mTBM: Tris-buffered medium; MTT: Thiazolyl blue; N: Nucleus; NCSU-23: North Carolina State University 23; PBS: Phosphate buffered saline; PBs: Polar bodies; pFF: Porcine follicular fluid; PI: Propidium iodide; PICSI: Physiological intracytoplasmic sperm injection; PN: Pronucleus; PVA: Polyvinyl alcohol; PVP: Polyvinylpyrrolidone;

SD: Standard deviation; TB: Trophoblast; V-W: Vitrification and warming; ZP: Zona pellucida

Acknowledgements
The authors thank the slaughterhouse "Los Arcos", Estado de Mexico for the donation of porcine ovaries. This publication represents partial fulfillment of the requirements for the degree of Doctor in Health and Biological Sciences for Fahiel Casillas.

Funding
This work was supported by CONACYT Scholarship to Fahiel Casillas (No. 302760).

Authors' contributions
Study design and direction: FC, MB, YD and SRM. Animal managing and experiments: FC. Analyzed the results and wrote the manuscript: FC, MB, YD, CC, AL, LJR and SR. All authors read and approved the final manuscript.

Competing interests
The authors declare that they have no competing interests.

Author details
[1]Departamento de Biología de la Reproducción, División de Ciencias Biológicas y de la Salud, Universidad Autónoma Metropolitana-Iztapalapa, 09340 CDMX, Mexico. [2]Doctorado en Ciencias Biológicas y de la Salud. Universidad Autónoma Metropolitana-Iztapalapa, 09340 CDMX, Mexico. [3]Departamento de Ciencias de la Salud, División de Ciencias Biológicas y de la Salud, Universidad Autónoma Metropolitana-Iztapalapa, 09340 CDMX, Mexico. [4]Departamento de Medicina y Cirugía Animal, Universidad de Murcia, 30100 Espinardo, Spain.

References
1. Dinnyes A, Liu J, Nedambale TL. Novel gamete storage. Reprod Fertil Dev. 2007;19:719–31.
2. García-Roselló E, Coy P, García-Vázquez FA, Ruiz S, Matás C. Analysis of different factors influencing the intracytoplasmic sperm injection (ICSI) yield in pigs. Theriogenology. 2006;66:1857–65.
3. Casillas F, Retana-Márquez S, Ducolomb Y, Betancourt M. New trends in assisted reproduction techniques: cryopreservation, in vitro fertilization, intracytoplasmic sperm injection and physiological intracytoplasmic sperm injection. Anat Physiol. 2015;5:184.
4. Edgar DH, Gook DA. A critical appraisal of cryopreservation (slow cooling versus vitrification) of human oocytes and embryos. Hum Reprod. 2012; 18(5):1–19. https://doi.org/10.1093/humupd/dms016.
5. Fahy GM, Wowk B, Wu J, Paynter S. Improved vitrification solutions based on the predictability of vitrification solution toxicity. Cryobiology. 2004;48:22–35.
6. Mahmoud KG, Scholkamy TH, Ahmed YF, Seidel GE Jr, Nawito MF. Effect of different combinations of cryoprotectants on in vitro maturation of immature buffalo (Bubalus bubalis) oocytes vitrified by straw and open-pulled straw methods. Reprod Dom Anim. 2012;45:565–71.
7. Somfai T, Men NT, Noguchi J, Kaneko H, Kashiwazaki N, Kikuchi K. Optimization of cryoprotectant treatment for the vitrification of immature cumulus-enclosed porcine oocytes: comparison of sugars, combinations of permeating cryoprotectants and equilibration regimens. J Reprod Dev. 2015;61:571–9.

8. Kuwayama M. Highly efficient vitrification for cryopreservation of human oocytes and embryos. The Cryotop method. Theriogenology. 2007;67:73–80.

9. Liang YY, Srirattana K, Phermthai T, Somfai T, Nagai T, Parnpai P. Effects of vitrification cryoprotectant treatment and cooling method on the viability and development of buffalo oocytes after intracytoplasmic sperm injection. Cryobiology. 2012;65:151–6.

10. Somfai T, Yoshioka K, Tanihara F, Kaneko H, Noguchi J, Kashiwazaki N, et al. Generation of live piglets from cryopreserved oocytes for the first time using a defined system for in vitro embryo production. PLoS One. 2014;9:e97731.

11. Vajta G. Vitrification of the oocytes and embryos of domestic animals. Anim Reprod Sci. 2000;60-61:357–64.

12. Casillas F, Teteltitla-Silvestre M, Ducolomb Y, Lemus AE, Salazar Z, Casas E, et al. Co-culture with granulosa cells improve the in vitro maturation ability of porcine immature oocytes vitrified with Cryolock. Cryobiology. 2014;69:299–304.

13. Zhang X, Miao Y, Zhao JG, Spate L, Bennett MW, Murphy CN, et al. Porcine oocytes denuded before maturation can develop to the blastocyst stage if provided a cumulous cell-derived coculture system. J Anim Sci. 2010;88:2604–10.

14. Wu G, Jia B, Quan G, Xiang D, Zhang B, Shao Q, Hong Q. Vitrification of porcine immature oocytes: association of equilibration manners with warming procedures, and permeating cryoprotectants effects under two temperatures. Cryobiology. 2017;75:21–7.

15. Casillas F, Ducolomb Y, Lemus AE, Cuello C, Betancourt M. Porcine embryo production following in vitro fertilization and intracytoplasmic sperm injection from vitrified immature oocytes matured with a granulosa cell co-culture system. Cryobiology. 2015;71:299–305.

16. McEvoy TG, Coull GD, Broadbent PJ, Hutchinson JSM, Speake BK. Fatty acid composition of lipids in immature cattle, pig and sheep oocytes with intact zona pellucida. J Rep Fertil. 2000;118:163–70.

17. Nagashima H, Kashiwazaki N, Ashman RJ, Grupen CG, Seamark RF, Nottle MB. Removal of cytoplasmic lipid enhances the tolerance of porcine embryos to chilling. Biol Reprod. 1994;51:618–22.

18. Fernandez-Reyes F, Ducolomb Y, Romo S, Casas E, Salazar Z, Betancourt M. Viability, maturation and embryo development in vitro of vitrified immature and porcine oocytes. Cryobiology. 2012;64:261–6.

19. Fujihira T, Kishida R, Fukui Y. Developmental capacity of vitrified immature porcine oocytes following ICSI, effects of cytochalasin B and cryoprotectants. Cryobiology. 2004;49:286–90.

20. Santos RM, Barreta MH, Frajblat M, Cucco DC, Mezzalira JC, Bunn S, et al. Vacuum-cooled liquid nitrogen increases the developmental ability of vitrified-warmed bovine oocytes. Ciencia Rural. 2006;36:1501–6.

21. Mavrides A, Morroll D. Bypassing the effect of zona pellucida changes on embryo formation following cryopreservation of bovine oocytes. Europ J Obstet Gynecol and Reprod Biol. 2005;118:66–70.

22. Rojas C, Palomo MJ, Albarracin JL, Mogas T. Vitrification of immature and in vitro matured pig oocytes: study of distribution of chromosomes, microtubules, and actin microfilaments. Cryobiology. 2004;49:211–20.

23. Catt WJ, Rhodes SL. Comparative intracytoplasmic sperm injection (ICSI) in human and domestic species. Reprod Fertil Dev. 1995;7:161–7.

24. Flaherty SP, Payne D, Swann NJ, Mattews CD. Aetiology of failed and abnormal fertilization after intracytoplasmic sperm injection. Hum Reprod. 1995;10:2623–9.

25. García-Mengual E, García-Roselló E, Alfonso J, Salvador I, Cebrian-Serrano A, Silvestre MA. Viability of ICSI oocytes after caffeine treatment and sperm membrane removal with triton X-100 in pigs. Theriogenology. 2011;79:1658–66.

26. Hewitson L, Simerly C, Dominko T, Schatten G. Cellular and molecular events after in vitro fertilization and intracytoplasmic sperm injection. Theriogenology. 2000;53:95–104.

27. Kato Y, Nagao Y. Effect of polyvinylpyrrolidone on sperm function and early embryonic development following intracytoplasmic sperm injection in human assisted reproduction. Reprod Med Biol. 2012;11:165–76.

28. Li X, Hamano K, Qian XQ, Funauchi K, Furudate M, Minato Y. Oocyte activation and parthenogenetic development of bovine oocytes following intracytoplasmic sperm injection. Zygote. 1999;7:233–7.

29. Shirazi A, Ostad-Hosseini E, Ahmadi E, Heidari B, Shams-Esfandabadi N. In vitro development competence of ICSI-derived activated ovine embryos. Theriogenology. 2009;71:342–8.

30. Xian-Hong T, Li-Min W, Ren-Tao J, Li-Hua L, Hong-Bing L, Yu-Sheng L. Fertilization rates are improved after IVF if the corona radiata is left intact in vitrified–warmed human oocytes. Hum Reprod. 2012;27:3208–14.

31. De-Yi L. Could using the zona pellucida bound sperm for intracytoplasmic sperm injection (ICSI) enhance the outcome of ICSI? Asian J Androl. 2011;13:197–8.

32. Black M, Liu DY, Bourne H, Baker HW. Comparison of outcomes of conventional intracytoplasmic sperm injection (ICSI) and ICSI using sperm bound to the zona pellucida of immature oocytes. Fertil Steril. 2010;93:672–4.

33. Mokánszki A, Tóthné EV, Bondár B, Tándor Z, Molnár Z, Jakab A, et al. Is sperm hyaluronic acid binding ability predictive for clinical success of intracytoplasmic sperm injection: PICSI vs. ICSI? Syst Biol Reprod Med. 2014;60:348–54.

34. Parmegiani L, Cognigni GE, Ciampaglia W, Pocognoli P, Marchi F, Filicori M. Efficiency of hyaluronic acid (HA) sperm selection. J Assist Reprod Genet. 2010;27:13–6.

35. Park CY, Uhm SJ, Song SJ, Kim KS, Hong SB, Chung KS, et al. Increase of ICSI efficiency with hyaluronic acid binding sperm for low aneuploidy frequency in pig. Theriogenology. 2005;64:1158–69.

36. Tienthai P, Kjellen L, Pertroft H, Suzuki K, Rodriguez-Martinez H. Localization and quantitation of hyaluronan and sulfated glycosaminoglycans in the tissues and intraluminal fluid of the pig oviduct. Reprod Fertil Dev. 2000;12:173–82.

37. Huszar G, Jakab A, Sakkas D, Ozenci CC, Cayil S, Delpiano E. Fertility testing and ICSI sperm selection by hyaluronic acid binding: clinical and genetic aspects. Reprod BioMed Online. 2007;14:650–3.

38. Huszar G, Ozenci CC, Cayil C, Zavaczki Z, Hansch E, Vigue L. Hyaluronic acid binding by human sperm indicates cellular maturity, viability, and unreacted acrosomal status. Fertil Steril. 2003;79:1616–24.

39. Abeydeera LR, Wang WH, Prather RS, Day BN. Maturation in vitro of pig oocytes in protein-free culture media: fertilization and subsequent embryo development in vitro. Biol Reprod. 1998;58:1316–20.

40. Tajima K, Orisaka M, Yata H, Goto K, Hosokawa K, Kotsuji F. Role of granulosa and theca cell interactions in ovarian follicular maturation. Microsc Res Tech. 2006;69:450–8.

41. Abeydeera LR, Day BN. In vitro fertilization of pig oocytes in a modified tris-buffered medium: effect of BSA, caffeine and calcium. Theriogenology. 1997;48:537–44.

42. Abeydeera LR. In vitro fertilization and embryo development in pigs. Reprod Suppl. 2001;50:159–73.

43. Sánchez-Osorio J, Cuello C, Gil MA, Parrilla I, Maside C, Almiñana C, et al. Vitrification and warming of in vivo-derived porcine embryos in a chemically defined medium. Theriogenology. 2010;73:300–8.

44. Hernández-Pichardo JE, Ducolomb Y, Romo S, Kjelland ME, Fierro R, Casillas F, et al. Pronuclear formation by ICSI using chemically activated ovine oocytes and zona pellucida bound sperm. J Anim Sci Biotech. 2016;7:65.

45. Casas E, Bonilla E, Ducolomb Y, Betancourt M. Differential effects of herbicides atrazine and fenoxaprop-ethyl, and insecticides diazinon and malathion, on viability and maturation of porcine oocytes in vitro. Toxicol in Vitro. 2010;24:224–30.

46. Martino A, Pollard JW, Leibo SP. Effect of chilling bovine oocytes on their developmental competence. Mol Reprod Dev. 1996;45:503–12.

47. Suzuki T, Saha S, Sumantri C, Takagi M, Boediono A. The influence of polyvinylpyrrolidone on freezing of bovine IVF blastocysts following biopsy. Cryobiology. 1995;32:505–10.

48. Wei Y, Fan J, Li L, Liu Z, Li K. Pretreating porcine sperm with lipase enhances developmental competence of embryos produced by intracytoplasmic sperm injection. Zygote. 2016;4:594–602.

49. Huszar G. Hyaluronic acid binding-mediated sperm selection for ICSI. In: Gardner DK, Weissman A, Howles CM, Shoham Z, editors. Textbook of assisted reproductive techniques. London; 2011. p. 122–34. https://doi.org/10.3109/9781841849713.009.

50. Morrell JM, Rodriguez-Martínez H. Practical applications of sperm selection techniques as a tool for improving reproductive efficiency. Vet Med Int. 2010; https://doi.org/10.4061/2011/894767.

51. Javed A, Mozafari F, Ashwini LS, Ganguly D. Commentary: physiological intracytoplasmic sperm injection (PICSI), an alternative to the standard ICSI procedure. MOJ Anat Physiol. 2015; https://doi.org/10.15406/mojap.2015.01.00009.

52. Suzuki K, Eriksson B, Shimizu H, Nagai T, Rodríguez-Martinez H. Effect of hyaluronan on monospermic penetration of porcine oocytes fertilized in vitro. Int J Androl. 2000;23:13–21.

53. Ulbrich SE, Schoenfelder M, Thoene S, Einspanier R. Hyaluronan in the bovine oviduct-modulation of synthases and receptors during the estrous cycle. Mol Cell Endocrinol. 2004;214:9–18.

54. Henkel R. Sperm preparation: state-of-the-art-physiological aspects and application of advanced sperm preparation methods. Asian J Androl. 2012;14:260–9.

55. Somfai T, Dinnyes A, Sage D, Marosan M, Carnwath JW, Ozawa M, et al. Development to the blastocyst stage of parthenogenethically activated in vitro matured porcine oocytes after solid surface vitrification (SSV). Theriogenology. 2006;66:415–22.

56. Begin I, Bhatia B, Baldassarre H, Dinnyes A, Keefer CL. Cryopreservation of goat oocytes and in vivo derived 2- to 4- cell embryos using the cryoloop (CLV) and solid-surface vitrification (SSV) methods. Theriogenology. 2003;59: 1839–50.

57. Gupta MK, Uhm SJ, Lee HT. Cryopreservation of immature and in vitro matured porcine oocytes by solid surface vitrification. Theriogenology. 2007; 67:238–48.

58. Somfai T, Noguchi J, Kaneko H, Nagai M, Ozawa M, Kashiwazaki N, et al. Production of good-quality porcine blastocysts by in vitro fertilization of follicular oocytes vitrified at the germinal vesicle stage. Theriogenology. 2010;73:147–56.

59. Bedaiwy MA, Falcone T, Mohamed MS, Aleem AA, Sharma RK, Worley SE, et al. Differential growth of human embryos in vitro: role of reactive oxygen species. Fertil Steril. 2004;82:593–600.

60. Mahmoud KGM, El-Sokary MMM, Kandiel MMM, Abou El-Roos MEA, Sosa GMS. Effects of cysteamine during in vitro maturation on viability and meiotic competence of vitrified buffalo oocytes. Iran J Vet Res. 2016;17:165–70.

61. Somfai T, Ozawa M, Noguchi J, Kaneko H, Karja NWK, Farhudin M, et al. Developmental competence of in vitro-fertilized porcine oocytes after in vitro maturation and solid surface vitrification: effect of cryopreservation on oocyte antioxidative system and cell cycle stage. Cryobiology. 2007;55:115–26.

62. Wu C, Rui R, Dai J, Zhang C, Ju S, Xiao-Lu BX, et al. Effects of cryopreservation on the developmental competence, ultrastructure and cytoskeletal structure of porcine oocytes. Mol Rep Dev. 2006;73:1454–62.

63. Godard NM, Pukazhenthi BS, Wildt DE, Comizzoli P. Paracrine factors from cumulus-enclosed oocytes ensure the successful maturation and fertilization in vitro of denuded oocytes in the cat model. Fertil Steril. 2009;91:2051–60.

64. Yu-Hung L, Jiann-Loung H, Kok-Min S, Lee-Wen H, Heng-Ju C, Chii-Ruey T. Effects of growth factors and granulosa cell co-culture on in-vitro maturation of oocytes. Rep Biomed Onl. 2009;19:165–70.

65. Appeltant R, Somfai T, Santos ECS, Dang-Nguyen TQ, Nagai T, Kikuchi K. Effects of vitrification of cumulus-enclosed porcine oocytes at the germinal vesicle stage on cumulus expansion, nuclear progression and cytoplasmic maturation. Rep Fertil Dev. 2017;29:2419–29.

66. Egerszegi I, Somfai T, Nakai M, Tanihara F, Noguchi J, Kaneko H, et al. Comparison of cytoskeletal integrity, fertilization and developmental competence of oocytes vitrified before or after in vitro maturation un a porcine model. Cryobiology. 2013;67:287–92.

67. Appeltant R, Beek J, Vandenberghe L, Maes D, Soom AV. Increasing the cAMP concentration during in vitro maturation of pig oocytes improves cumulus maturation and subsequent fertilization in vitro. Theriogenology. 2015;83:344–52.

68. Romar R, Coy P, Rath D. Maturation conditions and boar affect timing of cortical reaction in porcine oocytes. Theriogenology. 2012;78:1126–39.

69. García-Mengual E, Silvestre MA, Salvador I, Cebrian-Serrano A, García-Rosello E. Male pronucleus formation sfter ICSI: effect of oocyte cysteine or sperm triton X-100 treatments. Czech J Anim Sci. 2015;60:241–9.

70. Che L, Lalonde A, Bordigon V. Chemical activation of parthenogenetic and nuclear transfer porcine oocytes using ionomycin and strontium chloride. Theriogenology. 2007;67:1297–304.

71. Kolbe T, Holtz W. Intracytoplasmic injection (ICSI) of in vivo or in vitro matured oocytes with fresh ejaculated or frozen-thawed epididymal spermatozoa and additional calcium.Ionophore activation in the pig. Theriogenology. 1999;52:671–82.

72. Nakai M, Ozawa M, Maedomari N, Noguchi J, Kaneko H, Ito J, Onishi A, Kashiwazaki N, Kikuchi K. Delay in cleavage of porcine embryos after intracytoplasmic sperm injection (ICSI) shows poorer embryonic development. J Reprod Dev. 2014;60:256–9.

73. Vatzias G, Hagen DR. Effects of porcine follicular fluid on oviduct-conditioned media on maturation and fertilization of porcine oocytes in vitro. Biol Reprod. 1999;60:42–8.

74. Majumdar G, Majumdar A. A prospective randomized study to evaluate the effect of hyaluronic acid sperm selection on the intracytoplasmic sperm injection outcome of patients with unexplained infertility having normal semen parameters. J Assist Reprod Genet. 2013;30:1471–5.

75. Burrel V, Klooster K, Barker CM, Pera RR, Mayers S. Abnormal early cleavage events predict early embryo demise: sperm oxidative stress and early abnormal cleavage. Sci Rep. 2014;4:6598.

76. Neri QV, Lee B, Rosenwaks Z, Machaca K, Palermo GD. Understanding fertilization through intracytoplasmic sperm injection (ICSI). Cell Cal. 2014;55:24–37.

77. Erberelli RF, Salgado RM, Mendes-Pereira DH, Wolff P. Hyaluronan-binding system for sperm selection enhances pregnancy rates in ICSI cycles associated with male factor infertility. JBRA Assist Reprod. 2017;21:2–6.

78. Worrilow KC, Eid S, Woodhouse D, Perloe M, Smith S, Witmyer J, et al. Use of hyaluronan in the selection of sperm for intracytoplasmic sperm injection (ICSI): significant improvement in clinical outcomes-multicenter, double-blinded and randomized controlled trial. Hum Reprod. 2013;28:306–14.

79. Yagci A, Murk W, Stronk J, Huszar G. Spermatozoa bound to solid state hyaluronic acid show chromatin structure with high DNA chain integrity: an acridine orange fluorescence study. J Androl. 2010;31:566–72.

22

Comparison of serum pools and oral fluid samples for detection of porcine circovirus type 2 by quantitative real-time PCR in finisher pigs

Gitte Blach Nielsen[1]* ⓘ, Jens Peter Nielsen[2], John Haugegaard[1], Sanne Christiansen Leth[3], Lars E. Larsen[4], Charlotte Sonne Kristensen[5], Ken Steen Pedersen[6], Helle Stege[2], Charlotte K. Hjulsager[4] and Hans Houe[2]

Abstract

Background: Porcine circovirus type 2 (PCV2) diagnostics in live pigs often involves pooled serum and/or oral fluid samples for group-level determination of viral load by quantitative real-time polymerase chain reaction (qPCR). The purpose of the study was to compare the PCV2 viral load determined by qPCR of paired samples at the pen level of pools of sera (SP) from 4 to 5 pigs and the collective oral fluid (OF) from around 30 pigs corresponding to one rope put in the same pen. Pigs in pens of 2 finishing herds were sampled by cross-sectional (Herd 1) and cross-sectional with follow-up (Herd 2) study designs. In Herd 1, 50 sample pairs consisting of SP from 4 to 5 pigs and OF from around 23 pigs were collected. In Herd 2, 65 sample pairs consisting of 4 (SP) and around 30 (OF) pigs were collected 4 times at 3-week intervals.

Results: A higher proportion of PCV2-positive pens (86% vs. 80% and 100% vs. 91%) and higher viral loads (mean difference: 2.10 and 1.83 log(10) PCV2 copies per ml) were found in OF versus SP in both herds. The OF cut-off value corresponding to a positive SP (>3 log(10) PCV2 copies per ml) was estimated to 6.5 and 7.36 log(10) PCV2 copies per ml for Herds 1 and 2, respectively. Significant correlations between SP and OF results were found in Herd 1 (rho = 0.69) and the first sampling in Herd 2 (rho = 0.39), but not for the subsequent consecutive 3 samplings in Herd 2.

Conclusions: The proportion and viral loads of PCV2 positive pens were higher in collective OF (including up to 30 pigs) compared to SP (including 4–5 pigs) of the same pens. Also, OF seemed to detect the PCV2 infection earlier with OF values just below 6.5 (Herd 1) and 7.36 (Herd 2) log(10) being associated with a negative SP for the same pen. Nevertheless, a statistically significant correlation between SP and OF could not be found for all sampling time points, probably due to a high within-pen variation in individual pig viral load becoming very evident in SP of only four or five pigs. Consequently, the results imply that OF is well suited for detecting presence of PCV2 but less so for determining the specific viral load of pigs in a pen.

Keywords: Diagnostics, Finishers, Oral fluid, Pooling, Porcine circovirus type 2, Serum

* Correspondence: gitte.blach.nielsen@merck.com
[1]MSD Animal Health Nordic, Havneholmen 25, 1561 Copenhagen V, Denmark
Full list of author information is available at the end of the article

Background

Porcine circovirus type 2 (PCV2), a circular, single-stranded, non-enveloped DNA virus has been demonstrated to be present in almost all commercial swine herds worldwide [1, 2]. PCV2 is the essential infectious agent involved in post-weaning multi-systemic wasting syndrome (PMWS) in pigs [3, 4]. The virus has been detected in serum and tissues (lymph nodes, lung, tonsil, kidney, liver, heart) and is shed in a variety of secretions (nasal, oral, fecal, urinary) [5–7]. In serum, individual viral loads above 7 log(10) PCV2 copies per ml serum have been associated with occurrence of clinical signs [8–10]. Currently, however, infection with PCV2 most commonly leads to subclinical infections that still negatively impact production parameters resulting in economic losses for the farmer [11]. Thus, the average daily gain has been found significantly reduced in pigs with viral loads as low as 4.3–5.3 log(10) PCV2 copies per ml serum [12].

Vaccination provides an effective tool to control PCV2 infections [13–17] but is an extra cost. Valid diagnostic tests enabling determination of the PCV2 viral load in a specific herd are therefore crucial when deciding whether or not to vaccinate. Furthermore, in cases of subclinical infections or infection with non-specific clinical signs, methods to confirm the diagnosis without euthanasia of pigs are highly preferable. For this purpose, virus detection in serum samples by quantitative real-time polymerase chain reaction (qPCR) has been widely used. To save laboratory costs in clinical swine practice, it has furthermore become increasingly popular to pool serum samples and then interpret the result as being representative for the age group sampled. Serum samples and nasal swabs have been suggested to be more suitable for evaluating PMWS status for a group of pigs than for individuals [9] and pooled samples could be a further development of this. However, it was later concluded that qPCR testing of pooled serum samples was not sufficiently reliable for diagnosis of PMWS at herd level but might be useful for determination of viral loads [18].

In the last 10 years, oral fluid sampling has gained growing interest as an even more cost and time-saving method while also considering animal welfare. The sampling procedure consists of hanging a cotton rope in a pen for the pigs to chew on, followed by wringing of the rope to release the oral fluid. The method was initially described in 2008 [19, 20], and the suitability of oral fluids for diagnosing different porcine pathogens by PCR such as PRRSV, swine influenza virus, foot-and-mouth disease virus, African and classical swine fever viruses as well as *Haemophilus parasuis* and *Streptococcus suis* has since been demonstrated [20–23]. Also for PCV2, qPCR of oral fluid has been proven valid for detection of infection [19, 24–26].

Some previous studies have compared detection and load of PCV2 by PCR in serum and oral fluid. A fair agreement between individual PCV2-positive serum and oral fluid samples (kappa = 0.24) but a poor agreement between pooled serum and oral fluid collected from pen-housed pigs (kappa = 0.001, 8–15 pigs per pen) has been found [27]. Another study reported that in 57 oral fluid samples of 3 PCV2-inoculated pens, 56 samples were PCV2-positive, whereas all 19 oral fluid samples in one pen of negative control pigs were PCV2-negative. Consequently, a sensitivity of 98% and a specificity of 100% of oral fluid were calculated [25, 28]. A very recent study found a higher proportion of PCV2-positive pens when PCR-analysis was done on oral fluid (11–23 pigs per pen) compared to pooled serum (2–4 pigs) and a relatively high, but non-significant, correlation (r = 0.76) between viral loads in the two sample types [29]. A similar correlation (r = 0.78) between viral loads in oral fluid (20–30 pigs per pen) and pooled serum (5 pigs) was found to be significant in another study [24]. One small experimental study reported a difference in the median viral loads between oral fluid and serum of around 1 log(10) based on 10 repeated samplings of the same pen [30]. A similar difference between mean viral loads in oral fluid and pooled serum samples at one sampling time point (including 40 pens) has been mentioned briefly elsewhere [29].

The inconclusive and limited number of studies regarding the association between viral loads in pooled serum and oral fluid at pen level and possible differences between PCR-assays require further elucidation by including additional herds/samples for the comparison. Moreover, since both oral fluid and pooled serum sampling are done with the purpose of diagnosing PCV2 infection in a group of pigs, determination of the oral fluid viral load corresponding to a positive serum pool is relevant for practical validation of oral fluid as a substitute for serum pools. Consequently, the objectives of this study were to: 1) determine the oral fluid viral load cut-off agreeing best with a PCV2-positive serum pool and 2) compare viral loads of PCV2 in serum pools and collective oral fluid from pigs in the same pen.

Methods

Herds

Serum and oral fluid samples were collected in 2 PCV2-infected finishing herds (Herd 1 and 2). Neither of the herds experienced clinical signs attributable to PCV2 infection (wasting, dyspnea or enlarged lymph nodes) [11]. Herd 1 was a conventional herd known to be seropositive for porcine reproductive and respiratory syndrome virus (PRRSv) and samples were collected in August 2010. Herd 2 was a specific-pathogen-free herd (free from *Mycoplasma hyopneumoniae*, *Actinobacillus pleuropneumoniae* type 2 + 6 + 12 and PRRSv) and samples were collected between September 2014 and July 2015 as a part of a larger field trial. None of the herds vaccinated against PCV2 prior to initiation of sampling, but in the field trial in Herd 2, half of the finishers were vaccinated during sample collection as a part of a PCV2 vaccine trial. However, only PCV2-qPCR results from the non-vaccinated group were included in the present study and an overview of the serum results have been presented briefly elsewhere [31].

Sample size calculations

At the time of sampling in Herd 1 (August 2010), no previous studies had estimated the correlation coefficient between serum pools and oral fluid samples and the interest of the study was therefore to determine whether or not a correlation existed. Therefore, the sample size calculation was based on detecting a correlation coefficient equal to or higher than 0.4 at a significance level of 95% and a power of 0.8 corresponding to a sample size of 47 [32]. In Herd 2 (where the primary purpose was to detect a difference in feed conversion rate between vaccinated and control pigs), a sample size of 65 pens was estimated [31], which in terms of correlation between serum and oral fluid corresponded to detecting a significant correlation at a 95% level with a power of 0.8, if the correlation coefficient was equal to or higher than 0.34 [32].

Study design

The study design in Herd 1 was cross-sectional with all samples collected from pigs of 3 different age groups in one day. The study design in Herd 2 was cross-sectional with follow-up consisting of totally 4 repeated samplings of the same pigs/pens at 3-week intervals. Serum and oral fluid were collected simultaneously at each sampling.

Selection of study units

The study unit was the pen. Herd 1 had a total of 64 pens of which 50 were randomly (with age-stratification) selected for sampling [33]. In Herd 2, all pens with non-vaccinated finishers in 14 finishing batches were sampled, corresponding to a total number of 65 pens, each sampled 4 times. Pigs for blood sampling within the pens were selected as every n[th] pig in the pen depending on the number of pigs per pen, assuring that 5 or 4 pigs per pen were selected in Herd 1 and 2, respectively. In Herd 2, the same 4 pigs per pen were bled at the 4 consecutive sampling time points (unless death or early removal had occurred, in which case a substitute pig was randomly selected).

Blood sampling

Blood samples were collected from the cranial vena cava in plain tubes. In Herd 1, the blood samples were transported directly to the laboratory after sampling and refrigerated overnight. In Herd 2, samples were kept refrigerated overnight and were shipped to the laboratory by mail the following day.

At the laboratory, blood samples were centrifuged to separate serum. Equal amounts of serum from each of the 4/5 pigs per pen were pooled prior to PCV2-qPCR analysis, resulting in one serum PCV2 copy number (viral load) per pen. Thus, serum viral loads refer to qPCR-results from pooled serum samples.

Oral fluid sampling

Sampling of oral fluid was performed as previously described [19]. Briefly, a cotton rope, fixed to the pen railings, was presented to the pigs allowing them to chew on it, thereby transferring oral fluid to the rope. Thirty min later, ropes were collected in individual plastic bags and wringed to release the oral fluid for later qPCR-analysis. Based on numerous observations during sampling, it was estimated that more than 80% of the pigs in a pen contributed to the oral fluid sample. Storage and shipment of oral fluid samples to the laboratory were as described for the blood samples.

Quantification of PCV2 in oral fluid and serum by qPCR

The oral fluids collected in both herds were grey and dirty in appearance, probably reflecting fecal contamination. Feces as well as saliva can contain PCR inhibitors [34–36] and if these are present during qPCR-analysis, underestimation of quantitative levels or false-negative results may occur. To eliminate the effect of potential PCR inhibitors in oral fluid, the samples were centrifuged and diluted 1:10 in nuclease-free water[1] prior to DNA extraction. The applicability of this pre-extraction dilution was confirmed by testing 5 naturally PCV2-positive oral fluid samples and 5, initially PCV2-negative, oral fluid samples spiked 1:100 with PCV2 virus isolate. Evaluation was performed by comparison of Ct-values and PCR efficiencies calculated from 10-fold dilution series of extracted DNA and tested for PCV2 as described below.

DNA extraction from all oral fluid samples and the serum samples from Herd 2 was performed with a commercially available extraction kit[2] using 200 μl serum or 200 μl oral fluid diluted 1:10 in nuclease free water[1]. DNA extraction from serum from Herd 1 was performed differently[3] but internal laboratory validation was performed by testing 78 samples using both methods. On average, the results obtained by the two methods were very similar with an average difference of 0.2 log(10) PCV2 copies per ml serum (range 0.0–1.6).

The serum and oral fluid samples were tested for PCV2-DNA by qPCR essentially as previously described [37]. During the testing of some of the oral fluid samples from Herd 2 an inhibition of the qPCR was revealed, probably due to a fava bean feed ingredient. Therefore, the DNA extracted from these samples were tested both undiluted and diluted 1:10 in nuclease-free water[1] to avoid false negative test results. Oral fluid viral loads were subsequently corrected according to the extra dilutions. The qPCR-assay had a detection limit of 10^3 and a quantification range of 3.3×10^4–3.3×10^9 PCV2 copies per ml [37]. Because the oral fluid was diluted 10 times prior to DNA extraction, the minimum concentration that could be detected in the samples was 10 times higher for OF compared to serum (10^4 versus 10^3). Samples were considered positive when the viral load was above the detection limit.

Statistical analyses

All PCV2 viral loads were analyzed on a log-transformed scale. Comparison of PCV2 viral loads in serum and oral fluid was made separately for Herd 1 and 2, and because the same pens were repeatedly sampled in Herd 2, and hence could not be considered independent, each sampling time point in Herd 2 was also analyzed separately. Viral loads below the assay detection limit were included in the statistical analyses with a value of 0, since the true distribution of these was unknown and excluding the observations would reduce the actual variation and thereby bias the results.

Descriptive statistics consisted of frequency distributions, graphical illustrations and summary statistics. Evaluation of agreement between serum and oral fluid PCV2 viral loads was done both on a dichotomous (PCV2-positive/negative) and a quantitative scale. On a dichotomous scale, the oral fluid cut-off value for obtaining the best agreement with a PCV2-positive serum result (above the test detection limit of 3 log(10) PCV2-copies per ml serum) was estimated by drawing a receiver operating characteristic (ROC)-curve for all possible oral fluid cut-off values against a serum value fixed at the assay detection limit. Best agreement was defined as the oral fluid cut-off value where relative sensitivity and relative specificity were maximized simultaneously. The terms 'relative sensitivity' and 'relative specificity' were used, since the serum result could not be considered 'gold standard' in the classical sense but rather a 'reference standard' (as in a study from 2003 [38]). All sample pairs (serum and oral fluid collected from the same pen) in Herd 1 and sample pairs from the first sampling in Herd 2 were used for this purpose, since only those included more than one PCV2-negative serum result. On a quantitative scale, the viral loads in serum and oral fluid were compared and the correlation coefficients estimated. Due to the non-normal distribution of serum and oral fluid PCV2 viral loads, nonparametric tests were used (paired Wilcoxon-test and Spearman's rank correlation test). All statistical analyses

were performed in R [39] with a significance level set at 0.05. However, due to multiple comparisons, the significance level was adjusted by the Bonferroni method. Finally, in order to evaluate an eventual effect of the number of pigs per pen at sampling on the oral fluid viral loads, two linear regressions with oral fluid viral load as the outcome were performed, one for each herd. For Herd 1, serum pool viral load and number of pigs per pen were included as explanatory variables. For Herd 2, also sampling number and the interaction between pigs per pen at sampling and sampling number were included as additional explanatory variables. Model selection was based on a backwards elimination procedure, also with a significance level of 0.05 for keeping variables in the models. The final models´ distribution of residuals was assessed visually for normality.

Results

In total, 310 serum and oral fluid sample pairs were collected. Of these, 50 sample pairs were from Herd 1 with 4–5 pigs bled per pen with a mean of 23 pigs per pen (range: 5–33) and 260 sample pairs (65 pens sampled 4 times) were from Herd 2 with 4 pigs bled per pen with a mean of 29 pigs per pen (range: 9–32). The number of pigs per pen reflects the maximum number of pigs contributing to the oral fluid sample.

Agreement between serum pools and oral fluid for classification of pens into PCV2 positive/negative

Classification of sample pairs into PCV2 positive and PCV2 negative based on the test detection limit is shown in Table 1. In Herd 1, 80% of serum pools and 86% of oral fluid samples were PCV2 positive, whereas totally in Herd 2, 91% of serum pools and 100% of oral fluid samples were PCV2 positive. Of

Table 1 Distribution of serum and oral fluid samples below (negative) versus above (positive) the PCV2-qPCR test detection limit for finishing pigs in 2 herds

Sampling			Serum Positive	Serum Negative
Herd 1 (n = 50) 1	Oral fluid	Positive	39	4
		Negative	1	6
Herd 2 (n = 65) 1	Oral fluid	Positive	43	22
		Negative	0	0
2	Oral fluid	Positive	65	0
		Negative	0	0
3	Oral fluid	Positive	64	1
		Negative	0	0
4	Oral fluid	Positive	65	0
		Negative	0	0
Total			277	33

the 23 negative serum pools in Herd 2, 22 were negative at the first sampling.

The 2 ROC-curves (one for Herd 1 and one for the first sampling in Herd 2) for evaluation of best agreement between serum and oral fluid concerning a PCV2-positive serum result are displayed in Fig. 1. The cut-off value for oral fluid associated with the best agreement with a PCV2-positive serum result was estimated to be 6.5 and 7.36 log(10) PCV2 copies per ml serum for Herd 1 and 2, respectively (Table 2).

Comparison of serum and oral fluid PCV2 viral loads

Figure 2 contains plots of the serum and oral fluid sample pairs from both herds at each sampling time point. As the sampling in Herd 2 was longitudinal, the evolution with time of serum and oral fluid viral loads are additionally shown in Figs. 3 and 4, respectively. Summary statistics of and estimated Spearman's correlation coefficients between sample pairs by herd and sampling time point are displayed in Table 3. A pairwise comparison of the quantitative viral loads in serum and oral fluid showed a significantly higher number of PCV2 copies in oral fluid compared to serum for both herds and at all sampling time points. The overall mean differences between oral fluid and serum were 2.10 log(10) (1Q,3Q = 1.68, 2.63) and 1.83 (1Q,3Q = 0.88, 2.11) for Herd 1 and 2, respectively. For Herd 1 and the first sampling in Herd 2, significant correlations between serum and oral fluid were found. However, no correlations were found for samplings 2, 3 and 4 in Herd 2.

Results from the linear regression models showed that oral fluid viral load was not significantly influenced by the number of pigs per pen when the viral load in serum (Herd 1 and 2) and sampling number (Herd 2) were also included in the models.

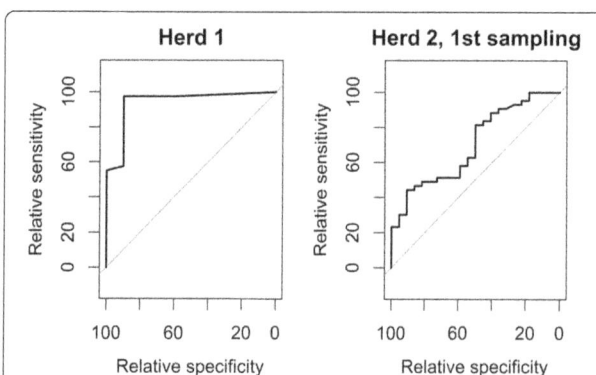

Fig. 1 ROC curves from Herd 1 (left) and first sampling in Herd 2 (right) to estimate the oral fluid cut-off for obtaining the best agreement with a PCV2-positive serum pool result for finishing pigs

Discussion

Overall, both herds had a widespread PCV2 infection with moderate viral loads resulting in relatively few serum pools and even fewer oral fluid samples being negative. A relatively small number of serum pools had viral loads above 7 log(10), which fits well with the observation that no clinical signs clearly related to PCV2 infection were present in either of the 2 herds. This, however, also implies that generalizing results to herds with high viral loads and/or clinical signs of PCV2 infection should be done with caution. Only one sample pair had a positive serum PCV2 result (5.59 log(10) PCV2 copies per ml serum) and a negative oral fluid PCV2 result, which may reflect that not all blood-sampled pigs chewed on the rope. The estimated contribution to the oral fluid sample of more than 80% of the pigs in a pen is supported by a study reporting that 94% of pigs in a pen (pen size: 17–24 pigs) had chewed on the presented rope after 30 min [40].

As expected, a slightly higher proportion of oral fluid samples compared to serum were PCV2 positive which probably reflects that the likelihood of a positive result is higher when more animals are tested (4 or 5 pigs were bled versus up to 33 pigs contributing to the oral fluid sample). This is similar to previous findings concerning PCV2 [24, 29] and more general findings reporting increasing herd sensitivities at increasing pool sizes [41]. Alternatively, contamination of the rope with PCV2 present in feces could also explain the difference, as a previous study has shown a higher proportion of positive rectal swabs compared to serum samples from individual animals [9]. In Herd 2, this difference in positive proportions was only evident at the first sampling with 66% positive serum pools versus 100% positive oral fluid samples, probably reflecting a lower within-pen prevalence of PCV2 compared to the subsequent samplings, when the infection may have spread. Based on simple sample size calculations, with a 95% probability of finding at least one positive animal, 4 negative samples can be achieved even with a 50% disease prevalence, whereas a sample size of 20 (approximation of the pigs sampled by oral fluid) would detect disease at a prevalence below 10% [42]. Consequently, the risk of overlooking a PCV2 infection, when the within-pen prevalence is low, seems increased if serum samples from a few pigs, instead of oral fluid samples from many pigs, are used.

The estimated oral fluid cut-offs for best agreement (the highest possible relative sensitivity and specificity) with a PCV2-positive serum pool were fairly similar for Herd 1 and 2 (first sampling) with 6.5 and 7.36 log(10) PCV2 copies per ml oral fluid, respectively. However, the oral fluid cut-off was determined with a higher accuracy in terms of relative sensitivity and specificity for Herd 1 than for Herd 2, probably due to the lower

Table 2 Oral fluid cut-off value best agreeing with a PCV2-positive serum pool in finishers

Best agreement	Oral fluid cut-off (log(10))	Relative sensitivity (95% C.I.)	Relative specificity (95% C.I.)	Area under curve (95% C.I.)
Herd 1	6.50	0.98 (0.87;1.00)	0.90 (0.55;1.00)	0.941 (0.851;1.00)
Herd 2, 1st sampling	7.36	0.58 (0.42;0.73)	0.59 (0.36;0.79)	0.7 (0.567; 0.833)

variation between individual oral fluid results in Herd 1 compared to Herd 2 (first sampling) (see Fig. 2). This has previously been described as a well-known challenge in diagnostic test evaluation [43].

The viral loads in oral fluid were significantly higher compared to the matched serum pools. A difference of almost 2 log(10) PCV2 copies per ml sample was found in both herds, hence, substantially higher than the 1 log(10) reported by others [29, 30]. Whether this divergence is merely due to PCR-assay differences is unknown. As with the higher proportion of positives, a higher viral load in oral fluid was expected because far more pigs were sampled with oral fluid. Earlier studies

demonstrating a high variation of viral loads in serum between individual pigs within a group support this [18, 44]: In 10 animals in each of 5 different PMWS-negative farms, ranges between <4 (detection limit) and 8.7 log(10) PCV2 copies per ml serum within the same farm and age group were found [18]. And in a vaccination trial, a mean level of 6.1 log(10) and a standard deviation of 1.7 log(10) PCV2 copies per ml serum in 8 PCV2-positive control pigs were reported [44]. Consequently, the specific viral load found in a positive serum pool is prone to vary greatly, being very dependent upon which pigs happen to be selected for blood sampling as opposed to oral fluid sampling that includes nearly all pigs in a pen. The results

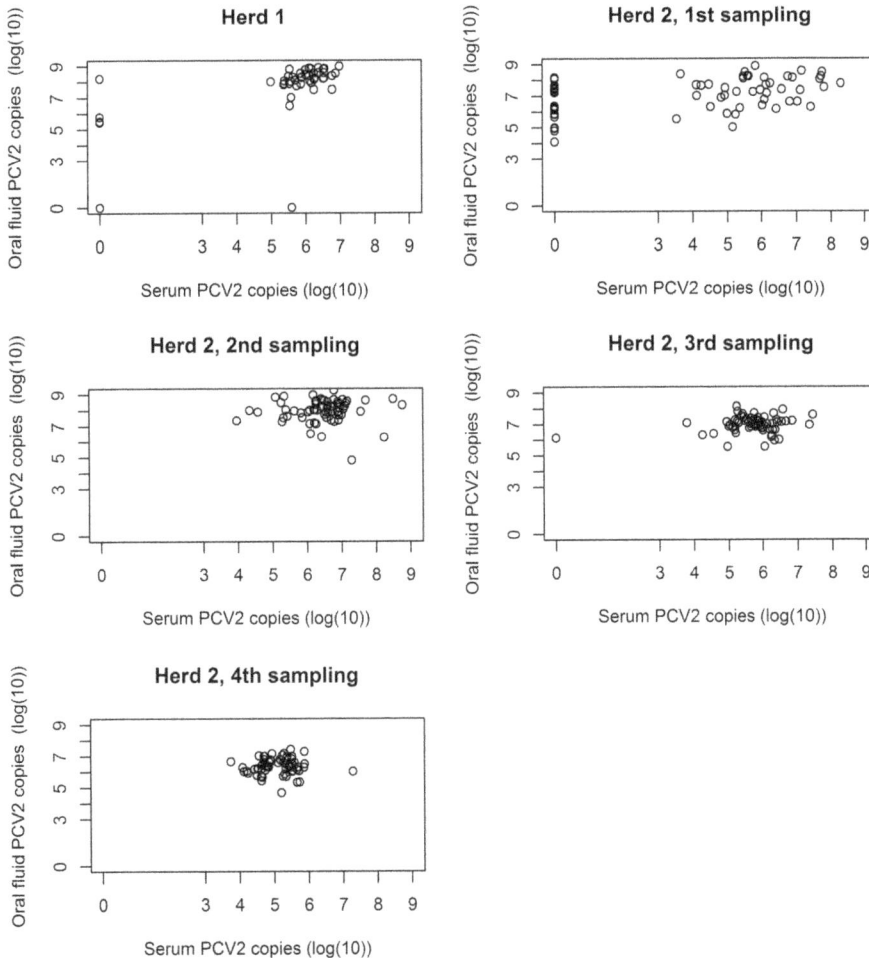

Fig. 2 Plots of serum pools and oral fluid sample pairs from finishing pigs for both herds and all samplings with serum pool viral loads on the x-axis and oral fluid viral loads on the y-axis

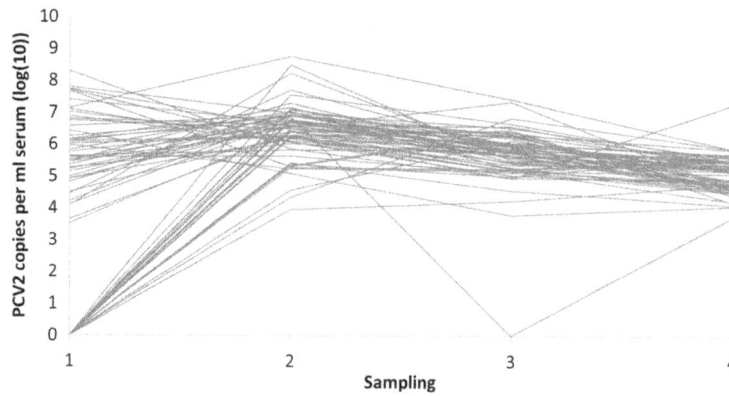

Fig. 3 Evolution with time in Herd 2 of PCV2 viral loads in serum pools. Samplings were done at 3-week intervals and each line represents one pen

from Herd 2 nicely demonstrate this when comparing Figs. 3 and 4 which show the evolution with time. Here, a higher variation between individual-pen serum viral loads compared to individual-pen oral fluid viral loads is generally seen.

Secondly, higher PCV2 viral loads may be present in oral fluid compared to the viral loads found in serum. Previous comparisons of serum and oral/tonsillar swabs found either no difference concerning prevalence of PCV2 positives [6, 45] and viral loads [6, 7] or a higher prevalence [7] and higher viral loads [45] in oral/tonsillar swabs compared to serum. Furthermore, in Herd 1, 2 pens contained only 5 pigs resulting in 100% of pigs being blood sampled. Still, the oral fluid PCV2 viral loads were higher than the serum viral loads with 8.07 and 7.03 log(10) in oral fluid versus 6.12 and 5.57 log(10) in serum.

A significant correlation between serum and oral fluid viral loads was found for Herd 1 and the first sampling in Herd 2, whereas no significant correlations were found for samplings 2, 3 and 4 in Herd 2. For Herd 1, the estimated correlation coefficient of 0.69 was comparable to the 0.76 and 0.78 previously reported [24, 29].

However, of these previously reported correlation coefficients, only the coefficient of 0.78 was found to be significant [24]. This was based on 18 pens sampled 5 consecutive times thus challenging the assumption of independency between observations and an analysis of time points individually, as in the current study, might have given a different result.

For the first sampling in Herd 2, the correlation coefficient, even though significant, was only estimated to 0.39, which may be due to the high number of negative serum pools. For samplings 2, 3 and 4 in Herd 2, no statistically significant correlations were found between serum pools and oral fluid. A higher proportion of pigs in the pen were blood sampled in Herd 1 (~ 20%) compared to Herd 2 (~14%), which would seem like a plausible explanation, but the results from the linear regression models showed that the number of pigs per pen at sampling did not influence the oral fluid viral load when the serum viral load (Herd 1 and 2) and sampling number (Herd 2) were accounted for. Another explanation could be the higher variation in positive serum viral loads for all samplings in Herd 2 compared to Herd

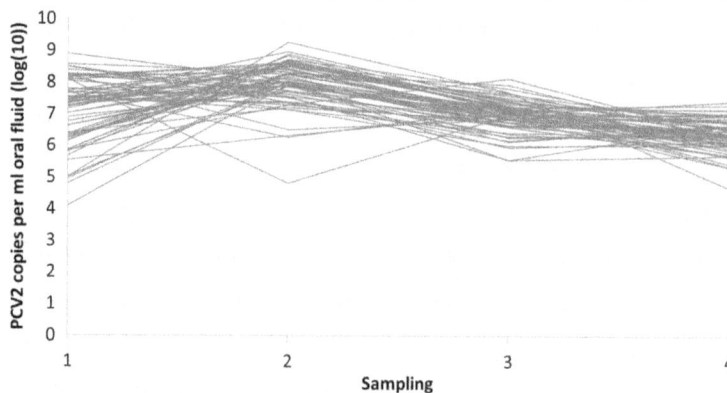

Fig. 4 Evolution with time in Herd 2 of PCV2 viral loads in oral fluid. Samplings were done at 3-week intervals and each line represents one pen

Table 3 Summary statistics of PCV2 viral loads and estimated Spearman's correlation coefficients (ρ) between oral fluid and serum pools from two finishing herds

PCV2 viral load	Sampling no.	Sample type	Mean	Median	Standard deviation	Min	Max	Wilcoxon (p-value)[c]	Spearman's correlation	
									ρ	p-value[c]
Herd 1	1	Serum[a]	4.82	5.86	2.47	0	6.97	<0.001	0.69	<0.001
(n = 50)		OF[b]	6.92	8.13	2.92	0	8.99			
Herd 2	1	Serum	3.89	4.99	2.96	0	8.29	<0.001	0.39	0.001
(n = 65)		OF	7.09	7.37	1.07	4.1	8.89			
	2	Serum	6.43	6.51	0.86	3.96	8.76	<0.001	0.14	0.278
		OF	7.98	8.03	0.73	4.80	9.26			
	3	Serum	5.69	5.79	0.96	0	7.43	<0.001	0.04	0.725
		OF	6.97	7.03	0.51	5.56	8.13			
	4	Serum	5.09	5.19	0.56	3.74	7.28	<0.001	0.08	0.524
		OF	6.37	6.37	0.51	4.67	7.43			

[a]Serum = serum pool, [b]OF = oral fluid, [c]significance level is 0.005 due to Bonferroni correction

1 (Fig. 2) which could reduce the likelihood of finding a significant correlation between serum and oral fluid, if it existed. Nevertheless, with the datasets included in this study, a cut-off for oral fluid corresponding to the established cut-off regarding clinical signs for serum of 7 log(10) PCV2 copies per ml serum [8–10] could not be determined.

Conclusions

In conclusion, a slightly higher proportion of PCV2 positive pens and higher viral loads were found with oral fluid as sample material compared to serum pools. Furthermore, oral fluid seemed to detect a PCV2 infection earlier with viral loads as high as 7 log(10) being associated with a negative serum pool for the same pen. Nevertheless, a statistically significant correlation between serum pools and oral fluid samples could not be found for all sampling time points, probably due to a high within-pen variation in individual pig viral load becoming very evident in serum pools including only four or five pigs in a pen of around 30. Hence, from a practitioner's point of view, oral fluid might be better suited to identify presence or not of the pathogen than to determine the specific viral load.

Endnotes

[1]UltraPure™ DNase/RNase-Free Distilled Water, Invitrogen, Nærum, Denmark.

[2]QIAamp DNA Mini Kit automated on QIAcube extraction robot, QIAGEN, Copenhagen, Denmark.

[3]QIAsymphony Virus/Bacteria Mini Kit, protocol Pathogen complex 200 without IC V2, with elution in 110 μl elution buffer, automated on QIASymphony extraction robot, QIAGEN, Copenhagen, Denmark.

Acknowledgements
The authors would like to thank herd owners for hospitality and cooperation, veterinary students (Berit Rasmussen, Thomas Kusk, Martin Rasmussen, Christian Bonnerup Møller, Emil Hjerrild, Simon Smed Sørensen), Lise Kirstine Kvisgaard, Jesper Schak Krog, Bjarne Ellegaard, Anette Rasmussen, Susanne Gram, Torben Adel Larsen and Karsten Nielsen for practical help on the farms, veterinarians Erik Dam Sørensen and Andreas Birch for establishing contact to trial farms and Matthew James Denwood and Søren Saxmose Nielsen for input regarding statistics. Furthermore, the authors would like to thank Peter Astrup and Bjarne Ellegaard for general discussions during the study. Finally, Rika Jolie is thanked for proof-reading.

Funding
This work was economically supported by the Danish Agency for Science Technology and Innovation [case number 0604-02976B] and MSD Animal Health, Denmark. The funders did not try to inflict any bias regarding the design, conduction, statistical evaluation or interpretation of the study or the study results.

Authors' contributions
Conception of the study: GBN, JPN, JH, SCL, LEL, CSK, KSP, HS, CKH, HH. Design of the study: GBN, JPN, JH, SCL, HH. Acquisition and analysis of data: GBN and SCL. Interpretation of data: GBN, JPN, JH, LEL, CSK, KSP, HH. Drafting the manuscript: GBN, JPN, JH, LEL, CKH, HH. All authors read, critically revised and approved the final manuscript.

Competing interests
At the time of submission of this article, John Haugegaard and the corresponding author are employed by MSD Animal Health, Denmark, the company partly sponsoring this work as mentioned above. However, the employment did not inflict any bias regarding the study and the work was conducted during the corresponding author's enrolment as Industrial PhD student at the University of Copenhagen.

Author details

[1]MSD Animal Health Nordic, Havneholmen 25, 1561 Copenhagen V, Denmark. [2]Department of Veterinary and Animal Sciences, University of Copenhagen, Grønnegårdsvej 2+8, 1870 Frederiksberg C, Denmark. [3]Porcus Veterinary Pig Practice, Ørbækvej 276, 5220 Odense, SØ, Denmark. [4]National Veterinary Institute, Henrik Dams Allé, Bygning 205B, 2800 Kgs. Lyngby, Denmark. [5]SEGES Pig Research Centre, Vinkelvej 11, 8620 Kjellerup, Denmark. [6]Ø-vet A/S, Køberupvej 33, 4700 Næstved, Denmark.

References

1. Patterson AR, Opriessnig T. Epidemiology and horizontal transmission of porcine circovirus type 2 (PCV2). Anim Health Res Rev. 2010;11(2):217–34.
2. Rose N, Opriessnig T, Grasland B, Jestin A. Epidemiology and transmission of porcine circovirus type 2 (PCV2). Virus Res. 2012;164:78–89.
3. Grau-Roma L, Fraile L, Segales J. Recent advances in the epidemiology, diagnosis and control of diseases caused by porcine circovirus type 2. Vet J. 2011;187:23–32.
4. Tomas A, Fernandes LT, Valero O, Segales J. A meta-analysis on experimental infections with porcine circovirus type 2 (PCV2). Vet Microbiol. 2008;132:260–73.
5. Harding JCS, Baker CD, Tumber A, McIntosh KA, Parker SE, Middleton DM, Hill JE, Ellis JA, Krakowka S. Porcine circovirus-2 DNA concentration distinguishes wasting from nonwasting pigs and is correlated with lesion distribution, severity and nucleocapsid staining intensity. J Vet Diagn Investig. 2008;20:274–82.
6. Patterson AR, Ramamoorthy S, Madson DM, Meng XJ, Halbur PG, Opriessnig T. Shedding and infection dynamics of porcine circovirus type 2 (PCV2) after experimental infection. Vet Microbiol. 2011;149:91–8.
7. Segales J, Calsamiglia M, Olvera A, Sibila M, Badiella L, Domingo M. Quantification of porcine circovirus type 2 (PCV2) DNA in serum and tonsillar, nasal, tracheo-bronchial, urinary and faecal swabs of pigs with and without postweaning multisystemic wasting syndrome (PMWS). Vet Microbiol. 2005;111:223–9.
8. Brunborg IM, Moldal T, Jonassen CM. Quantitation of porcine circovirus type 2 isolated from serum/plasma and tissue samples of healthy pigs and pigs with postweaning multisystemic wasting syndrome using a TaqMan-based real-time PCR. J Virol Methods. 2004;22:171–8.
9. Grau-Roma L, Hjulsager CK, Sibila M, Kristensen CS, López-Soria S, Enøe C, Casal J, Bøtner A, Nofrarías M, Bille-Hansen V, Fraile L, Baekbo P, Segalés J, Larsen LE. Infection, excretion and seroconversion dynamics of porcine circovirus type 2 (PCV2) in pigs from post-weaning multisystemic wasting syndrome (PMWS) affected farms in Spain and Denmark. Vet Microbiol. 2009;135:272–82.
10. Olvera A, Sibila M, Calsamiglia M, Segales J, Domingo M. Comparison of porcine circovirus type 2 load in serum quantified by a real time PCR in postweaning multisystemic wasting syndrome and porcine dermatitis and nephropathy syndrome naturally affected pigs. J Virol Methods. 2004;117:75–80.
11. Segales J. Porcine circovirus type 2 (PCV2) infections: clinical signs, pathology and laboratory diagnosis. Virus Res. 2012;164:10–9.
12. López-Soria S, Sibila M, Nofrarías M, Calsamiglia M, Manzanilla EG, Ramírez-Mendoza H, Mínguez A, Serrano JM, Marín O, Joisel F, Charreyre C, Segalés J. Effect of porcine circovirus type 2 (PCV2) load in serum on average daily weight gain during the postweaning period. Vet Microbiol. 2014;174:296–301.
13. Fort M, Sibila M, Perez-Martin E, Nofrarias M, Mateu E, Segales J. One dose of a porcine circovirus 2 (PCV2) sub-unit vaccine administered to 3-week-old conventional piglets elicits cell-mediated immunity and significantly reduces PCV2 viremia in an experimental model. Vaccine. 2009;27:4031–7.
14. Fraile L, Sibila M, Nofrarías M, López-Jimenez R, Huerta E, Llorens A, López-Soria S, Pérez D, Segalés J. Effect of sow and piglet porcine circovirus type 2 (PCV2) vaccination on piglet mortality, viraemia, antibody titre and production parameters. Vet Microbiol. 2012;161:229–34.
15. Kixmöller M, Ritzmann M, Eddicks m, Saalmüller A, Elbers K, Fachinger V. Reduction of PMWS-associated clinical signs and co-infections by vaccination against PCV2. Vaccine. 2008;26:3443–51.
16. Kristensen CS, Baadsgaard NP, Toft N. A meta-analysis comparing the effect of PCV2 vaccines on average daily weight gain and mortality rate in pigs from weaning to slaughter. Prev Vet Med. 2011;98:250–8.
17. Segales J, Urniza A, Alegre A, Bru T, Crisci E, Nofrarias M, Lopez-Soria S, Balasch M, Sibila M, Xu Z, Chu H-J, Fraile L, Plana-Duran J. A genetically engineered chimeric vaccine against porcine circovirus type 2 (PCV2) improves clinical, pathological and virological outcomes in postweaning multisystemic wasting syndrome affected farms. Vaccine. 2009;27:7313–21.
18. Cortey M, Napp S, Alba A, Pileri E, Grau-Roma L, Sibila M, Segalés J. Theoretical and experimental approaches to estimate the usefulness of pooled serum samples for the diagnosis of postweaning multisystemic wasting syndrome. J Vet Diagn Investig. 2011;23:233–40.
19. Prickett JR, Wonil K, Simer R, Yoon KJ, Zimmerman J. Oral-fluid samples for surveillance of commercial growing pigs for porcine reproductive and respiratory syndrome virus and porcine circovirus type 2 infections. J Swine Health Prod. 2008;16(2):86–91.
20. Prickett J, Simer R, Christopher-Hennings J, Yoon K-J, Evans RB, Zimmerman JJ. Detection of porcine reproductive and respiratory syndrome virus infection in porcine oral fluid samples: a longitudinal study under experimental conditions. J Vet Diagn Investig. 2008;20:156–63.
21. Costa G, Oliveira S, Torrison J. Detection of Actinobacillus pleuropneumoniae in oral-fluid samples obtained from experimentally infected pigs. J Swine Health Prod. 2012;20(2):78–81.
22. Decorte I, Steensels M, Lambrecht B, Cay AB, Regge ND. Detection and isolation of swine influenza A virus in spiked oral fluid and samples from individually housed, experimentally infected pigs: Potential role of porcine oral fluid in active Influenza A virus surveillance in swine. PLoS ONE. 2015;10(10):e0139586.
23. Grau FR, Schroeder ME, Mulhern EL, MT MI, Bounpheng MA. Detection of African swine fever, classical swine fever and foot-and-mouth disease viruses in swine oral fluids by multiplex reverse transcription real-time polymerase chain reaction. J Vet Diagn Investig. 2015;27(2):140–9.
24. Kim W-I. Application of oral fluid sample to monitor porcine circovirus-2 infection in pig farms. J Vet Clin. 2010;27(6):704–12.
25. Prickett JR, Johnson J, Murtaugh MP, Puvanendiran S, Wang C, Zimmerman JJ, Opriessnig T. Prolonged detection of PCV2 and anti-PCV2 antibody in oral fluids following experimental inoculation. Transboundary Emerging Dis. 2011;58:121–7.
26. Ramirez A, Wang C, Prickett JR, Pogranichniy R, Yoon K-J, Main R, Johnson JK, Rademacher C, Hoogland M, Hoffmann P, Kurtz A, Kurtz E, Zimmerman J. Efficient surveillance of pig populations using oral fluids. Prev Vet Med. 2012;104:292–300.
27. Van Cuong N, Carrique-Mas J, Thu HTV, Hien ND, Hoa NT, Nguyet LA, Anh PH, Bryant JE. Serological and virological surveillance for porcine reproductive and respiratory syndrome virus, porcine circovirus type 2 and influenza a viruses among smallholder swine farms of the Mekong Delta, Vietnam J Swine Health Prod 2014;22(5):224–231.
28. Opriessnig T, Prickett JR, Madson DM, Shen H-G, Juhan NM, Pogranichniy RM, Meng X-J, Halbur PG. Porcine circovirus type 2 (PCV2)-infection and re-inoculation with homologous or heterologous strains: virological, serological, pathological and clinical effects in growing pigs. Vet Res. 2010;41:31.
29. Oliver-Ferrando S, Segales J, López-Soria S, Callén A, Merdy O, Joisel F, Sibila M. Evaluation of natural porcine circovirus type 2 (PCV2) subclinical infection and seroconversion dynamics in piglets vaccinated at different ages. Vet Res. 2016;47:121.
30. Steinrigl A, Revilla-Fernández S, Schmoll F, Sattler T. Detection of porcine reproductive and respiratory syndrome virus and porcine circovirus type 2 in blood and oral fluid collected with GenoTube swabs. Berl Münch Tierärztl Wochenschr. 2016;129:437–43.
31. Nielsen GB, Nielsen JP, Haugegaard J, Denwood MJ, Houe H. Effect of vaccination against sub-clinical porcine circovirus type 2 infection in a high-health finishing pig herd: a randomised clinical field trial. Prev Vet Med. 2017;141:14–21.
32. Hulley SB, Cummings SR, Browner WS, Grady D, Newman TB. Designing clinical research: an epidemiologic approach. 4th edition, Philadelphia, PA: Lippincott Williams & Wilkins; 2013;Appendix 6C:79. Found at. www.sample-size.net

33. Random.org – True Random Number Service. https://www.random.org/. Accessed Summer 2010.

34. Chittick WA, Stensland WR, Prickett JR, Strait EL, Harmon K, Yoon K-J, Wang C, Zimmerman JJ. Comparison of RNA extraction and real-time reverse transcription polymerase chain reaction methods for the detection of porcine reproductive and respiratory syndrome virus in porcine oral fluid specimens. J Vet Diagn Investig. 2011;23:248–53.

35. Ochert AS, Boulter AW, Birnbaum W, Johnson NW, Teo CG. Inhibitory effect of salivary fluids on PCR: potency and removal. Genome Res. 2012;3.365–8.

36. Schrader C, Schielke A, Ellerbroek L, Johne R. PCR inhibitors – occurrence, properties and removal. J Appl Microbiol. 2012;113:1014–26.

37. Hjulsager CK, Grau-Roma L, Sibila M, Enøe C, Larsen L, Segales J. Inter-laboratory and inter-assay comparison on two real-time PCR techniques for quantification of PCV2 nucleic acid extracted from field samples. Vet Microbiol. 2009;133:172–8.

38. Klausen J, Huda A, Ekeroth L, Ahrens P. Evaluation of serum and milk ELISAs for paratuberculosis in Danish dairy cattle. Prev Vet Med. 2003;58:171–8.

39. R: A language and environment for statistical computing, version 3.3.2. R Foundation for Statistical Computing, Vienna, Austria. URL http://www.R-project.org\; 2016.

40. Seddon YM, Guy JH, Edwards SA. Optimising oral fluid collection from groups of pigs: effect of housing system and provision of ropes. Vet J. 2012; 193:180–4.

41. Christensen J, Gardner IA. Herd-level interpretation of test results for epidemiologic studies of animal diseases. Prev Vet Med. 2000;45:83–106.

42. Houe H, Ersbøll AK, Toft N (eds.). Introduction to veterinary epidemiology. 1st Edition, Biofolia, Frederiksberg 2004:113–117.

43. Ransohoff DF, Feinstein AR. Problems of spectrum and bias in evaluating the efficacy of diagnostic tests. The New England Journal of Medicine, Special article. 1978:926–30.

44. O'Neill KC, Shen HG, Lin K, Hemann M, Beach NM, Meng XJ, Halbur PG, Opriessnig T. Studies on Porcine circovirus type 2 vaccination of 5-day-old piglets. Clin Vaccine Immunol. 2011:1865–71.

45. Patterson AR, Madson DM, Halbur PG, Opriessnig T. Shedding and infection dynamics of porcine circovirus type 2 (PCV2) after natural exposure. Vet Microbiol. 2011;149:225–9.

Permissions

List of Contributors

Joan Pujols
IRTA, Centre de Recerca en Sanitat Animal (CReSA, IRTA-UAB), Campus de la Universitat Autònoma de Barcelona, 08193 Bellaterra, Barcelona, Spain

Joaquim Segalés
UAB, Centre de Recerca en Sanitat Animal (CReSA, IRTA-UAB), Campus de la Universitat Autònoma de Barcelona, 08193 Bellaterra, Barcelona, Spain Departament de Sanitat i Anatomia Animals, Universitat Autònoma de Barcelona (UAB), 08193 Bellaterra, Barcelona, Spain

Javier Polo and Carmen Rodríguez
APC EUROPE, S.A. Avda, Sant Julià 246-258, Pol. Ind. El Congost, E-08403 Granollers, Spain

Joy Campbell and Joe Crenshaw
APC Inc., 2425 SE Oak Tree Court, Ankeny, IA 50021, USA

Satomi Tani and Yuzo Koketsu
School of Agriculture, Meiji University, Higashi-mita 1-1-1, Tama-ku, Kawasaki, Kanagawa 214-8571, Japan

Carlos Piñeiro
PigCHAMP Pro Europa S.L., c/Santa Catalina 10, 40003 Segovia, Spain

Annette Backhans, Marie Sjölund and Ulf Emanuelson
Department of Clinical Sciences, Swedish University of Agricultural Sciences, SE-750 07 Uppsala, Sweden

Marie Sjölund
Department of Animal Health and Antimicrobial Strategies, National Veterinary Institute, SE-751 89 Uppsala, Sweden

Ann Lindberg
Department of Epidemiology and Disease Control, National Veterinary Institute, SE-751 89 Uppsala, Sweden

Anja Joachim
Institute of Parasitology, University of Veterinary Medicine Vienna, Veterinaerplatz 1, A-1210 Wien, Austria

Carolin Holling and Elisabeth grosse Beilage
University of Veterinary Medicine Hannover, Field Station for Epidemiology, Büscheler Str. 9, D-49456 Bakum, Germany

Beatriz Vidondo and Christina Nathues
Veterinary Public Health Institute, Vetsuisse Faculty, Schwarzenburgstrasse 155, CH-3097 Liebefeld, BE, Switzerland

Corinne Arnold, Patricia Scheer and Myriam Harisberger
SUISAG, Division SGD, Sempach, Switzerland

Gertraud Schüpbach-Regula
Veterinary Public Health Institute, Vetsuisse Faculty, University of Bern, Bern, Switzerland

Patricia Hirsiger, Julia Malik and Xaver Sidler
Department for Farm Animals, Division of Swine Medicine, Vetsuisse Faculty, University of Zurich, Zurich, Switzerland

Peter Spring and Judith Peter-Egli
Berne University of Applied Sciences, HAFL - Agricultural Sciences, Zollikofen, Switzerland

Minna Haimi-Hakala, Outi Hälli, Tapio Laurila, Claudio Oliviero, Olli Peltoniemi and Mari Heinonen
Department of Production Animal Medicine, University of Helsinki, Paroninkuja 20, 04920 Saarentaus, Finland

Mirja Raunio-Saarnisto
Finnish Food Safety Authority Evira, Seinäjoki, Finland

Tiina Nokireki, Taina Laine, Suvi Nykäsenoja and Kirsti Pelkola
Finnish Food Safety Authority Evira, Mustialankatu 3, 00790 Helsinki, Finland

Joaquim Segales and Marina Sibila
Centre de Recerca en Sanitat Animal (CReSA, IRTA-UAB), Campus de la Universitat Autònoma de Barcelona, 08193 Bellaterra, Spain

Joaquim Segales
Departament de Sanitat i Anatomia Animals, Facultat de Veterinària, UAB, 08193 Bellaterra, Barcelona, Spain

Katie M. Cottingim, Pedro E. Urriola and Gerald C. Shurson
Department of Animal Science, University of Minnesota, St. Paul, MN 55108, USA

Harsha Verma, Fernando Sampedro and Sagar M. Goyal
Department of Veterinary Population Medicine, University of Minnesota, St. Paul, MN 55108, USA

Joaquin Morales, Alberto Manso, Laura de Frutos and Carlos Piñeiro
PigCHAMP Pro Europa S.L. c, Santa Catalina, 10, Segovia, Spain

Andre Dereu and Niels Wuyts
Zoetis Inc, Hoge Wei 10, 1930 Zaventem, Belgium

Edgar G. Manzanilla
Teagasc, Pig Development Department, Moorepark, Fermoy, Co Cork, Ireland

Guillermo Cano and Alberto Morillo
Tests and Trials S.L., Monzon, Spain

Marcia Oliveira Cavalcanti and Christian Kraft
Boehringer Ingelheim Veterinary Research Center GmbH & Co. KG, Hannover, Germany

Francois-Xavier Orveillon and Oliver Gomez-Duran
Boehringer Ingelheim Animal Health GmbH, Ingelheim, Germany

Jeremy Kroll
Boehringer Ingelheim Vetmedica Inc., Ames, IA, USA

Mate Zoric and Per Wallgren
Department of Animal Health and Antimicrobial Strategies, National Veterinary Institute, SE-751 89 Uppsala, Sweden

Mate Zoric and Per Wallgren
Department of Clinical Sciences, Faculty of Veterinary Medicine and Animal Sciences, Swedish University of Agricultural Sciences, Uppsala, Sweden

Ulla Schmidt and Anna Wallenbeck
Department of Animal Breeding and Genetics, Swedish University of Agricultural Sciences, Box 7023SE-750 07 Uppsala, Sweden

Luuk Kaalberg
De Graafschapdierenartsen bv, Schimmeldijk 1 Vorden, 7251 MX Vorden, The Netherlands

Victor Geurts
MSD Animal Health, Wim de Korverstraat 35, 5831 AN Boxmeer, The Netherlands

Rika Jolie
Merck Animal Health, 2 Giralda Farms, Madison, NJ 07940, USA

Gerald Reiner
Department of Veterinary Clinical Sciences, Swine Clinic, Justus-Liebig-University, Frankfurter Strasse 112, 35392 Giessen, Germany

Heiko Nathues, Guillaume Fournie, Dirk U. Pfeiffer and Katharina D. C. Stärk
Veterinary Epidemiology, Economics and Public Health Group, Royal Veterinary College London, Hawkshead Lane, Hatfield, Hertfordshire AL97TA, UK

Heiko Nathues
Clinic for Swine, Vetsuisse Faculty, University of Berne, Bremgartenstrasse 109a, 3012 Bern, Switzerland

Barbara Wieland
International Livestock Research Institute, Addis Ababa, Ethiopia

Erik Grandemange and Pierre-Alexandre Perrin
Vetoquinol SA, Research and Development Centre, B.P. 189, 70204 Lure Cedex, France

Dejean Cvejic, Miriam Haas and Klaus Hellmann
Klifovet AG, Geyerspergerstr 27, D-80689 Munich, Germany

Tim Rowan
Rowdix Ltd, Folly Hall, Cawton, York YO62 4LW, UK

Merel Postma and Jeroen Dewulf
Veterinary Epidemiology Unit, Department of Reproduction, Obstetrics and Herd Health, Faculty of Veterinary Medicine, Ghent University, Salisburylaan 133, 9820 Merelbeke, Belgium

Annette Backhans and Marie Sjölund
Department of Animal Health and Antimicrobial Strategies, National Veterinary Institute, SVA, SE-751 89 Uppsala, Sweden

Annette Backhans, Marie Sjölund and Ulf Emanuelson
Department of Clinical Sciences, Swedish University of Agricultural Sciences, Uppsala, Sweden

Lucie Collineau and Katharina D. C. Stärk
SAFOSO AG, Waldeggstrasse 1, CH-3097 Liebefeld, Switzerland

Lucie Collineau and Catherine Belloc
UMR1300 BioEpAR, LUNAM Université, Oniris, INRA, BP40706, F-44307 Nantes, France

Svenja Loesken and Elisabeth grosse Beilage
Field Station for Epidemiology, University of Veterinary Medicine Hannover, Büscheler Straße 9, D-49456 Bakum, Germany

Elisabeth Okholm Nielsen
Danish Agriculture and Food Council, Axeltorv 3, DK-1609 Copenhagen V, Denmark

Didier Duivon, Martial Rigaut and David Roudaut
MSD Santé Animale, 7, rue Olivier de Serres - Angers Technopole, C.S. 17144, 49071 Beaucouzé cedex, France

Isabelle Corrégé and Anne Hémonic
IFIP, La Motte au Vicomte, 35650 Le Rheu, France

Rika Jolie
MSD Animal Health, 2 Giralda Farms, Madison, NJ 07940, USA

Anja Joachim and Bärbel Ruttkowski
Institute of Parasitology, Department of Pathobiology, University of Veterinary Medicine Vienna, Veterinaerplatz 1, A-1210 Vienna, Austria

Daniel Sperling
CEVA Santé Animale, 10 avenue de la Ballastière, 33500 Libourne, France

Jeremy Kroll
Boehringer Ingelheim Animal Health, 2412 South Loop Dr, Ames, IA 50010, USA

Mike Piontkowski
Boehringer Ingelheim Animal Health, 2621 North Belt Highway, St. Joseph, MO 64506, USA

Poul H. Rathkjen, Francois-Xavier Orveillon and Oliver G. Duran
Boehringer Ingelheim Vetmedica GmbH, Binger Straße 173, 55216 Ingelheim, Germany

Christian Kraft
Boehringer Ingelheim Veterinary Research Center GmbH & Co. KG, Bemeroder Str. 31, 30559 Hannover,Germany

Vojislav Cvjetković
Ceva Tiergesundheit GmbH, Kanzlerstraße 4, 40472 Düsseldorf, Germany

Sabine Sipos
Veterinary Practice Schwertfegen, Schwertfegen 2, 3040, Neulengbach, Austria

Imre Szabó
Ceva-Phylaxia, Co., Szállás u.5, Budapest 1107, Hungary

Wolfgang Sipos
Clinic for Swine, University of Veterinary Medicine Vienna, Veterinärplatz 1, 1210 Vienna, Austria

Fahiel Casillas, Lizbeth Juárez-Rojas and Socorro Retana-Márquez
Departamento de Biología de la Reproducción, División de Ciencias Biológicas y de la Salud, Universidad Autónoma Metropolitana-Iztapalapa, 09340 CDMX, Mexico

Fahiel Casillas
Doctorado en Ciencias Biológicas y de la Salud. Universidad Autónoma Metropolitana-Iztapalapa, 09340 CDMX, Mexico

Miguel Betancourt, Yvonne Ducolomb and Alma López
Departamento de Ciencias de la Salud, División de Ciencias Biológicas y de la Salud, Universidad Autónoma Metropolitana-Iztapalapa, 09340 CDMX,Mexico

Cristina Cuello
Departamento de Medicina y Cirugía Animal, Universidad de Murcia, 30100 Espinardo, Spain

Gitte Blach Nielsen and John Haugegaard
MSD Animal Health Nordic, Havneholmen 25, 1561 Copenhagen V, Denmark

Jens Peter Nielsen, Helle Stege and Hans Houe
Department of Veterinary and Animal Sciences, University of Copenhagen, Grønnegårdsvej 2+8, 1870 Frederiksberg C, Denmark

Sanne Christiansen Leth
Porcus Veterinary Pig Practice, Ørbækvej 276, 5220 Odense, SØ, Denmark

Lars E. Larsen and Charlotte K. Hjulsager
National Veterinary Institute, Henrik Dams Allé, Bygning 205B, 2800 Kgs. Lyngby, Denmark

Charlotte Sonne Kristensen
SEGES Pig Research Centre, Vinkelvej 11, 8620 Kjellerup, Denmark

Ken Steen Pedersen
Ø-vet A/S, Køberupvej 33, 4700 Næstved, Denmark

Index

www.ingramcontent.com/pod-product-compliance
Lightning Source LLC
Chambersburg PA
CBHW082037190326
41458CB00010B/3396